Generative Intelligence in Healthcare

This book explores the intersection of artificial intelligence and healthcare with a focus on generative intelligence. The book will introduce the concept of generative intelligence and its transformative potential in patient care, showcasing applications that go beyond conventional AI approaches.

Generative Intelligence in Healthcare: Transforming Patient Care with AI Creativity delves into the use of generative models for personalized medicine, data analytics, and predictive modelling, providing real-world examples of how AI creativity can revolutionize treatment strategies and diagnostic processes. It focuses on the origin and basics of generative AI, generative AI models, and possible areas in healthcare where generative AI can work. It discusses how generative AI model will help healthcare providers automatically generate prescriptions, discharge summaries, and patient conditions. The unique strength of this book lies in its comprehensive examination of ethical considerations and regulatory frameworks, ensuring a responsible and transparent integration of generative intelligence in healthcare. By addressing current challenges and envisioning future directions, this book serves as a valuable resource for healthcare professionals, researchers, and policymakers seeking to harness the full potential of AI creativity to enhance patient outcomes.

The book is written for graduate students, researchers, and professionals in biomedical engineering, electrical engineering, signal process engineering, biomedical imaging, and computer science.

Artificial Intelligence for Sustainable Engineering and Management

Sachi Nandan Mohanty
School of Computer Science & Engineering (SCOPE), VIT-AP University, Amaravati, Andhra Pradesh, India

Deepak Gupta

Artificial intelligence is shaping the future of humanity across nearly every industry. It is already the main driver of emerging technologies like big data, robotics and IoT, and it will continue to act as a technological innovator for the foreseeable future. Artificial intelligence is the simulation of human intelligence processes by machines, especially computer systems. Specific applications of AI include expert systems, natural language processing, speech recognition and machine vision. The future of business intelligence combined with AI will see the analysis of huge quantities of contextual data in real-time. So, the tool will quickly capture customer needs and priorities and do what is needed.

Generative Intelligence in Healthcare: Transforming Patient Care with AI Creativity
Edited by Sakshi Gupta, Umesh Gupta, Moolchand Sharma, and Kamal Malik

Artificial Intelligence: Technical and Societal Advancements
Edited by Utku Kose and Mustafa Umut Demirezen

AI for Climate Change and Environmental Sustainability
Edited by Suneeta Satpathy, Satyasundara Mahapatra, Nidhi Agarwal, and Sachi Nandan Mohanty

Green Metaverse for Greener Economies
Edited by Sukanta Kumar Baral, Richa Goel, Tilottama Singh, and Rakesh Kumar

Healthcare Analytics and Advanced Computational Intelligence
Edited by Sushruta Mishra, Meshal Alharbi, Hrudaya Kumar Tripathy, Biswajit Sahoo, and Ahmed Alkhayyat

AI in Agriculture for Sustainable and Economic Management
Edited by Sirisha Potluri, Suneeta Satpathy, Santi Swarup Basa, and Antonio Zuorro

Deep Learning in Biomedical Signal and Medical Imaging
Edited by Ngangbam Herojit Singh, Utku Kose, and Sarada Prasad Gochhayat

https://www.routledge.com/AI-for-Sustainable-Engineering-and-Management-series/book-series/AISEM

Generative Intelligence in Healthcare

Transforming Patient Care with AI Creativity

Edited by Sakshi Gupta, Umesh Gupta, Moolchand Sharma, and Kamal Malik

CRC Press
Taylor & Francis Group
Boca Raton London New York

CRC Press is an imprint of the
Taylor & Francis Group, an **informa** business

Designed cover image: © Shutterstock

First edition published 2025
by CRC Press
6000 Broken Sound Parkway NW, Suite 300, Boca Raton, FL 33487-2742

and by CRC Press
4 Park Square, Milton Park, Abingdon, Oxon, OX14 4RN

CRC Press is an imprint of Taylor & Francis Group, LLC

ISBN: 978-1-032-88740-1 (hbk)
ISBN: 978-1-032-88742-5 (pbk)
ISBN: 978-1-003-53948-3 (ebk)

DOI: 10.1201/9781003539483

Typeset in Times
by Apex CoVantage, LLC

Dr. Sakshi Gupta *would like to dedicate this book to her parents, who now watch over her from heaven. A heartfelt thanks to her family members, including her husband, Mr. Ashish Gupta, and kids, Mohak Gupta and Anika Gupta, and in-laws for their continuous steadfast love, support, and belief. I also thank the publisher and my other co-editors for their belief in this project and tireless efforts in bringing this work to life. Above all, I thank God for His grace and guidance throughout this journey. Without You, none of this would be possible,*

Dr. Umesh Gupta *would like to dedicate this book to his mother, Smt. Prabha Gupta and his father, Sh. Mahesh Chandra Gupta for their constant support and motivation, and his family members, including his wife, Ms. Umang Agarwal, and Son Avaya Gupta. I also thank the publisher and my other co-editors for believing in my abilities. Before beginning and after finishing my endeavor, I must appreciate the Almighty God, who provides me with the means to succeed.*

Dr. Moolchand Sharma *would like to dedicate this book to his father, Sh. Naresh Kumar Sharma and his mother, Smt. Rambati Sharma for their constant support and motivation, and his family members, including his wife, Ms. Pratibha Sharma, and Son Dhairya Sharma. I also thank the publisher and my other co-editors for believing in my abilities.*

Dr. Kamal Malik *would like to dedicate this book to her father, Sh. Ashwani Malik, her mother, Smt. Shakuntla Malik and her brother, Dr. Shiv Malik, for their constant support and motivation; I would also like to give my special thanks to the publisher and my other co-editors for believing in my abilities. Above all, a humble thanks to the Almighty for this accomplishment.*

Contents

About the Editors

Sakshi Gupta is presently working as an assistant professor at the School of Computer Application, Manav Rachna International Institute of Research and Studies, Faridabad, Haryana. She received her PhD from the Birla Institute of Technology Mesra, Ranchi, and MCA from Gautam Buddha Technical University, Lucknow, Uttar Pradesh. Her areas of interest include the Internet of Things, mobile ad-hoc networks, body area networks, machine learning, and deep learning. She has published in more than 14 referred journals, including SCI and Scopus-indexed journals, and she has published many conference papers and book chapters. She also has three published patents. She also works as reviewer for many conferences and Springer journals. Dr. Sakshi has also attended various technical conferences/workshops/faculty development programs.

Umesh Gupta is currently an associate professor at the School of Computer Science Engineering and Technology at Bennett University, Greater Noida, India. He received a doctor of philosophy (PhD) (machine learning) from the National Institute of Technology, Arunachal Pradesh, India. He was awarded a gold medalist for his master of engineering (ME) from the National Institute of Technical Teachers Training and Research (NITTTR), Chandigarh, India, and bachelor of technology (BTech) from Dr APJ, Abdul Kalam Technical University, Lucknow, India. He has more than 15 years of work experience in academics and research. His research interests include support vector machine, extreme learning machine, random vector functional link, machine learning, and deep learning approaches. He has published over 50 referred journal and conference papers of international repute. His scientific research has been published in reputable international journals and conferences, including SCI-indexed and Scopus-indexed journals like *Applied Soft Computing* (Elsevier) and *Applied Intelligence* (Springer), each of which is a peer-reviewed journal. His publications have more than 535 citations, with an h-index of 11 and an i10-index of 12 on Google Scholar. He is a senior member of IEEE (SMIEEE) and an active member of ACM, CSTA, and other scientific societies. He has also reviewed papers for many scientific journals and conferences in the US and abroad. He led sessions at the International Conference (ICICC-2022, 2023, 2024), the International Conference on Data Analytics and Management (ICDAM 2022, 2023), the 3rd International Conference on Computing and Communication Networks (ICCCN 2022, 2023, 2024), and other international conferences like Springer ETTIS 2022 and 2023. He is currently supervising two PhD students. He is the co-principal investigator (co-PI) of two major research projects. He published four patents in the years 2021–2023. He also published four books with Springer, CRC.

Moolchand Sharma is currently an assistant professor in the Department of Computer Science and Engineering at the Maharaja Agrasen Institute of Technology, GGSIPU, Delhi. He has published scientific research papers in reputed international journals and conferences, including SCI-indexed and Scopus-indexed journals such as *Cognitive Systems Research* (Elsevier), *Physical Communication* (Elsevier), *Intelligent Decision Technologies: An International Journal, Cyber-Physical*

Systems (Taylor & Francis Group), *International Journal of Image & Graphics* (World Scientific), *International Journal of Innovative Computing and Applications* (Inderscience), and *Innovative Computing and Communication Journal* (scientific peer-reviewed journal). He has authored/co-authored chapters with international publishers like Elsevier, Wiley, and De Gruyter. He has authored/edited four books with national/international-level publishers (CRC Press, Bhavya Publications). His research areas include artificial intelligence, nature-inspired computing, security in cloud computing, machine learning, and search engine optimization. He is associated with various professional bodies like IEEE, ISTE, IAENG, ICSES, UACEE, and the Internet Society and holds life membership in Universal Innovators Research Lab and others. He possesses teaching experience of more than nine years. He is the co-convener of the ICICC, DOSCI, ICDAM & ICCCN Springer Scopus Indexed conference series and ICCRDA-2020 Scopus Indexed IOP Material Science & Engineering conference series. He is also the organizer and co-convener of the International Conference on Innovations and Ideas towards Patents (ICIIP) series. He is also the advisory and TPC committee member of the ICCIDS-2022 Elsevier SSRN Conference. He is also a reviewer for many reputed journals like Springer, Elsevier, IEEE, IEEE JBHI, Wiley, Taylor & Francis Group, IJEECS, and World Scientific Journal and many Springer conferences. He also served as a session chair at many international Springer conferences. He completed his PhD at DCR University of Science & Technology, Haryana, in June 2024. He completed his postgraduate in 2012 from SRM University, NCR Campus, Ghaziabad, and graduated in 2010 from KNGD Modi Engineering College, GBTU.

Kamal Malik is currently working as a professor in CSE at the School of Engineering and Technology at CTU Ludhiana, Punjab, India. She has published scientific research papers in reputed international journals, including SCI- and Scopus-indexed journals. Apart from this, she has attended many national and international conferences of repute like Springer and Elsevier in India. Her major areas of research are artificial intelligence, machine learning, deep learning, data analytics, computational neurosciences, and bio-inspired computing. She has more than 13 years of rich academic and research experience. Her passion is to teach ever-evolving computer science engineering and enlighten students in emerging domains like machine learning, data science, business analytics, cloud computing, Internet of Things, and blockchain and to inculcate critical thinking among students. She is the Editor of many journals for Springer, Elsevier, and so on. She has also edited one book, *Techniques of Computational Neurosciences*, with the publishers Taylor & Francis. She is also the Deputy Director of the MOOC Cell at CTU.

Contributors

Adithya V
School of Computer Science and Applications
REVA University
India

Naved Ahmad
Department of Computer Science
Jamia Hamdard University
New Delhi, India

Mehtab Alam
Department of Computer Science
Jamia Hamdard University
New Delhi, India

Deghinmotei Alfred-Ugbenbo
Faculty of Pharmaceutical Sciences
Bayelsa Medical University
Yenagoa, Bayelsa State, Nigeria

Anshika
Department of Pharmacy
Bharat Institute of Technology
Meerut, India

Subhranil Das
UPES, Dehradun
Uttarakhand, India

Sonali Deshpande
Computer Science & Engineering Department
MIT SoC, MIT Art, Design and Technology University
Pune, India

Sreedeep Dey
Bioequivalence Study Centre, Department of Pharmaceutical Technology
Jadavpur University
Kolkata, India

Ogola-Emma Ebitimitula
Faculty of Pharmaceutical Sciences
Bayelsa Medical University
Yenagoa, Bayelsa State, Nigeria

Iram Fatima
Manav Rachna international Institute of Research and Studies
Faridabad Haryana, India

Ritu Gautam
Department of Computer Science & Applications
Amity University
Noida, India

Poonam Suraj Gham
KJ College of Engineering and Management Research
Pune, India

Priyanshi Goyal
School of Pharmacy
Mangalayatan University
Aligarh, India

Mayuresh Gulame
MIT Art Design and Technology University
Pune, India

Jaishree Jain
Department of Computer Science and Engineering
Ajay Kumar Garg Engineering College
Ghaziabad (U.P.), India

Updesh Kumar Jaiswal
Department of Computer Science and Engineering
Ajay Kumar Garg Engineering College
Ghaziabad (U.P.), India

Amulya Jindal
Department of Pharmaceutical Technology
Meerut Institute of Engineering and Technology
Meerut, India

Prableen Kaur
Department of Computer Applications
GMN College
Ambala Cantt, Ambala, India

Ihtiram Raza Khan
Department of Computer Science
Jamia Hamdard University
New Delhi, India

Nilima Kulkarni
Computer Science & Engineering Department
MIT SoC, MIT Art, Design and Technology University
Pune, India

Anoop Kumar
Department of Pharmaceutical Technology
Meerut Institute of Engineering and Technology
Meerut, India

Rashmi Kumari
Bennett University
Greater Noida, Uttar Pradesh, India

Ankit Lodhi
Department of Pharmaceutical Technology
Meerut Institute of Engineering and Technology
Meerut, India

Amena Mahmoud
Faculty of Computers and Information
Kafrelsheikh University
Kafr El-Sheikh Governorate, Egypt

Mainuddin
Amity Institute of Pharmacy
Amity University
Greater Noida, India

Abhay Narayana
National Institute of Technology
Calicut, India

Odangowei Inetiminebi Ogidi
Faculty of Basic Medical Sciences
Bayelsa Medical University Yenagoa
Bayelsa State, Nigeria

Jayashri D. Palkar
KJ College of Engineering and Management Research
Pune, India

Vijaya S. Patil
MIT Art Design and Technology University
Pune, India

Aarti P. Pimpalkar
MIT Art Design and Technology University
Pune, India

Rajeev Ranjan
School of Computer Science and Applications
REVA University, India

Ketan Sarvakar
Ganpat University
Ganpat Vidyanagar, North Gujarat, INDIA

G. Sasikala
School of Computer Science and Applications
REVA University
India

Kartik Sharma
Department of Pharmaceutical Technology
Meerut Institute of Engineering and Technology
Meerut, India

Manik Sharma
Department of Computer Science & Applications
DAV University
Jalandhar, India

Raghwendra Kishore Singh
SR University
Warangal, India

Sreenivasan M
National Institute of Technology
Calicut, India

Yadvendra Singh Thenuan
School of Pharmacy
Mangalayatan University
Aligarh, India

Nilesh N. Thorat
MIT Art Design and Technology University
Pune, India

Deepak Tomar
SRM Institute of Science and Technology
Delhi-NCR Campus, Modinagar, Ghaziabad
Uttar Pradesh, India

Nisha Varghese
Department of Computer Science
Christ University
India

Introduction

The book *Generative Intelligence in Healthcare: Transforming Patient Care with AI Creativity* serves as an innovative exploration into the intersection of artificial intelligence and healthcare, penned by leading experts in the field. This groundbreaking book navigates the cutting-edge landscape where technology and creativity converge to revolutionize patient care. Delving into the realms of generative artificial intelligence (AI), the authors present a compelling vision of how creativity can be harnessed to address complex healthcare challenges. From personalized treatment plans to predictive diagnostics, the book offers a comprehensive journey through the transformative potential of AI in healthcare. Through a blend of insightful analysis, real-world case studies, and forward-thinking strategies, this book guides healthcare professionals, technologists, and enthusiasts alike, ushering them into the era of generative intelligence where innovation meets compassion in the pursuit of enhanced patient well-being.

The future scope of the book extends beyond the boundaries of conventional AI applications, exploring the ongoing advancements in generative AI that promise to revolutionize patient care. The book aims to equip readers with the knowledge and tools necessary to navigate the evolving landscape of AI in healthcare by delving into the latest algorithms, models, and practical implementation strategies. Emphasizing patient-centric approaches, it anticipates a future where generative intelligence tailors treatments, improves outcomes, and enhances overall healthcare experiences. The ethical considerations surrounding the use of AI in healthcare are also addressed, emphasizing responsible practices and mitigating biases. The book envisions collaborative efforts across disciplines, fostering partnerships between AI experts, healthcare professionals, and policymakers to accelerate the global impact of generative intelligence. As technology evolves, the book explores emerging trends, including augmented reality, virtual reality, and the Internet of Medical Things, and their synergies with generative intelligence. Moreover, it envisions an educational paradigm that prepares the workforce for the challenges and opportunities at the intersection of AI and healthcare. In essence, the book not only serves as a comprehensive guide to the current landscape but also as a forward-looking beacon guiding readers through the transformative journey of generative intelligence in shaping the future of patient care.

SCOPE OF THE BOOK

Generative Intelligence in Healthcare: Transforming Patient Care with AI Creativity embarks on a comprehensive exploration of the expansive scope within the convergence of artificial intelligence and healthcare. The book's scope extends across various dimensions, beginning with an in-depth analysis of generative AI's current state and its healthcare applications. It ventures into the intricacies of advanced algorithms and models, shedding light on how these technologies can revolutionize diagnostics, treatment planning, and patient outcomes.

A pivotal aspect of the book's scope lies in its emphasis on practical implementation strategies. It offers a detailed roadmap for integrating generative intelligence into existing healthcare systems, navigating regulatory frameworks, and addressing real-world challenges. By providing actionable insights, the book becomes a practical guide for healthcare professionals, technologists, and decision-makers seeking to harness the transformative power of AI creativity.

The collaborative nature of the book extends across disciplines, envisioning partnerships between AI experts, healthcare professionals, researchers, and policymakers. It outlines how these collaborations can catalyze innovation, address healthcare disparities, and contribute to the global impact of generative intelligence. In anticipation of emerging technologies, the book explores the synergy between generative intelligence and cutting-edge trends like augmented reality, virtual reality, and the Internet of Medical Things. It outlines how these technologies can complement and enhance the capabilities of AI in healthcare.

Furthermore, the book considers the future educational landscape, recognizing the need for a skilled workforce capable of navigating the complexities at the intersection of AI and healthcare. It envisions educational initiatives and training programs to equip professionals with the knowledge and expertise required to leverage generative intelligence effectively. The scope of the book is ambitious, aiming to provide a comprehensive and accessible resource for scientists, researchers, practitioners, professionals, and educators interested in the transformative applications of generative AI in the dynamic and evolving field of healthcare.

Preface

We are delighted to launch our book entitled *Generative Intelligence in Healthcare: Transforming Patient Care with AI Creativity* under the book series Artificial Intelligence for Sustainable Engineering and Management, CRC Press, Taylor & Francis Group. The value of the book is in exploring the intersection of artificial intelligence and healthcare with a focus on generative intelligence. The book will introduce the concept of generative intelligence and its transformative potential in patient care, showcasing applications that go beyond conventional AI approaches. It delves into the use of generative models for personalized medicine, data analytics, and predictive modelling, providing real-world examples of how AI creativity can revolutionize treatment strategies and diagnostic processes. Essentially, this book not only imparts knowledge but also functions as a practical guide, empowering readers to apply advanced strategies and contribute meaningfully to the transformative advancements in medical and biomedical research.

The unique strength of this book lies in its comprehensive examination of ethical considerations and regulatory frameworks, ensuring a responsible and transparent integration of generative intelligence in healthcare. By addressing current challenges and envisioning future directions, this book serves as a valuable resource for healthcare professionals, researchers, and policymakers seeking to harness the full potential of AI creativity to enhance patient outcomes. This book will focus on the origin and basics of generative AI, generative AI models, and possible areas in which generative AI can work. However, the focus will be on the integration of generative AI and the healthcare sector to enhance the user experience. A generative AI model can assist healthcare providers by automatically creating prescriptions, discharge summaries, and detailed reports of patient conditions. Around 50 full-length chapters were received. Amongst these, 14 chapters have been included in this volume. All the chapters submitted were peer-reviewed by at least two independent reviewers and provided with a detailed review proforma. The comments from the reviewers were communicated to the authors, who incorporated the suggestions in their revised manuscripts. The recommendations from two reviewers were considered while selecting chapters for inclusion in the volume. The exhaustiveness of the review process is evident, given the large number of chapters received addressing a wide range of research areas. The stringent review process ensured that each published chapter met the rigorous academic and scientific standards.

We would also like to thank the authors of the published chapters for adhering to the schedule and incorporating the review comments. We extend our heartfelt acknowledgment to the authors, peer reviewers, committee members, and production staff whose diligent work shaped this volume. We especially want to thank our dedicated peer reviewers who volunteered for the arduous and tedious step of quality checking and critiquing the submitted chapters.

1 Drug Discovery and Development with Generative Artificial Intelligence

Odangowei Inetiminebi Ogidi, Deghinmotei Alfred-Ugbenbo, and Ogola-Emma Ebitimitula

LIST OF ABBREVIATIONS

ADMET	adsorption, distribution, metabolism, excretion, toxicity
ADME	adsorption, distribution, metabolism, excretion
AI	artificial intelligence
AIF	apoptosis-inducing factor
ANNs	artificial neural networks
BERT	bidirectional encoder representations from the transformers
CASP	Critical Assessment of Protein Structure Prediction
CLMs	chemical language models
CNN	convolutional neural network
CYP450	cytochrome 450
DDR 1	discoidin domain receptor 1
DL	deep learning
EGFR	epidermal growth factor receptor
GAI	generative artificial intelligence
GANs	generative adversarial networks
GENTRL	generative tensorial reinforcement learning
GPT	generative pretrained transformer
LLMS	large language models
ML	machine learning
MM	molecular mechanics
MOSE	molecular sets
NLP	natural language models
NLP	natural language processing
QM	quantum mechanical
R&D	research and development

DOI: 10.1201/9781003539483-1

RL	reinforcement learning
RNNs	recurrent neural networks
RXR	retinoid X receptor
SAMPN	self-attention message passing graph neural network
SAR	structure-activity relationship
SBDD	structure-based drug design
SMILE	simplified molecular input line entry system
VAEs	variational autoencoders

1.1 INTRODUCTION

The development of novel pharmaceuticals necessitates a significant investment of time and capital. An abysmal success rate has been exacerbated by fear of rejection and uncertainty. The pharmaceutical sector is experiencing a decline in productivity as a result of the increasing costs of drug research and market introduction, as discovered by Paul et al. (2010) and DiMasi et al. (2016). Thierer et al. (2017), Coeckelbergh (2020), Collins and Moons (2019), and von Ungern-Sternberg (2017) all observe that AI has significantly enhanced computer vision, autonomous vehicles, and robotics as a result of more potent processing hardware and enhanced deep learning (DL) algorithms.

AlphaGo and AlphaGo Zero, two AI programmes developed by DeepMind, are proficient Go players. These algorithms have advanced to the stage where they can surpass top-tier human competitors in competitive environments, per Singh et al. (2017) and Chao et al. (2018). AlphaFold was created by DeepMind to address the complex and enduring biological issue of protein folding. According to Service (2020), AlphaFold 2 was the most effective method in the 14th Critical Assessment of Protein Structure Prediction (CASP). It is evident that AI has the potential to significantly accelerate the pace of inquiry, which could subsequently transform fundamental research.

Healthcare professionals are investigating and implementing the potential pharmaceutical applications of AI in light of these promising discoveries. A number of pharmaceutical companies have either initiated their own AI initiatives in-house or formed partnerships with AI startups and universities. Artificial intelligence techniques have only recently been implemented in a variety of biological and drug development research domains. To anticipate biologically active compounds, for example, they have been training deep neural networks with transcriptional data (Aliper et al. 2016). Additionally, artificial intelligence has been implemented to generate innovative small molecule medicinal leads (Mamoshina et al. 2016).

AI is currently revolutionising the drug discovery process at every stage, as indicated by recent research. This process encompasses a variety of activities, including the selection of trial participants, synthesis planning, target selection, ligand generation, repurposing of existing medications, and predictions regarding the physicochemical and biological properties of molecules. Two of the numerous prerequisites that each potential medication candidate must satisfy are production feasibility and adsorption, distribution, metabolism, excretion, and toxicity (ADMET). Consequently, the development of medications is contingent upon the accurate prediction of molecular properties. Computer studies can be employed to evaluate and improve the molecular properties that are anticipated, thereby reducing research and development (R&D) expenses prior to conducting costly animal and clinical trials. It was demonstrated that the inhibition of human cytochrome 450 (CYP450) can be predicted using a multitask deep autoencoder, which may reduce undesirable effects and medication interactions (Li et al. 2018). The logP and aqueous solubility of small compounds were predicted by Tang and colleagues using a deep self-attention message-passing graph neural network (SAMPN) (2020).

Additionally, they acquired a wealth of knowledge regarding the interpretability issue in deep learning through the utilisation of their SAMPN model, which effectively identified the primary structural characteristic of the attribute they were attempting to learn. This could also be achieved through the use of artificial neural networks (ANNs) that have been trained to predict chemical characteristics. Stokes et al. (2020) employed a deep neural network that employs molecular graphs to forecast the antibiotic activity of compounds that are structurally distinct from existing antibiotics. Subsequently, they implemented experiments to validate their predictions. Nevertheless, these techniques have several substantial disadvantages. For instance, they require extensive training datasets and neural networks that are adept at acquiring molecular grammar, chemical properties, molecular attributes, and conceptual representations of molecules. It is also important to note that the prediction-based method is unable to produce novel molecules when the chemical library does not contain the essential or foundational components. This is the point at which generative AI (GAI) is implemented.

Generative adversarial intelligence is an AI technique that employs deep learning to produce novel and distinctive information. GAI tools are capable of comprehending the complexities and patterns in their training data, which enables them to produce new data that aligns with the user's expectations. This data can be either an enhanced version of the extant data or a similar replica. The data's representation in a variety of media, such as text, images, audio, video, and chemical compounds, can be informed by the patterns learned from the training data. Currently, the GAI system is using user prompts to generate material. In contrast to traditional AI systems, GAI (an acronym for "generative artificial intelligence") can analyse data and make predictions using pattern recognition. The capacity of GAI models to create new compounds is one of the most attractive parts of GAI-driven drug development. Engaging in De-Novo molecular generation involves the production of novel molecular structures that possess the desired properties. Consequently, feature-predicting neural networks are frequently implemented in GAI models.

Popova et al. (2018) devised the system ReLeaSE, which serves as an illustration. It combines a deep generative neural network for the purpose of generating novel compounds with the desired physicochemical and biological properties with a neural network for predicting molecular properties. Nevertheless, Popova et al.'s GAI model remains unsupported by experimental data. After training their GAI model with natural product data, Merk et al. (2018a) created a ligand generation algorithm. Experimental validation as novel retinoid X receptor (RXR) modulators followed the creation of these newly synthesised compounds. Insilico Medicine, with headquarters in both New York and Hong Kong, has achieved a major scientific breakthrough in the battle against fibrosis. To find new DDR1 kinase inhibitors, the generative tensorial reinforcement learning (GENTRL) GAI model was developed. To ensure their efficacy, GENTRL chemicals underwent biological testing. By going from an in silico to successful preclinical phase in just 21 days, the researchers accomplished an unprecedented feat (Zhavoronkov et al. 2019).

Reinforcement learning (RL) methods were employed by a team of researchers, including Korshunova et al. (2021), to create novel EGFR inhibitors. A combination of real-time incentives, the policy gradient algorithm, experience replay, and transfer learning constituted these methodologies. The inhibitors' efficacy was subsequently verified through experimental validation (Korshunova et al. 2021). The remarkable applications of GAI models offer potential for enhancing the genesis of novel therapeutic substances. The examples provided here illustrate the potential effectiveness of a medication development process that is GAI driven. It is emphasised that there is currently no silver bullet for AI-driven drug discovery. It may be required to make significant adjustments to the hyperparameters, GAI frameworks, and model training, among other things, in order to achieve optimal performance in an AI-driven drug development project. The primary challenges in the development of AI-driven medications are the absence of a consistent mathematical framework, the limited availability of sufficient data, and the numerous iterations of trial and error. Furthermore, the efficacy of any of the GAI models previously mentioned is exceedingly unlikely to persist in the event that the objective is altered, due to the intricacy of biological systems.

Shifting the focus from A1 may result in the predictor and generator lacking adequate data to generate compounds with therapeutic characteristics. The quantity and calibre of the data employed to train the model determine its predictive, classificatory, or outcome-generating capacities. Despite being widely discussed among deep learning specialists (Salakhutdinov 2015), researchers in medicinal chemistry have not fully utilised GAI frameworks (Lavecchia 2019). Despite its lack of discussion in the scientific community, GAI-driven drug development is rapidly emerging as a promising and efficient approach for generating novel molecules. The procedure involves training AI models, making predictions about molecular properties, generating novel drug-like chemicals, synthesising virtual laboratories, and verifying biological data. Instead of relying on unpredictable luck, this chapter provides a comprehensive description of current endeavours to surmount these challenges by examining different general artificial intelligence frameworks, with a particular emphasis on their use in drug development, recent accomplishments, and setbacks. The "Recent Advances" section contains extensive details on multiple medications currently undergoing clinical trials. The utilisation of generative artificial intelligence facilitated the detection and recognition of these chemical substances (Gupta et al. 2024).

1.2 GENERATIVE ARTIFICIAL INTELLIGENCE OVERVIEW

Incoming data may be assessed for patterns and insights by AI models, which may then execute a variety of tasks. Deep learning and machine learning (ML) are two examples of this. Among these activities are the following: data clustering, data synthesis (from inputs), numerical output prediction (regression), and data categorisation. A significant number of these positions are classified as either computer vision or natural language processing. Chemical graphs, which illustrate chemical structures,

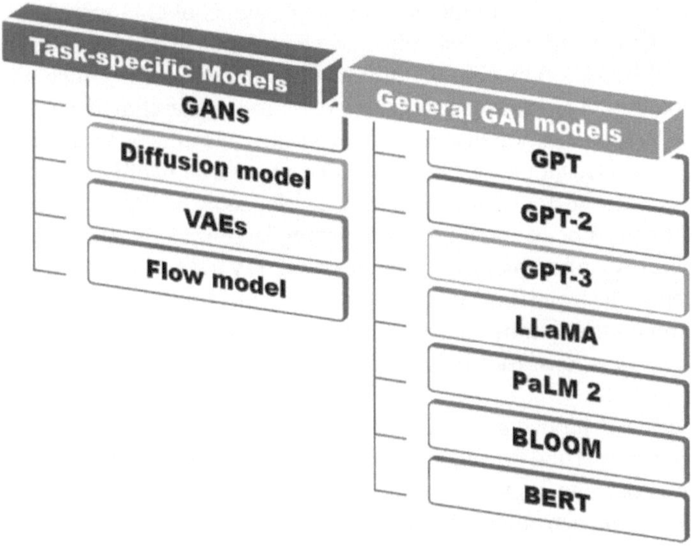

FIGURE 1.1 Types of generative artificial intelligence models.

as well as other images and medical images, are all subject to analysis in computer vision using convolutional neural network (CNN) models. In contrast, RNN models are employed in natural language processing (NLP) to analyse sequential data, such as strings that represent chemical structures or text. The recent success of large language models (LLMs) has sparked significant interest in the potential of GAI models to generate or construct distinctive datasets, such as photos, audio, phrases, films, and chemical compounds. The output may be an enhanced version of the inputs or an exact replica, contingent upon the task at hand and the GAI model's output.

By utilising the LLM (GPT-4) as its primary motivation, ChatGPT is intended to replicate human speech patterns and is taught accordingly. Similar to other LLM-based GAI models, this model was trained using extensive text and code datasets. As a result, it is capable of producing new content, translating languages, generating text that is comparable to its training data, and providing pertinent responses to inquiries from humans. ChatGPT is currently the most sophisticated language emulator capable of simulating spoken communication. GAI technologies/models (Figure 1.1) created a transformer architecture by utilising extensive online text datasets for training. Midjourney and DALL-E 2 are two notable private products in the sector of general artificial intelligence. While DALL-E 2 lets people create new images with text-to-graphics suggestions, Midjourney is an AI programme that can do the same thing and more (Shen et al. 2023; Editorials 2023; Patel et al. 2023).

It was noted earlier that the conventional method of developing new drugs has been time consuming and costly. However, the industry has undergone a significant transformation since GAI was introduced. The GAI method has the potential to revolutionise the industry by automating a multitude of laborious and repetitive processes that are associated with the development of medications. A new paper provides a comprehensive explanation of the potential applications of GAI models to generate therapeutic ideas by utilising extant biological and chemical data. Pharma by Insilico Medicine and BioNeMo by NVIDIA are two examples of cutting-edge pharmaceutical technologies. The pharmaceutical business uses general artificial intelligence tools for medication creation in a variety of contexts, one of which is artificial intelligence and related technologies. One generative adversarial intelligence platform that the pharmaceutical sector uses is BioNeMo, developed by NVIDIA and hosted in the cloud. For the purpose of training and deploying large-scale biomolecular language models, this HPC infrastructure was built. Using NVIDIA cloud APIs, researchers can easily build, test, and implement AI models for biomolecular prediction and generation. Through the simplification of GAI integration into biomolecule and protein structures and functions, BioNeMo accelerates the synthesis of new compounds for drug development.

Pharmaceutical products such as PandaOmics, Chemistry42, and inClinico are three components of the AI platform that are designed to perform specific duties. PandaOmics is a technology that was developed by iPanda and utilises network analysis to identify the activation or inhibition of specific pathways. Furthermore, it is capable of identifying pathways that involve dysregulated biochemical processes by establishing connections between related genes. PandaOmics facilitates the identification of novel targets by employing multi-omics techniques. PandaOmics generates a prioritised list of potential biological targets for each condition or subtype. Subsequently, it prioritises target theories based on their safety, capacity to interact with biologics and small molecules, and degree of originality. A potential objective score is produced by this approach. The company claims that Chemistry42 is a specialised platform that assists users in identifying novel compounds that are similar to lead. This automated and scalable methodology is exclusively dedicated to the development of De-Novo drugs. The discovery procedure can be completed in as little as one week. Chemistry42 employs generative artificial intelligence to produce innovative, drug-like compounds with precisely customised properties.

In order to accomplish this, we implement an extensive array of molecular components and compounds. Chemistry42 has established criteria for the molecular structure, chemical complexity, ease of synthesis, and stability of novel compounds in biological systems. Before comparing a newly synthesised molecule to other compounds in institutional and commercial databases, it is possible to assess its unique properties, including physicochemical parameters, binding scores, and drug-likeness traits, by annotating it. Data analysis on the inClinico platform can be employed to make predictions regarding the likelihood of clinical trial success. Mountains of data regarding the individuals under investigation, their health, the trials themselves, and the researchers themselves are employed by the methodology.

1.3 THE ROLE OF GAI IN DRUG DISCOVERY AND DEVELOPMENT PROCESSES

Pharmaceutical research and development has come a long way in the past 40 years, resulting in a complex and comprehensive process that encompasses drug discovery,

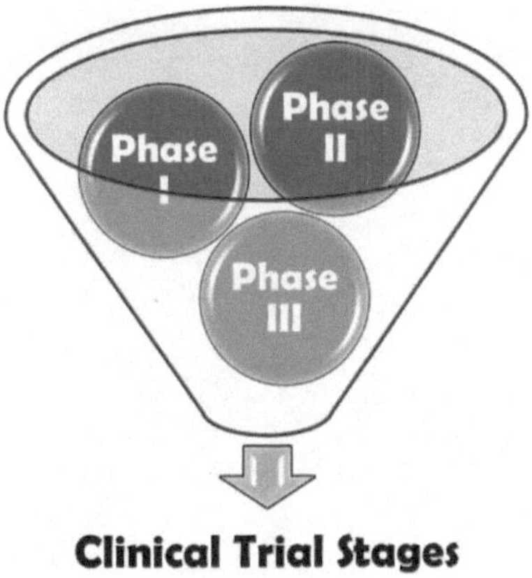

FIGURE 1.2 Stages of clinical trials.

clinical trials, and, ultimately, production certification from regulatory bodies. The drug development process, which encompasses the identification of targets, the optimisation of lead molecules, and the identification of promising compounds, typically requires approximately three years and a total of $500 million to be completed. It is followed by preclinical testing and clinical investigations. In clinical trials, there are three distinct stages: Phase I, Phase II, and Phase III (Figure 1.2). The compound's efficacy, safety, and dose requirements are all determined, and any adverse side effects are monitored. This phase is a significant investment of time and money, typically requiring approximately seven years and costing billions. After the effective conclusion of clinical trials, the subsequent step is to obtain authorisation from the appropriate regulatory bodies, such as the FDA or the EMA, to commence production. The subsequent phase involves obtaining approval to distribute or market the chemical. The final stage of this process typically requires approximately $50 million and lasts for a year or two (Zhang et al. 2022). In summary, the pharmaceutical industry's medicine development process is characterised by a significant amount of financial commitment and rigour, which are evident from the commencement of preliminary research to the release of the product to the market (Zhang et al. 2022). The roles of GAI in the drug discovery and development process are illustrated in Figure 1.3.

1.3.1 Identification and Validation of Targets

Generative AI has the ability to revolutionise traditional methods in the early stages of drug development by examining large and complicated biological datasets including genomes, transcriptomics, and proteomics. Artificial intelligence models can find and verify novel molecular targets involved in disease progression by employing complex algorithms. Because of their complex patterns and interactions, these targets are typically hard to spot using conventional analysis approaches. These

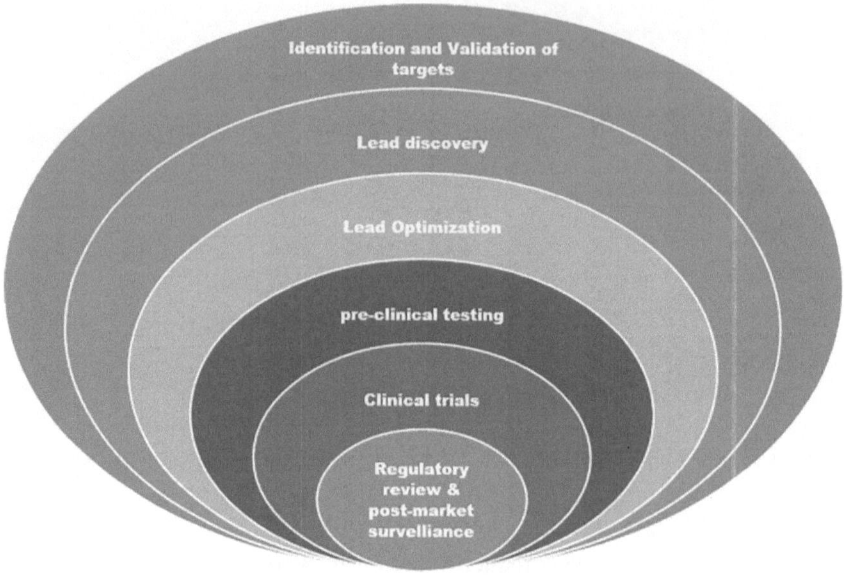

FIGURE 1.3 Roles of GAI in drug discovery and development.

models can use cutting-edge methods like reinforcement learning and deep learning to predict the biological activities and interactions of potential targets with high accuracy. Because of this, we can find possible chemical possibilities more efficiently (Moustaqil et al. 2020).

1.3.2 Lead Discovery

Generative adversarial networks (GANs), recurrent neural networks, and variational autoencoders (VAEs) improve generative AI's lead detection capabilities in comparison to conventional chemical screening methods (Rayhan 2024). When it comes to the modelling and suggestion of novel chemical compounds with targeted pharmacokinetic and pharmacodynamic characteristics, these AI frameworks truly excel. By iteratively enhancing the chemical structures to increase binding affinity and specificity, generative AI-driven models can substantially reduce the time and resources required to identify suitable lead compounds. This significantly simplifies the process of identifying new prospects.

1.3.3 Lead Optimisation

Generative AI-driven models can reduce side effects, optimise therapeutic efficacy, and improve pharmacological characteristics during the lead optimisation phase. Improving the precision of these forecasts through the use of QM/MM simulations paves the way for the methodical creation of candidates with the safest and most effective profiles (de Souza Neto et al. 2020).

1.3.4 Preclinical Testing

By applying predictive analytics to the study of prospective drugs' pharmacological and toxicological features, generative AI can make preclinical testing more efficient and predictable. If artificial intelligence models are capable of accurately predicting adverse reactions and therapeutic efficacy by analysing intricate biological data, the necessity for conventional in vitro and in vivo tests will diminish. The clinical data's dependability is enhanced by the ability to predict outcomes, which also expedites the process of clinical development (Mak et al. 2023).

1.3.5 Clinical Trials

The introduction of generative AI has the potential to revolutionise the selection of clinical trial participants, study design, and data analysis. By employing sophisticated language models to analyse vast quantities of patient data in order to identify the most promising candidates for recruitment, clinical trial success rates are enhanced. AI-powered platforms with generative capabilities can improve adaptive trial designs by enabling the real-time dynamic adjustment of trial parameters. Additionally, AIF facilitates the continuous monitoring of trial data, which aids in the early detection of efficacy and adverse effects (Bordukova et al. 2024).

1.3.6 Regulatory Review and Post-Market Surveillance

Artificial intelligence can enhance the efficiency and comprehensiveness of regulatory assessment by automating the accumulation and evaluation of submission dossiers. The efficacy of pharmaceuticals in real populations is perpetually evaluated through the use of artificial intelligence technologies after they are released to the market. Algorithms of this nature are capable of identifying adverse drug reactions and monitoring the efficacy of treatments in real time. The health of patients is protected by this real-time monitoring capability, which guarantees that clinical and regulatory responses to emergent safety concerns are promptly implemented (Mehran et al. 2004). Generative AI significantly improves decision-making and streamlines and expedites each phase of the drug development process. This results in the successful development of innovative medications. The healthcare industry is significantly affected by the extensive implementation of artificial intelligence, which enhances the quality of medicine and results in superior patient outcomes.

1.4 BLUEPRINT FOR USING GENERATIVE AI IN DRUG DISCOVERY AND DEVELOPMENT

The application of generative AI's novel solutions, which expedite and optimise the process, might dramatically alter the course of drug discovery. The use of generative AI could significantly impact numerous areas of medicinal research, including but not limited to biomarker discovery, compound library expansion, molecule generation, drug optimisation, drug design, and ADME property prediction (Figure 1.4).

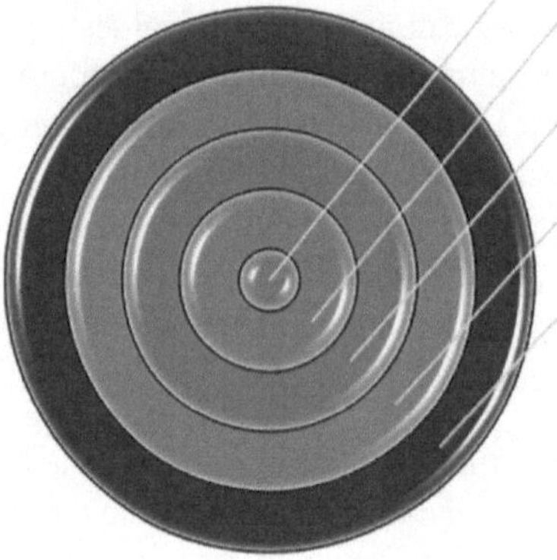

FIGURE 1.4 Blueprint for using GAI in drug discovery and development.

All of these applications highlight how generative AI can outperform current methods in pharmaceutical R&D, which could lead to a dramatic shift in the industry.

1.4.1 Drug Optimisation

The optimisation stage of medication formulation may be significantly altered by generative AI, which introduces sophisticated computational tools for modifying chemical structures. The objective of this AI application is to suggest modifications to existing drug molecules in order to enhance the therapeutic efficacy, safety features, and critical pharmacological qualities, such as binding affinity and solubility. It incorporates generative AI into drug development and conducts an exhaustive study of the vast chemical space to rapidly evaluate and predict the repercussions of molecular alterations. Generative AI systems that implement intricate algorithms can anticipate the toxicity, target interaction, ADME characteristics, and overall impact of molecular-level modifications on medicinal substances. This instrument simplifies the process of iteratively improving drugs, which can be both time consuming and expensive.

Additionally, this AI-driven approach enables the computational analysis of a broader spectrum of potential modifications, in contrast to conventional experimental methods. Generative AI employs deep learning models, including convolutional neural networks and generative neural networks (GNNs), to simulate and forecast the results of molecular modifications (Jing et al. 2018). In order to accomplish this, we leverage the existing knowledge of molecular dynamics and the interactions between drugs and receptors. The strategy has considerably reduced the risks associated with the development of new pharmaceutical drugs. Generative AI facilitates a more informed decision-making process during the development of new pharmaceuticals by rapidly assessing the efficacy and potential adverse effects of modified molecules. This results in a reduction in the optimisation time and an increase in the success rate of medication candidates in clinical trials.

1.4.2 De-Novo Drug Design

The De-Novo drug generation process could be greatly enhanced by generative AI's ability to generate novel therapeutic options. In order to accomplish this, we employ massive language models to assess and enhance these compounds by considering critical parameters such as safety profiles, selectivity for specific biological targets, and chemical feasibility. The initial step involves the meticulous selection of data, which is typically sourced from publicly available sources. The focus is on compounds that exhibit promising properties for future research. Property-based filtering and categorisation techniques are implemented by generative AI to enhance the dataset and establish the foundation for further model training. As part of this effort, which aims to improve understanding of molecular structures and characteristics, improved feature representation methods like SMILES and graph-based representations are crucial.

The focus moves to generative model development when the first phase ends. The selection and refinement of these models is the first step in the inception-to-development process of novel compounds. In the optimisation phase, we use property prediction models and reinforcement learning approaches to make the machine better at recommending molecular entities with optimised profiles. This phase is distinguished by its dynamic character. The primary objective is to identify a method of navigating the immense chemical space that is both more innovative and efficient than current methods. This will facilitate the identification of compounds that exhibit significant potential as therapeutic agents. The generative approach, which is the foundation of this methodology, has also piqued the interest of researchers.

It employs sophisticated deep learning algorithms to comprehend the probability distribution of chemical data, thereby constructing unique molecules that are customised to possess specific properties. This method is particularly well suited for the application of SBDD and property-based design due to its capacity to produce molecules in both two- and three-dimensional forms (Lima et al. 2016). The ability of AI-driven design to construct compounds that preferentially interact with target proteins, taking into account the structural properties of both the ligands and proteins, is a testament to its revolutionary power in drug development. As a consequence of these advancements, two distinct methodologies for compound generation have emerged: structure oriented and ligand oriented. The objective of each method is to develop compounds that exhibit improved selectivity and binding to particular proteins. The manufacturing of medicinal pharmaceuticals is about to enter a new era.

1.4.3 Compound Library Expansion

The development of analogues and derivatives of known molecules could be revolutionised by generative AI, which offers a fresh perspective on chemical library expansion in pharmaceutical research. The first step is to use advanced machine learning methods to thoroughly examine the structure-activity relationships (SARs) of all the compounds in the library (Guha 2013). Generative AI may anticipate modifications that enhance desirable attributes, including efficacy, reduced toxicity, or improved pharmacokinetic profiles, by investigating the impact of structural variations on molecular biological activity. The process of generating new chemical structures is enhanced by AI-generated suggestions, which enables the compound library to expand with variants that may not be feasible with more traditional methods. The diversity of molecules that are amenable to further investigation is significantly expanded by this new class of chemicals. Identifying compounds that are expected to have safety and efficacy benefits simplifies their integration into drug research. This enables scientists to rapidly design and evaluate these molecules, thereby transitioning from theoretical frameworks to real, testable candidates. Consequently, the compound library is perpetually enhanced and expanded through the iterative process of drug development, which entails synthesis, prediction, and experimental validation cycles. The process of identifying and optimising lead compounds can be continuously refined to significantly improve the efficiency and time-savings of drug development operations.

1.4.4 Predicting ADME Properties

By utilising a variety of deep learning techniques tailored to comprehend the complex biological processes that medications go through in the body, generative AI has the ability to greatly improve the prediction of ADME qualities in drug candidates. Transformer models, RNNs, CNNs, and GNNs are leading the charge in this groundbreaking development (Huang et al. 2021). One of the primary criteria for selecting these models is their ability to manage and evaluate extensive datasets that describe drug pharmacokinetics. Convolutional neural networks are capable of conducting a comprehensive analysis of molecular structures and accurately predicting the impact of these structures on drug absorption and distribution in the body due to their exceptional ability to identify patterns in geographical data. By interpreting intricate molecular visual or structural representations, CNNs may accurately predict ADME results. Sequential data processing efficacy is one of the numerous advantages of RNNs. This is the reason they are so beneficial for simulating the complex pathways of drug metabolism and excretion.

The arrangement of these structures is crucial for comprehending the progression of a medication through its metabolic pathways, as it enables the preservation of information from previous inputs. Generative neural networks (GNNs) offer a sophisticated approach to capturing the dynamic interactions of molecule elements. This property is essential for the investigation of the complex network of molecular interactions and their impact on the distribution and interaction of drugs within the body. Transformer models have garnered recognition for their capacity to manage densely linked data, which has been demonstrated in their application in pharmacological discovery and their success in NLP. They are capable of conducting a comprehensive analysis of intricate chemical structures or metabolic activities, identifying patterns that regulate the ADME characteristics of drugs in various biological contexts (Huang et al. 2021). The pharmacokinetic behaviours of a medicine can be predicted with great precision and complexity by generative AI through the use of these advanced deep learning techniques. The drug discovery process can be more effectively directed towards candidates with favourable ADME characteristics as a result. In addition to speeding up the discovery of promising medicinal molecules, this innovative approach may improve the safety and effectiveness of new pharmaceuticals.

1.4.5 Discovery of Biomarkers

Biomarker discovery stands to benefit greatly from generative AI's ability to shed light on the origins, progression, and therapeutic efficacy of a wide range of diseases. Biomarkers are essential in many areas of medicine due to their distinctive molecular signatures; for example, they help with improving diagnostic accuracy, finding new therapeutic targets, and creating more targeted treatments. The intrinsic complexity of biological data, characterised by its high dimensionality and the intricate interaction of genetic and environmental factors, presents a significant difficulty in the accurate identification of biomarkers. The discovery of biomarkers is a challenging procedure. The advanced and all-encompassing language models used by generative AI give it the ability to discover complex linkages and patterns that would be missed by conventional analysis techniques. One area where deep neural networks really shine is in representing complex and nonlinear associations between genes and their phenotypic effects. Biomarkers that show a person's reactivity to treatment or their vulnerability to a disease can be found using this approach. It is possible to train generative models like GANs and VAEs to reproduce a broad variety of biological data. By creating synthetic data points, this could help find new biomarkers, which could improve our understanding of disease processes (Hong et al. 2019).

Machine learning classifiers can use supervised learning techniques to correctly categorise individuals according to the presence of particular biomarkers, which can improve patient stratification and the identification of possible therapy targets. Accelerating the identification of biomarkers and laying the groundwork for the creation of precise and personalised therapeutic interventions are both made possible by generative AI's ability to efficiently assess and extract crucial knowledge from complicated biological datasets. Improved, patient-specific medicines may be on the horizon, thanks to the abundance of data that could be uncovered by this innovative method of studying disease causes. That being the case, it may herald a new age in precision medicine, which may lead to dramatic improvements in patient outcomes.

1.5 CHALLENGES AND OPPORTUNITIES OF GAI IN DRUG DISCOVERY AND DEVELOPMENT

The pharmaceutical development sector is significantly impacted by AI, as it enables scientists to create new compounds from the ground up. The global pharmaceutical industry remains primarily driven by small molecules (Bickerton et al. 2012). This implies that GAI technologies will likely remain in existence for an extended period and will likely alter the method by which we discover and develop new medications. Growing evidence suggests that GAI can be used to explore chemically uncharted territories. In the case of CLMs, the fundamental rationale for this is the versatility and ease of use of molecular strings, as well as the numerous tasks they are capable of conducting. The integration of medicinal chemistry knowledge and enhancements in LLMs/NLP algorithms is expected to result in enhanced drug discovery capabilities in GAI. GAI's future is promising; however, numerous challenges must be surmounted before it can be implemented extensively in the development of medications. It is a common practice to optimise fundamental measures, such as molecular weight, octanol-water partitioning coefficient, or quantitative drug-likeness estimation, when evaluating GAI models (Renz et al. 2019).

The development of compounds that meet specific criteria, as well as the exact behaviour and destiny of these compounds within biological systems, may result in oversimplifications if the complexities of actual drug development are disregarded (Merk et al. 2018b; Moret et al. 2021). The quality of the molecules produced is not thoroughly assessed by existing De-Novo design standards, such as GuacaMol (Brown et al. 2019) and MOSES (Polykovskiy et al. 2020), which enable the comparison of independently developed techniques. Experimental validation is considered the most effective method for assessing the quality of novel ideas due to the challenges posed by computational concerns. Only a small number of potential GAI applications have been documented thus far (Li et al. 2020; Grisoni et al. 2021; Moret et al. 2021). In order to ensure the successful implementation of general artificial intelligence in practical scenarios, it is imperative that experts in medicinal chemistry, cheminformatics, and deep learning collaborate.

Van Tilborg et al. (2022) discovered that automated synthesis platforms can be a viable alternative for expediting the De-Novo design process that GAI initiated, despite their limitations in terms of the chemical space that can be accessed for synthesis. Despite their application in comprehending the molecular architectures of pharmaceutical complexes, BERT and GPT models have had minimal impact on the development of medicines. The computational prediction of DTIs is an additional challenge. However, the absence of annotated data complicates the process of training models that operate on larger molecules, such as proteins or peptides. However, this discipline would make significant progress if LLMs were capable of reading protein and peptide sequences in the same way as text. Additionally, the most effective therapy combinations for complex diseases can now be predicted by utilising the most recent deep learning advancements to comprehend the relationship between genetic modifications and minute compounds. For instance, this serves as an illustration of the construction of GAI models by incorporating data from gene expression and chemical structure, two interconnected yet distinct domains. Similar to the construction of LLMs, the process of constructing large CLMs involves training the model with examples from the literature. It is anticipated that conditional generation algorithms will continue to play an increasingly significant role in the future. These strategies have the potential to address the deficiencies of current scoring systems, such as non-additivity and activity cliffs, by developing compounds that are tailored to meet specific needs (Kwapien et al. 2022; Özçelik et al. 2022). Volkov et al. (2022) assert that structure-based design has not yet explored the potential of creating novel macromolecular targets.

This approach is intended to generate molecules that possess electrostatic and geometric properties that enable them to bond to specific sites. Graff et al. (2021) suggest that the current protein-ligand affinity databases may have biases and constraints that contribute to the failure of structure-based De-Novo design in practice. Understudied disciplines such as polypharmacology and selectivity would be significantly impacted if specific aspects of De-Novo design could be precisely controlled. In addition to the substantial expense of establishing a GAI, there are biassed GAI models to address. It is imperative to conduct a comprehensive evaluation of drug candidates that have been developed using biassed models. These candidates may be ineffective, entail risks, or even expose the biases of the experts. Cloud computing can resolve the issue of elevated processing costs. Cloud computing has enabled scientists to access vast quantities of computational power without the need to invest in costly equipment. Resolution of the data insufficiency issue and reduction of the time and cost required to train GAI models are both feasible. We have already proven that federated learning, active learning, and transfer learning offer an alternative approach. Another alternative is to experiment with various data augmentation methods. This implies that GAI models are more resilient to the effects of data noise bias. Future applications of GAI models are expected to be enhanced by few-shot learning techniques combined with large-scale pre-trained CLMs (Gao and Coley 2020).

Krenn et al. (2022) assert that CLMs will be significantly more beneficial in the drug development process once they improve their ability to suggest synthesisable molecules. The introduction of more complex molecular entities, such as peptides and proteins, including non-natural amino acids, into chemical languages is a promising prospect for the extension of GAI tools in chemistry. Bender and Cortés-Ciriano (2021) examined potential SELFIES enhancements in order to address the deficiencies of current molecular string representations. These concepts have the potential to influence the future development of DeepSMILES and SMILES. GAI models are anticipated to become more significant as novel drugs are developed. GAI will enhance the efficiency and cost-effectiveness of medicine discovery by expediting the research of unexplored chemical regions and the development and evaluation of intriguing new scientific concepts. The day will come when AI researchers, chemists, and biologists collaborate to develop state-of-the-art algorithms that incorporate authentic scientific data. Therefore, they have the ability to acquire critical information regarding human biology through the use of AI. A comprehensive assessment of the present state of AI-driven drug discovery and the constraints that restrict its full potential has been conducted, as cited by Bender et al. (Gao and Coley 2020; Bender and Cortés-Ciriano 2021). The subsequent two articles (Zhang et al. 2023) offer a comprehensive examination of the reasons artificial intelligence is demonstrating increased advantages in fields beyond chemistry and biology, specifically in the field of medication discovery.

1.6 FUTURE PROSPECTS

Innovations in artificial general intelligence have had a major impact on the creation of new pharmaceuticals. This chapter takes a look at GAI models as they are right now and how they could help find new drugs. Implementing recurrent neural networks, standard convolutional neural networks, and graphical neural networks in molecular generators could improve their performance. A variational inference strategy is used by algorithms such as GAN and VAE. Differentiating itself from variational inference, reinforcement learning may make real-time adjustments to processes to produce targeted molecules. The integration of state-of-the-art transformers and cutting-edge GAI methods with LLMs has the potential to significantly enhance drug development. In order to surmount this constraint and develop the ability to synthesise new molecules with the desired properties, GAI models require large and diverse datasets of compounds. Despite the algorithm's current advancements and rapid enhancements, it is evident that GAI has a promising future in drug discovery. Nevertheless, the process of obtaining access to these databases can be both time consuming and expensive. In order to fully leverage general artificial intelligence, it is imperative to develop novel techniques, as is the case in other disciplines where AI has advanced, despite the fact that there are numerous methods for addressing insufficient data. Research into a variety of AI applications, including computer vision, autonomous vehicles, and natural language processing, can be advantageous to the development of AI-based pharmaceuticals. The fundamental algorithms, which are typically universally applicable, must be refined to accommodate the unique requirements of chemical compounds and biological macromolecules.

Modern technologies are enabling an increasing number of scientists to recognise the numerous advantages of parallel and distributed computing. Additionally, the utility of GAI models in drug development is contingent upon their interpretability. In order to comprehend the process by which the model generates particular compounds, it is imperative that researchers be acquainted with its internal mechanisms. In order for GAI models to function effectively, the data must be highly dependable. This is due to the presence of a variety of noise and imperfections in the training data that is utilised to train these models. GAI models have the potential to revolutionise the discovery of medications, despite their limitations. These models have the potential to enhance efficacy and reduce the overall costs of medicine development by automating the production of novel molecules. It is anticipated that technology and GAI models will play a critical role in future drug development endeavours as they continue to advance. In due course, data scarcity, erroneous model interpretation, bias, and high processing costs will be resolved. No doubt, the development of medications will be transformed by GAI. We aspire to make significant progress in the development of compounds that have the potential to save lives by integrating them with established methodologies.

1.7 CONCLUSION

Integrating generative AI into healthcare, particularly in drug discovery, signifies a significant change from conventional methods to a more adaptable, effective, and individualised approach. This investigation illustrates that the drug discovery process can be substantially expedited by generative AI, which commences with target identification and concludes with post-market surveillance. This not only expedites the process but also enhances the precision and efficacy of the production of new medicinal substances. Generative AI can facilitate the development, optimisation, and evaluation of prospective therapeutic options by employing sophisticated large language models. It utilises extensive databases to conduct research in a wide range of chemical disciplines, demonstrating exceptional creativity and breadth. This investigation has the potential to identify promising therapeutic compounds that would have been difficult to identify using conventional drug discovery methods. According to market projections, the economic implications of this technological transition are expected to be substantial, as generative AI applications in drug development are anticipated to experience a significant increase in valuation.

Nevertheless, there is still a significant amount of work that must be accomplished in order to fully harness the maximum capabilities of generative AI in the field of drug development. Key obstacles involve the effective management of disparate and isolated data ecosystems, the representation of diverse biological data across many modes, and the mitigation of physician bias and stereotyping. These challenges highlight the fragile nature of incorporating AI into this discipline and the complex structure of biomedicine. Our research suggests that implementing a methodical approach to utilising generative AI could be advantageous for the pharmaceutical industry. This strategy enables a more customised approach to treatment, highlighting the technology's capacity to improve lead optimisation, identify biomarkers, and expand chemical libraries. Furthermore, it emphasises the significance of novel data collection techniques and regulatory structures that can facilitate the expanding capabilities of generative AI. Last, generative AI holds significant potential in both the healthcare and pharmaceutical sectors. The proponents of this concept envision a future in which medical treatments are customised to suit the unique needs and characteristics of each patient, with improved efficiency and affordability. In order to achieve this objective and enhance the accuracy of clinical outcomes in precision medicine, it is imperative to address the aforementioned challenges and fully harness the potential of generative AI. Collaboratively, researchers, medical experts, and politicians will influence the healthcare business of the future by disseminating and fully actualising the advantages of this state-of-the-art technology.

REFERENCES

Aliper, A., S. Plis, A. Artemov, A. Ulloa, P. Mamoshina, and A. Zhavoronkov. 2016. Deep learning applications for predicting pharmacological properties of drugs and drug repurposing using transcriptomic data. *Mol. Pharm.* 13: 2524–2530. https://doi.org/10.1021/acs.molpharmaceut.6b00248

Bender, A., and I. Cortés-Ciriano. 2021. Artificial intelligence in drug discovery: What is realistic, what are illusions? Part 1: ways to make an impact, and why we are not there yet. *Drug Discov. Today* 26: 511–524. https://doi.org/10.1016/j.drudis.2020.12.009

Bickerton, G.R., G.V. Paolini, J. Besnard, S. Muresan, and A.L. Hopkins. 2012. Quantifying the chemical beauty of drugs. *Nat. Chem.* 4: 90–98. https://doi.org/10.1038/nchem.1243

Bordukova, M., N. Makarov, R. Rodriguez-Esteban, F. Schmich, and M.P. Menden. 2024. Generative artificial intelligence empowers digital twins in drug discovery and clinical trials. *Expert Opin. Drug Discov.* 19(1): 33–42.

Brown, N., M. Fiscato, M.H.S. Segler, and A.C. Vaucher. 2019. GuacaMol: Benchmarking models for de novo molecular design. *J. Chem. Inf. Model.* 59: 1096–1108. https://doi.org/10.1021/acs.jcim.8b00839

Chao, X., G. Kou, T. Li, and Y. Peng. 2018. Jie Ke versus AlphaGo: A ranking approach using decision making method for large-scale data with incomplete information. *Eur. J. Operational Res.* 265: 239–247. https://doi.org/10.1016/j.ejor.2017.07.030

Coeckelbergh, M. 2020. Artificial intelligence, responsibility attribution, and a relational justification of explainability. *Sci. Eng. Ethics* 26: 2051–2068. https://doi.org/10.1007/s11948-019-00146-8

Collins, G.S., and K.G.M. Moons. 2019. Reporting of artificial intelligence prediction models. *Lancet* 393: 1577–1579. https://doi.org/10.1016/S0140-6736(19)30037-6

de Souza Neto, L.R., J.T. Moreira-Filho, B.J. Neves, et al. 2020. In silico strategies to support fragment-to-lead optimization in drug discovery. *Front. Chem.* 8: 93.

DiMasi, J.A., H.G. Grabowski, and R.W. Hansen. 2016. Innovation in the pharmaceutical industry: New estimates of R&D costs. *J. Health Econ.* 47: 20–33. https://doi.org/10.1016/j.jhealeco.2016.01.012

Editorials, N. 2023. Tools such as ChatGPT threaten transparent science; here are our ground rules for their use. *Nature* 613: 10–1038. https://doi.org/10.1038/d41586-023-001911

Gao, W., and C.W. Coley. 2020. The synthesizability of molecules proposed by generative models. *J. Chem. Inf. Model.* 60: 5714–5723. https://doi.org/10.1021/acs.jcim.0c00174

Graff, D.E., E.I. Shakhnovich, and C.W. Coley. 2021. Accelerating highthroughput virtual screening through molecular pool-based active learning. *Chem. Sci.* 12: 7866–7881. https://doi.org/10.1039/d0sc06805e

Grisoni, F., B.J.H. Huisman, A.L. Button, et al. 2021. Combining generative artificial intelligence and on-chip synthesis for de novo drug design. *Sci. Adv.* 7: eabg3338. https://doi.org/10.1126/sciadv.abg3338

Guha, R. 2013. On exploring structure–activity relationships. *Methods Mol. Biol. Silico Models Drug Discov.* 81–94.

Gupta, U., A. Pranav, A. Kohli, S. Ghosh, and D. Singh. 2024. The contribution of artificial intelligence to drug discovery: Current progress and prospects for the future. In *Microbial Data Intelligence and Computational Techniques for Sustainable Computing.* Springer Nature Singapore, pp. 1–23.

Hong, S.H., S. Ryu, J. Lim, and W.Y. Kim. 2019. Molecular generative model based on an adversarially regularized autoencoder. *J. Chem. Inf. Model.* 60(1): 29–36.

Huang, D.Z., J.C. Baber, and S.S. Bahmanyar. 2021. The challenges of generalizability in artificial intelligence for ADME/Tox endpoint and activity prediction. *Expert Opin. Drug Discov.* 16(9): 1045–1056.

Jing, Y., Y. Bian, Z. Hu, L. Wang, and X.Q.S. Xie. 2018. Deep learning for drug design: An artificial intelligence paradigm for drug discovery in the big data era. *AAPS J.* 20: 1–10.

Korshunova, M., N. Huang, S. Capuzzi, et al. 2021. A bag of tricks for automated de novo design of molecules with the desired properties: Application to EGFR inhibitor discovery. *Theor. Comput. Chem.* https://doi.org/10.26434/chemrxiv.14045072.v1

Krenn, M., Q. Ai, S. Barthel, et al. 2022. SELFIES and the future of molecular string representations. *Patterns* 3: 100588. https://doi.org/10.1016/j.patter.2022.100588

Kwapien, K., E. Nittinger, J. He, C. Margreitter, A. Voronov, and C. Tyrchan. 2022. Implications of additivity and nonadditivity for machine learning and deep learning models in drug design. *ACS Omega* 7: 26573–26581. https://doi.org/10.1021/acsomega.2c02738

Lavecchia, A. 2019. Deep learning in drug discovery: Opportunities, challenges and future prospects. *Drug Discov. Today* 24: 2017–2032. https://doi.org/10.1016/j.drudis.2019.07.006

Li, X., Y. Xu, H. Yao, and K. Lin. 2020. Chemical space exploration based on recurrent neural networks: Applications in discovering kinase inhibitors. *J. Cheminf.* 12: 42–13. https://doi.org/10.1186/s13321-020-00446-3

Li, X., Y. Xu, L. Lai, and J. Pei. 2018. Prediction of human cytochrome P450 inhibition using a multitask deep autoencoder neural network. *Mol. Pharm.* 15: 4336–4345. https://doi.org/10.1021/acs.molpharmaceut.8b00110

Lima, A.N., E.A. Philot, G.H. Trossini, L.P.B. Scott, V.G. Maltarollo, and K.M. Honorio. 2016. Use of machine learning approaches for novel drug discovery. *Expert Opin. Drug Discov.* 11(3): 225–239.

Mak, K.K., Y.H. Wong, and M.R. Pichika. 2023. Artificial intelligence in drug discovery and development. In *Drug Discovery and Evaluation: Safety and Pharmacokinetic Assays.* Springer Nature Singapore, pp. 1–38.

Mamoshina, P., A. Vieira, E. Putin, and A. Zhavoronkov. 2016. Applications of deep learning in biomedicine. *Mol. Pharm.* 13: 1445–1454. https://doi.org/10.1021/acs.molpharmaceut.5b00982

Mehran, R., M.B. Leon, D.A. Feigal, et al. 2004. Postmarket approval surveillance: A call for a more integrated and comprehensive approach. *Circulation* 109(25): 3073–3077.

Merk, D., F. Grisoni, L. Friedrich, and G. Schneider. 2018a. Tuning artificial intelligence on the de novo design of natural-product-inspired retinoid X receptor modulators. *Commun. Chem.* 1: 68. https://doi.org/10.1038/s42004-018-0068-1

Merk, D., L. Friedrich, F. Grisoni, and G. Schneider. 2018b. De novo design of bioactive small molecules by artificial intelligence. *Mol. Inf.* 37: 1700153. https://doi.org/10.1002/minf.201700153

Moret, M., M. Helmstädter, F. Grisoni, G. Schneider, and D. Merk. 2021. Beam search for automated design and scoring of novel ROR ligands with machine intelligence. *Angew. Chem. Int. Ed.* 60: 19477–19482. https://doi.org/10.1002/anie.202104405

Moustaqil, M., Y. Gambin, and E. Sierecki. 2020. Biophysical techniques for target validation and drug discovery in transcription-targeted therapy. *Int. J. Mol. Sci.* 21(7): 2301.

Özçelik, R., D. van Tilborg, J. Jiménez-Luna, and F. Grisoni. 2022. Structure-based drug discovery with deep learning. *ChemBioChem* 24: e202200776. https://doi.org/10.1002/cbic.202200776

Patel, S.B., K. Lam, and M. Liebrenz. 2023. ChatGPT: Friend or foe. *Lancet Digit. Health* 5: e102. https://doi.org/10.1016/s2589-7500(23)00023-7

Paul, S.M., D.S. Mytelka, C.T. Dunwiddie, et al. 2010. How to improve R&D productivity: The pharmaceutical industry's grand challenge. *Nat. Rev. Drug Discov.* 9: 203–214. https://doi.org/10.1038/nrd3078

Polykovskiy, D., A. Zhebrak, B. Sanchez-Lengeling, et al. 2020. Molecular sets (MOSES): a benchmarking platform for molecular generation models. *Front. Pharmacol.* 11: 565644. https://doi.org/10.3389/fphar.2020.565644

Popova, M., O. Isayev, and A. Tropsha. 2018. Deep reinforcement learning for de novo drug design. *Sci. Adv.* 4: eaap7885. https://doi.org/10.1126/sciadv.aap7885

Rayhan, A. 2024. *Accelerating Drug Discovery and Material Design: Unleashing AI's Potential for Optimizing Molecular Structures and Properties*. Preprint, pp 1–23. https://doi.org/10.13140/RG.2.2.27695.30888

Renz, P., D. Van Rompaey, J.K. Wegner, S. Hochreiter, and G. Klambauer. 2019. On failure modes in molecule generation and optimization. *Drug Discov. Today Technol.* 32: 55–63. https://doi.org/10.1016/j.ddtec.2020.09.003

Salakhutdinov, R. 2015. Learning deep generative models. *Annu. Rev. Statistics Appl.* 2: 361–385. https://doi.org/10.1146/annurev-statistics-010814-020120

Service, R.F. 2020. 'The game has changed.' AI triumphs at protein folding. *Science* 370. Washington, DC, United States: American Association for the Advancement of Science.

Shen, Y., L. Heacock, J. Elias, et al. 2023. ChatGPT and other large language models are double-edged swords. *Radiol. Soc. North Am.* e230163. Oak Brook, Illinois, United States.

Singh, S., A. Okun, and A. Jackson. 2017. Artificial intelligence: Learning to play go from scratch. *Nature* 550: 336–337. https://doi.org/10.1038/550336a

Stokes, J.M., K. Yang, K. Swanson, et al. 2020. A deep learning approach to antibiotic discovery. *Cell* 180: 688–702. https://doi.org/10.1016/j.cell.2020.01.021

Tang, B., S.T. Kramer, M. Fang, Y. Qiu, Z. Wu, and D. Xu. 2020. A self-attention based message passing neural network for predicting molecular lipophilicity and aqueous solubility. *J. Cheminform.* 12: 15–19. https://doi.org/10.1186/s13321-020-0414-z

Thierer, A.D., A. Castillo O'Sullivan, and R. Russell. 2017. *Artificial Intelligence and Public Policy*. Arlington, VA, United States: Mercatus Research Paper.

van Tilborg, D., A. Alenicheva, and F. Grisoni. 2022. Exposing the limitations of molecular machine learning with activity cliffs. *J. Chem. Inf. Model.* 62: 5938–5951. https://doi.org/10.1021/acs.jcim.2c01073

Volkov, M., J.A. Turk, N. Drizard, et al. 2022. On the frustration to predict binding affinities from protein–ligand structures with deep neural networks. *J. Med. Chem.* 65: 7946–7958. https://doi.org/10.1021/acs. jmedchem.2c00487

von Ungern-Sternberg, A. 2017. Autonomous driving: Regulatory challenges raised by artificial decision-making and tragic choices. In *Research Handbook on the Law of Artificial Intelligenc*e. Cheltenham, United Kingdom: Edward Elgar.

Zhang, Y., H. Pei, S. Zhen, et al. 2023. Downregulated RBM5 enhances CARM1 expression and activates the PRKACA/GSK3β signaling pathway through alternative splicing-coupled nonsense-mediated decay. *Gastroenterol. Endosc.* 1: 139–143. https://doi.org/10.3390/cancers16010139

Zhang, Y., M. Luo, P. Wu, S. Wu, T.Y. Lee, and C. Bai. 2022. Application of computational biology and artificial intelligence in drug design. *Int. J. Mol. Sci.* 23(21): 13568.

Zhavoronkov, A., Y.A. Ivanenkov, A. Aliper, et al. 2019. Deep learning enables rapid identification of potent DDR1 kinase inhibitors. *Nat. Biotechnol.* 37: 1038–1040. https://doi.org/10.1038/s41587-019-0224-x

2 Generative Models for Image-to-Image Translation

Theoretical Insights, Methodological Frameworks, and Practical Applications

Rashmi Kumari, Subhranil Das, and Raghwendra Kishore Singh

2.1 INTRODUCTION

Image-to-image translation is one of the most important transformative fields, where the picture is converted into the single domain [1, 2]. This technique uses recent machine learning (ML) models to change certain visual characteristics like style, colour, or texture to complete the new image by preserving the original core meaning [3]. Image-to-image translation is a ML and computer vision approach which converts an image from one representation to another [4, 5]. In this approach, deep learning (DL) models are applied to learn the mappings between multiple visual domains for different transformations such as black-and-white pictures [6], transforming sketches into realistic images, and changing the image style. Image-to-image translation is adaptable due to its real-time applications in many industries, including relevance for many image domains in health and autonomous driving applications [7, 8].

2.1.1 Background

Image-to-image translation can be applied to image processing methods in earlier years which is dependent on extraction of features [9]. These approaches were limited in scope and accuracy because they required extensive human intervention and could not generalise across different image types. Image-to-image translation has progressed from basic image processing techniques based on manual feature extraction and heuristic criteria to sophisticated deep learning models capable of producing high-quality, realistic results. The rise of DL models such as convolutional neural networks (CNNs) and generative adversarial networks (GANs) has accelerated progress in the field of image-to-image translation [10, 11]. These technologies have

DOI: 10.1201/9781003539483-2

improved the quality and application of changes in the picture, which allows for more realistic outcomes.

Various key frameworks are applicable image-to-image translation, including convolutional neural networks, which are essential for feature extraction and representation learning. Generative adversarial networks are used for generating realistic images through adversarial training. The pix2pix framework utilises conditional GANs for paired image translation tasks. CycleGAN addresses unpaired image translation with cycle consistency loss [12]. The gradual emergence of CNNs excels, while the extraction of hierarchical features and GANs are introduced for revolutionising realistic image generation through adversarial training. The interpretation of CNNs is mainly of the features obtained from images by efficiently learning the information from images. Kumari et al. [13] introduced GANs, which mainly consist of two competing networks, the generator and the discriminator, which improve each other through adversarial training. Kumari et al. [14] created a framework where conditional GANs learn to map input to output images, which gives a versatile solution for paired image translation challenges. Zhu et al. [15] proposed CycleGAN, which uses cycle consistency loss to handle unpaired image translation, allowing models to learn mappings between domains without using paired samples.

2.1.2 Motivation

Image-to-image translation has it potential advantages over existing approaches. Key motivations include the following:

- Practical Impact: The technology has the potential to alter several disciplines, including healthcare, driverless vehicles, and the creative industries.
- Enhancing Creativity: Artists and designers can use image-to-image translation to push the limits of digital art and design.
- Improving ML Models: Image-to-image translation, which generates different synthetic data, can improve the performance and robustness of ML models.
- Solving Real-World Problems: Real-world applications for improved image translation algorithms include environmental monitoring, forensic investigation, and historical photo restoration.

2.1.3 Scope of the Study

The scope of this research includes a thorough assessment of image-to-image translation, including basic fundamental principles, different methodologies, and various applications in real-time scenarios.

2.2 FUNDAMENTALS OF IMAGE-TO-IMAGE TRANSLATION

Various applications of image-to-image translation are diverse and span medical imaging, autonomous driving, art and design, and augmentation of data. The basic network is the convolutional neural network [16, 17], which is specifically designed for processing grid-like data, such as images. These networks consist of convolutional layers, pooling layers, and fully connected layers that capture spatial hierarchies and features in images. They are mainly used for the classification of images, detection of objects, and extraction of features, which are foundational for image-to-image translation.

The introduction of CNNs represented a watershed moment in image processing. CNNs' capacity to learn hierarchical features from images has substantially increased the accuracy and efficiency of image analysis operations. In the 1980s–1990s, the initial development of CNNs and their application were applied to simple image recognition tasks. In 2002, the breakthrough with AlexNet demonstrated the power of deep CNNs on the ImageNet challenge.

The next common network type is a generative adversarial network, which is a class of ML frameworks involving two neural networks, the generator and the discriminator, that train simultaneously through adversarial processes [18, 19]. The generator creates synthetic images, and the discriminator evaluates the authenticity of images, distinguishing between real and generated images. Through adversarial training, GANs improve the quality and realism of generated images [20].

GANs were introduced by Ian Goodfellow et al. in 2014, which revolutionised image generation by introducing adversarial training [21]. The introduction of GANs demonstrated the ability to generate realistic images through adversarial learning.

The most recently used are conditional GANs (cGANs), a variant of GANs where the generator and discriminator are conditioned on additional information, such as class labels or input images. The function is to enable controlled image generation is crucial for tasks like pix2pix. Cycle consistency loss used in CycleGAN for ensuring the consistency in the pixels in the image. The function of a cGAN is to facilitate unpaired image-to-image translation by enforcing consistency in bidirectional mappings.

Recent years have seen continuous improvements and innovations in image-to-image translation, including multimodal translation, where different techniques like multimodal unsupervised image-to-image translation (MUNIT) generate diverse outputs for a given input [22]. In high-resolution translation, the models are capable of handling high-resolution images, enhancing the realism and applicability of translations [23].

2.2.1 Variants of GANs

Different GAN variations have been created to meet particular issues and applications in image-to-image translation. pix2pix and CycleGAN are two of the most common variations and are described in the following paragraphs.

2.2.1.1 pix2pix

pix2pix, developed by Isola et al. in 2016 [24], is a conditional GAN for paired image-to-image translation problems. It learns the mapping from the input domain to the target domain using paired training data, in which each input image corresponds to an output image.

pix2pix's generator is built on a U-Net architecture, while the discriminator is a PatchGAN. The structure of encoder and decoder of U-Net architecture ensures to preserve information during translation. Adversarial loss functions are used by pix-2pix that encourage the generator to produce realistic images. L1-loss is calculated for generating any image where the scores suggest better convergence, resulting in high-quality outputs.

2.2.1.2 CycleGAN

CycleGAN, introduced by Zhu et al. [25], introduced challenging concepts in image-to-image translation where paired training data is not applicable. The concept of cycle consistency is introduced, where the image has been translated from different domains and back to the original domain.

Two generators are employed by CycleGAN, one for each translation direction. Two discriminators are applied for CycleGAN, one per domain. The model enables bidirectional mapping for learning the translation between the two domains. The loss functions are adversarial loss, which are applied separately for both domains to encourage the generation of realistic images. Cycle consistency loss ensures that an image translated to another domain and back remains consistent with the original image.

2.2.2 Variational Autoencoders

Another sort of generative model is variational autoencoders (VAEs) [26], which create new data points using a probabilistic technique. Unlike GANs, VAEs explicitly model the training data's underlying distribution and produce new instances by sampling from it. In contrast to GANs' adversarial training, VAEs encode and decode inputs, maximising a variational lower limit for smoother, more understandable latent spaces.

The encoder maps the input image to a latent space, producing a mean and variance that define a Gaussian distribution. The decoder samples from this latent distribution to generate new images that resemble the input data. VAEs are very suitable for jobs that need both interpretability and representation learning. They generate a smooth latent space that enables meaningful interpolations between data points. Inputs are encoded into the latent space by calculating reconstruction loss score.

2.3 GENERATIVE MODELS FOR IMAGE-TO-IMAGE TRANSLATION

2.3.1 Introduction to Generative Models

Generative models are ML frameworks that can produce new data instances that are similar to the training data [27]. Unlike discriminative models, which are used for classification tasks (for example, identifying whether an image contains a cat), generative models can generate new data points, such as images, by learning the underlying distribution of the training data. Generative models are important in image-to-image translation because they teach how to change images from one domain to another while keeping fundamental attributes. This includes accurately translating the complex relationships and structures in the input data to the destination domain.

The pre-processing steps for generative models are normalisation, which ensures consistent pixel value ranges, improving training stability. Then, image sizes is adjusted to fit model input requirements while preserving important features. Finally, the image is converted between colour spaces for specific tasks like simplifying image complexity.

Data augmentation techniques are applied for the processed images for a particular application. In geometric transformations, rotation, translation, flipping, and scaling are applied to increase dataset variability. Colour jittering alters brightness, contrast, saturation, and hue to make models robust to colour variations. Noise injection adds noise to images to enhance model robustness. Random erasing masks parts of images to improve model resilience to occlusions.

2.3.2 Generative Adversarial Networks

Generative adversarial networks are one of the most popular generative models [28]. Generally, GANs are made up of two neural networks, a generator and a discriminator, that are trained concurrently via adversarial training. The generator creates the images, whereas the discriminator distinguishes real from fake images. Adversarial loss guides both through forward and backward passes.

- **Generator**: The generator's goal is to create realistic visuals from random noise or conditioned input (such as an image from another domain). It attempts to deceive the discriminator by producing visuals that are indistinguishable from actual ones.
- **Discriminator**: The discriminator's function is to tell the difference between real images from the training data and bogus images created by the generator. It gives feedback to the generator, directing it to improve its output.

The adversarial training process is analogous to a game in which the generator attempts to fool the discriminator, while the discriminator progressively improves its capacity to detect bogus images. This procedure continues until the generator produces images that are so lifelike that the discriminator cannot tell them apart from genuine ones.

2.3.2.1 Architecture of GANs

The basic architecture of GANs involves two key components:

1. **Generator Network**: Typically, a deep neural network creates a new image from random noise or a conditioned input image. In image-to-image translation jobs, the generator frequently employs topologies such as U-Net, which incorporate encoder-decoder structures and skip links to retain spatial information.
2. **Discriminator Network**: Another deep neural network that assesses image authenticity, judging whether they are genuine (from the training set) or fabricated (produced by the generator). The discriminator frequently uses convolutional layers to capture the images' high-level characteristics.

2.3.2.1.1 Working Principles of GANs

The working principles of GAN are divided into four main steps. The first step is that the generator creates an image from random noise or a conditioned input. The second step is to evaluate; the discriminator evaluates this image along with real images from the training set. In the next step, the discriminator provides feedback in the form of a loss function, indicating how realistic the generated image is. In the last step, the generator adjusts its parameters based on this feedback to produce more realistic images in the next iteration. This adversarial process continues, leading to the gradual improvement of the generator's ability to produce high-quality images.

In GANs, original loss uses binary cross-entropy to measure real vs. generated divergence. Improvements like LSGAN use mean squared error for stability, while WGAN employs Wasserstein distance for better gradient flow and mode stability. Reconstruction loss measures pixel differences in image reconstruction. MSE squares differences across pixels, while MAE averages absolute differences, both crucial for evaluating fidelity in image generation and restoration tasks [29]. In perceptual loss, features are used from pre-trained networks (e.g., VGGs) to compute loss based on perceptual differences rather than pixel-wise differences. For content and style loss, this loss is particularly relevant for style transfer tasks.

2.3.3 Applications of Image-to-Image Translation

2.3.3.1 Style Transfer

Style transfer is one of the common applications for image-to-image translation, where the content of one image (such as a photograph) is translated into the style for another image (such as the brush strokes of a painting). In this process, new images are produced by combining the structural elements of the original image by creating the critical aspects.

Deep neural networks are used in this method, which was developed by Gatys et al. [30], to separate and recombine content and style. Neural networks may produce stylised images by minimising a loss function that captures the difference between the original image's content representation and the style image's representation. Some of the applications are art creation where artists and designers employ style transfer to produce one-of-a-kind artworks, turning photographs into paintings in the manner of well-known artists such as Picasso or Van Gogh. Through the application of creative filters to live video feeds, style transfer can be leveraged in augmented reality apps to improve user experiences.

2.3.3.2 Super-Resolution

The term "super-resolution" describes the technique of increasing an image's resolution to make it crisper and more detailed [31]. This method is crucial for applications where low-resolution photos are the only ones available yet high-quality images are required. In the single image super-resolution (SISR) method, a single low-quality image is unsampled to a higher resolution using deep learning models like CNNs. Photorealistic high-resolution images can be produced from low-resolution inputs with considerable improvement thanks to models like super-resolution GAN (SRGAN). The major applications are as follows:

- **Medical Imaging**: improving medical scan (such as MRI and CT) resolution to aid in analysis and diagnosis.
- **Surveillance**: enhancing security camera footage to enable more precise identification and analysis.
- **Photography and Media**: improving the visual quality of low-resolution images and movies by upscaling them.
- **Photo Restoration**: replacing missing or deteriorating sections of old and damaged photos to restore them.
- **Object Removal**: removing undesired subjects or items from pictures and smoothly adding background information.
- **Content Creation**: creating fresh material in knowledge-void regions; helpful in creative fields like gaming and film design.

As shown in Figure 2.1, the technique of filling in missing or damaged areas of an image is called image inpainting. This method can be applied to repair damaged photos, eliminate extraneous items, and even produce believable content in places where data is lacking. GANs and other neural networks are used in modern inpainting techniques to forecast and create the missing portions of an image based on the surrounding context. Particularly effective models in this field are partial convolutions and context encoders.

2.3.3.3 Domain Adaptation

Domain adaptation models allow data to train a particular type of data derived from the primary data. Labelled data is abundant in a similar domain but remains scarce in the target domain. Domain adaptation is possible only by methods such as CycleGAN where paired instances are not required. While studying the preserved content, these models are able to translate images from the source domain to the target domain. The various applications include autonomous driving, where models are developed using synthetic data to function in actual driving situations, which improves the dependability and security of self-driving cars. In healthcare applications, the information

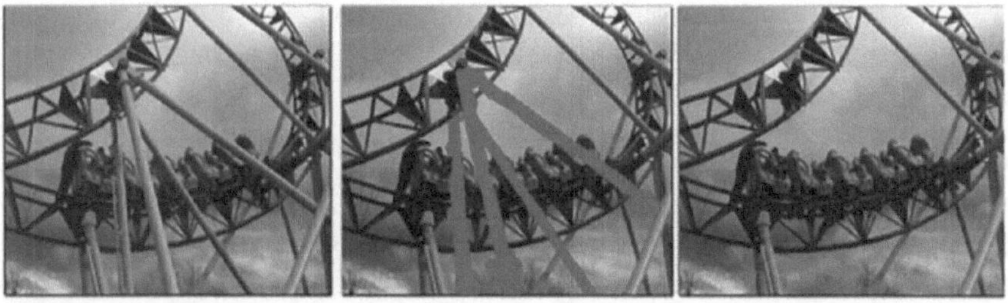

FIGURE 2.1 Inpainting example with image melding [32].

is transferred from one kind of medical imaging (MRI, for example) to another (CT, for example), which enables more advanced diagnostic instruments.

2.3.3.4 Medical Imaging

One of the applications in medical imaging is image synthesis, which creates medical images from several modalities such as MRI or CT scans to offer diagnostic data. The enhancement of the images increases the sharpness and quality of medical scans to enable more precise analysis. Also, segmentation and detection transform the photos into more analysed forms to improve image segmentation and detection tasks [33].

2.3.3.5 Autonomous Driving

In the field of autonomous driving, creating realistic training data for autonomous vehicles by translating simulated environments into more lifelike scenes helps in training robust driving models. Translating images from different driving conditions (e.g., sunny to rainy, day to night) to improve the adaptability and performance of autonomous driving systems is one of the examples of environment creation.

2.3.3.6 Satellite and Aerial Imagery

Resolution of the satellite images is used for monitoring geographical and environmental changes. Translating between different types of satellite images (e.g., optical to infrared) for comprehensive environmental monitoring is an example of image translation in satellite images [34].

2.3.3.7 Fashion and Retail

In the fashion and retail industry, translating clothing designs onto images of models to visualise how new clothes would look and enhancing online shopping experiences is a virtual try-on. Creating new fashion designs by translating sketches into photo-realistic images is a design creation [35].

2.4 CASE STUDIES AND PRACTICAL IMPLEMENTATIONS

2.4.1 Case Study 1: Style Transfer with CycleGAN

The task of style transfer in emojis involves converting emojis from one style (e.g., Apple) to another (e.g., Windows). This case study focuses on the implementation and evaluation of CycleGAN for the purpose of emoji style transfer, highlighting the dataset, model architecture, training process, implementation steps, and results.

There are 4,284 emojis in all in the dataset, divided almost evenly between Windows-style and Apple-style emojis. Every emoji has a 72 × 72–pixel RGB picture resolution. It's important to note that the databases are unpaired, which means that different Apple and Windows emojis do not directly correlate to one another.

Two models were employed in the study: DCGAN and CycleGAN. In deep convolutional GAN (DCGAN) architecture, a discriminator is used, a two-dimensional convolutional neural network containing four convolutional layers, each activated by ReLU after batch normalisation. Using 4 × 4 kernels with a stride of 2, the channel

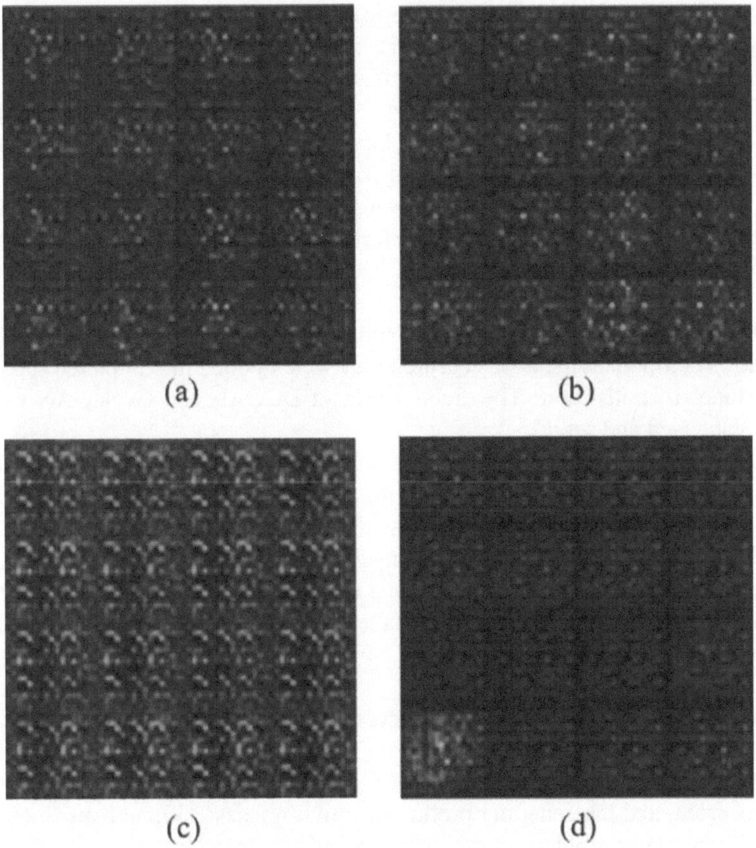

FIGURE 2.2 (a) Sample of generated images after 200 iterations; (b) with smaller learning rate in the discriminator; (c) Sample of generated images after 5200 images; (d) Sample of generated images after 5200 iterations with smaller learning rate in the discriminator [36].

sizes increase from 3 to 1 through 32, 64, and 128 channels. A generator consists of four ReLU-activated deconvolutional layers employing 4 × 4 kernels with stride 2 and padding 1, with channel sizes varying from 100 to 3 via 128 and 32 channels.

In CycleGAN architecture, generators appear as two style conversion generators (Apple to Windows and Windows to Apple) with the same architecture, each made up of:

- **Encoder:** Two convolutional layers with 4 × 4 kernels and stride 2 that go from 3 to 64 channels via 32 channels.
- **Transformation Block:** A residual block with a skip connection and 64 channels for the convolutional layer.
- **Decoder:** Using 4 × 4 kernels with stride 2, two deconvolutional layers reduce the number of channels from 64 to 3 through 32 channels.
- **Discriminators:** Two discriminators that share the DCGAN discriminator's architecture.

The training process involved several key steps and considerations. The loss functions were calculated as the sum of square losses, used by DCGAN and CycleGAN for training their generators and discriminators. To guarantee that an emoji would return to its original shape after being transformed to a different style and back again, CycleGAN also used a cycle consistency loss. The optimisation process consisted of the weights of the generators, and discriminators were updated using the Adam optimiser, with learning rates dynamically changed to avoid overfitting or mode collapse.

The implementation of the emoji-style transfer task using CycleGAN involved the following steps:

- **Data Preparation:** After loading and pre-processing the Apple and Windows emoji datasets, it was ensured they were divided into unpaired sets.
- **Model Initialisation:** The architectures of DCGAN and CycleGAN were established and set up.
- **Training DCGAN:** The original set of emojis designed by Apple was used to train the DCGAN generator. To lessen mode collapse problems, the discriminator's learning rate was adjusted.
- **Training CycleGAN:** Using the unpaired datasets, two CycleGAN generators and discriminators were trained by applying unpaired datasets. After cycle consistency loss, the effect of these two generators are affected by the standard of style transfer.

The simulation results of the training process were evaluated on these two models, as described in the following.

DCGAN Performance: When the DCGAN model was first trained, mode collapse occurred, and the generator produced similar images. Although mode collapse persisted as a major problem, results were marginally improved by varying the discriminator's learning rate.

CycleGAN Performance:

- **Without Cycle Consistency Loss:** The resulting images were less precise in transmitting styles and were noisy.
- **With Cycle Consistency Loss:** Significant improvements were made in the quality of style transfer, resulting in more precise and transparent style changes. Although they weren't as noticeable, problems like mode collapse and colour artefacts were noticed. Additionally, the cycle consistency loss improved the accuracy of style transfers and sped up model convergence.

2.4.2 Case Study 2: Super-Resolution Using GANs

In order to better understand how generative adversarial networks are applied to improve image resolution, this case study will concentrate on a survey [32] called "A Survey on Image Super-Resolution with Generative Adversarial Networks." Important details like the dataset, model architecture, training procedure, implementation methods, and outcomes are highlighted in the study.

Various datasets are used for super-resolution tasks in order to compare and test the effectiveness of various GAN-based models:

- **SET5 and SET14:** Typical super-resolution picture benchmarks have a limited quantity of high-resolution photographs.
- **Berkeley Segmentation Dataset (BSDS):** For assessing segmentation and border detection, variants such as *BSDS*100 and *BSDS*500 are employed.
- **Tsinghua-Tencent 100K:** Includes pictures of traffic signs for apps that use car view.
- **Caltech Pedestrian Detection Benchmark:** Used in car view videos to detect pedestrians.
- **Manga109:** A collection of Japanese manga images spanning multiple decades.
- **T91:** A dataset with high-resolution images for neural network training.
- **General100:** High-quality BMP images used for various image processing tasks.
- **CelebA:** A sizable collection of notes on celebrity photos.
- **Wider Face:** Designed especially for face benchmarking assignments
- **DIV2K:** A 2K picture collection of 1000 photos for super-resolution testing.
- **Flickr2K:** Includes 2650 high-quality photos taken from Flickr.
- **Outdoor Scene Training (OST):** Includes more than 10,000 photos gathered from search engines.
- **Urban100:** Includes pictures of urban landscapes and buildings.
- **ImageNet:** A sizable dataset used for object recognition tasks that contains more than 14 million photos.

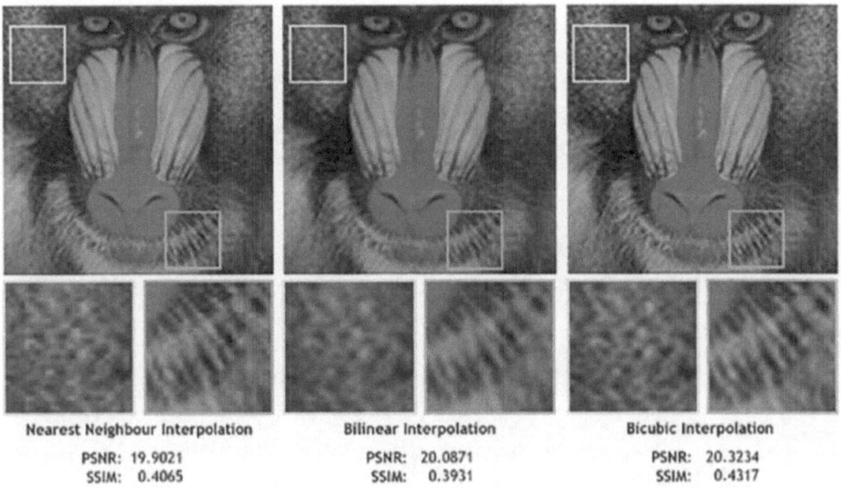

FIGURE 2.3 Quality comparisons of interpolation methods with peak signal-to-noise ratio (PSNR) and structural similarity index (SSIM) [37].

The generator (G) and discriminator (D) are the two main parts of generative adversarial networks. The discriminator's objective is to discern between the created and actual high-resolution images, whereas the generator's objective is to create high-resolution images from low-resolution inputs. Important models based on GANs are:

- **SRGAN:** SRGAN, which was first presented by Ledig et al., creates realistic high-resolution images by integrating content loss with adversarial loss in a perceptual loss function.
- **Enhanced SRGAN (ESRGAN):** Using residual-in-residual dense blocks (RRDBs), ESRGAN captures high-frequency information more efficiently than SRGAN. In order to improve image quality and stability, batch normalisation is removed.
- **Face Super-Resolution Models:** These models improve the small and hazy human faces by applying refinement and upsampling sub-networks in order to increase clarity.
- **Transferred GAN (TGAN):** By increasing the quality of satellite images, transfer learning model can be combined with batch normalization for demonstrating the versatility of the model.

The training process for GAN-based super-resolution models involves several stages:

- **Initialisation:** Initially, the generator generates low-resolution images that are easily distinguished from actual high-resolution photos by the discriminator.

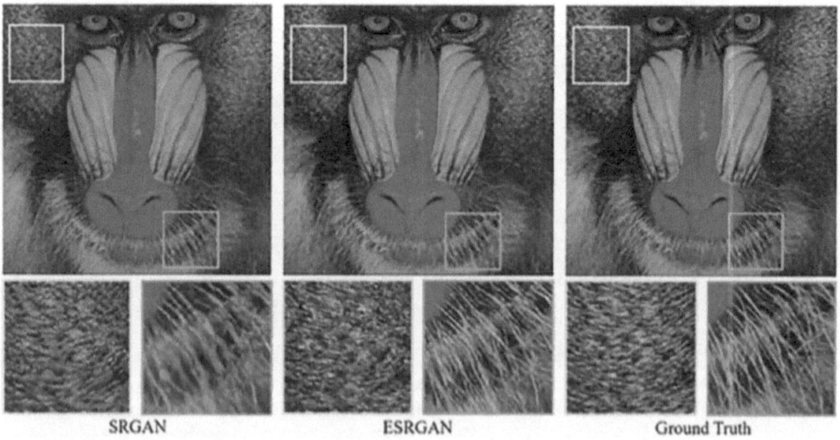

FIGURE 2.4 Visual details of state-of-the-art super-resolution methods SRGAN and ESRGAN [38].

- **Adversarial Training:** Concurrent training is done on the discriminator and generator. Realistic images are encouraged by the discriminator, which maximises the value of log(1 – D(G(z))), while the generator minimises it.
- **Loss Functions:** Various loss functions are used to improve the training process. Pixel-based loss measures pixel differences between generated and real images. Charbonnier loss is a variant of the L2 loss function providing robustness against outliers. Feature matching loss ensures the generated images retain low-frequency details. Texture matching loss focuses on maintaining realistic textures in the generated images.
- **Data Preparation:** Gather and prepare datasets, making sure each one has a matched set of high- and low-resolution photos as described in each step.
- **Model Setup:** Establish and configure the generator and discriminator architectures. Select the proper optimisation methods and loss functions.
- **Training:** Begin with adversarial training, iteratively updating the discriminator and generator. Modify learning rates and hyperparameters to stabilise training and avoid mode collapse.
- **Evaluation:** Assess the quality of the generated images using performance metrics like mean opinion score (MOS), structural similarity index (SSIM), and peak signal-to-noise Ratio (PSNR). Adjust the training regimen in light of the evaluation's findings.

GAN-based super-resolution models have shown significant improvements over traditional methods. While comparing SRGAN vs. ESRGAN, SRGAN established the groundwork for high-quality super-resolution, but ESRGAN performed better due to improvements in network architecture and loss functions, especially when managing textures and patterns inherent in natural images. Richardson et al. [39] developed a specialised method that showed that emphasising a face's distinctive features—such as its eyes or lips—improves results considerably and yields lifelike, finely detailed high-resolution photographs. Because they can be optimised without enhancing visual quality, traditional measurements like PSNR and SSIM might not accurately represent perceptual quality. MOS is seen to be a more dependable method of assessing perceptual enhancements. CycleGAN's use of cycle consistency loss produced better style transfer results, highlighting the significance of custom loss functions in producing better results.

2.4.3 Case Study 3: Image Inpainting with VAEs

This case study describes the dataset, model architecture, training procedure, processes involved in implementation, and outcomes as it assesses deep learning models for picture inpainting. Comparing models and evaluating how well they reconstruct images is the goal, from the first dataset analysis to the last model evaluation.

The Places2 dataset was the one used in this investigation. Because of its vast range of scenarios and high-resolution photos, this dataset is frequently used for training and testing inpainting models. However, the size of the dataset was decreased because of computing constraints.

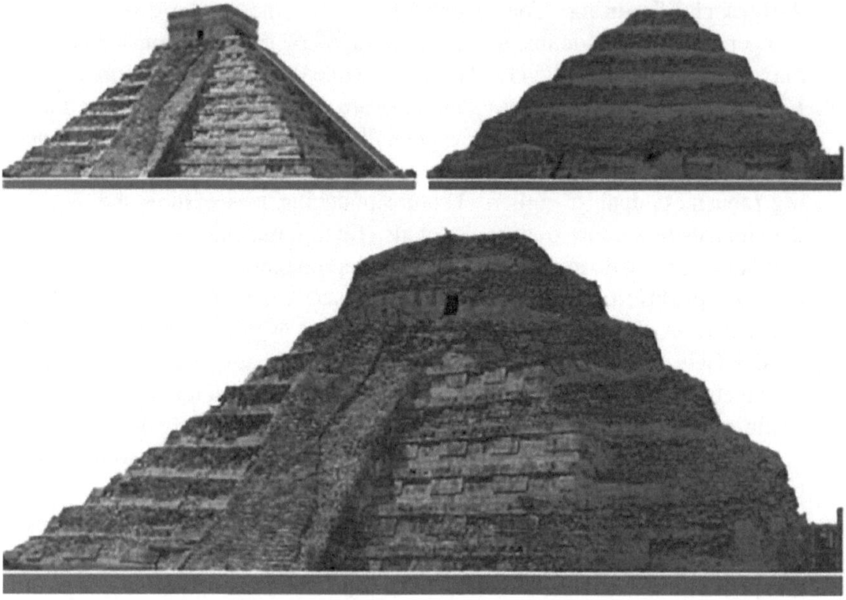

FIGURE 2.5 Image melding example [40].

The characteristics of the dataset are a range of sceneries, each offering rich contextual information helpful for inpainting tasks, included in the Places2 collection. Two types of masks were used for training. Line masking is applied for little flaws in the image by producing sporadic lines. Rectangular masking entails masking a portion of the image, say 10% or 20%, beginning at a random location. The goal of the project was to develop a modular framework that combines several deep learning models. The framework standardises feedback creation, making it simple to switch between and evaluate alternative models. The overall overview of the framework is the Building Blocks, which are utility scripts for creating masked images and dataset scripts are the main parts. Masking functions allows for both rectangle and line masking, which makes thorough model examination easier.

In generative adversarial networks, CycleGAN is used to learn mappings across two domains without the need for paired instances in order to transfer styles. The pix2pix model uses paired examples for image-to-image translation and other tasks. Variational autoencoders are used to create visuals through latent representation learning.

The computational power required for inpainting makes training the models difficult. PyTorch and TensorFlow libraries were combined to train the models, with the use of GPUs to expedite the process.

- **Data Preprocessing**: The recommended masking techniques were used throughout the preprocessing of the images.

- **Model Training**: In order to minimise loss functions, weights were adjusted iteratively over the dataset during the training phase.
- **Loss Functions**: A range of loss functions, such as perceptual loss and pixel-wise loss, were employed to guarantee superior inpainting outcomes.

The implementation involved several critical steps to ensure the models' successful execution and evaluation, which were applied in sequence.

- **Step 1: Data Preparation**: Preprocessing the Places2 dataset and applying masks.
- **Step 2: Model Setup**: Configuring the chosen models within the modular framework.
- **Step 3: Training**: Executing the training process with appropriate hyperparameters and utilising GPU acceleration.
- **Step 4: Evaluation**: Assessing the models using metrics like PSNR, SSIM, and Fréchet inception distance (FID).

Using various mask types, the models were evaluated on the validation dataset, and their performances were compared using the PSNR, SSIM, and FID scores, which are described in the following.

- **PSNR Results**:
  - **Line Mask**: The best-performing model achieved a PSNR of 32.143
  - **10% Mask**: The highest PSNR recorded was 26.148
  - **20% Mask**: The maximum PSNR noted was 22.508
- **SSIM Results**:
  - **Line Mask**: The highest SSIM value was 0.949
  - **10% Mask**: The top SSIM score was 0.911
  - **20% Mask**: The peak SSIM value was 0.826
- **FID Results**:
  - **Line Mask**: The best FID score achieved was 14.851
  - **10% Mask**: The lowest FID score was 26.202
  - **20% Mask**: The minimum FID noted was 40.449

2.5 CHALLENGES AND LIMITATIONS

2.5.1 Data Quality and Quantity

Quality of Data: The training data has a significant impact on image-to-image translation models. Appropriate labelling, diversity, and high-resolution datasets are essential for training any effective models. The performance of these models is affected by their low-resolution, noisy, and imperfect photographs. Inconsistencies in the dataset, such as different backdrops, lighting conditions, or angles, can also create biases and impair the generalisation capacity of the model [41].

Quantity of Data: Effective deep learning model training sometimes requires large-scale datasets. Overfitting, in which the model performs well on training data but badly on unknown data, can result from insufficient data. Large dataset collection and annotation, however, frequently need a lot of time and resources. Due to privacy considerations and the requirement for expert annotation, getting a sufficiently large and diverse dataset can be particularly difficult for many specialised applications, such as medical imaging.

Data Augmentation: Data augmentation, in which preexisting photos are altered (e.g., rotated, flipped, or cropped) to produce fresh training examples, is one method to lessen the restrictions of the data amount. Augmentation can strengthen the model's resilience, but it cannot take the place of truly broad and high-quality data [42, 43].

2.5.2 Computational Requirements

High Computational Costs: Deep learning model training requires a lot of computing power, particularly for generative models like GANs. For these models to train well, high-end GPUs or TPUs are necessary pieces of hardware. Depending on the quantity of the dataset and the model's complexity, the training procedure may take several days or even weeks.

Resource Limitations: Not every organisation or researcher has access to the required computational resources. This restriction may make it more difficult to design and test sophisticated models, which would benefit larger institutions more than smaller ones or lone researchers.

Inference Time: Certain models require processing power for inference after which they are trained, as a drawback for real-time applications. It is a struggle to optimise these models for faster inference without sacrificing accuracy [44–46].

2.5.3 Generalisation and Robustness

Overfitting: Overfitting has been considered one of the situations where the deep learning model performs well on training data but is unable to fit on new data. This is one of the primary training issues faced by these models. Translation of the images means that it can change it adaptively for different images in the target domain [46, 47].

Domain Adaptation: The optimal solutions obtained after training for one dataset perform better in other datasets in real-world scenarios. These models are resilient to changes in content, style, and image quality that they have not experienced before during training. Various strategies like transfer learning and domain adaptation can help in the improvement of generalisation.

Handling Different Occlusions and Artifacts: Image-to-image translation models are required to manage occlusions, where one item is partially dependent on another, which would prevent artifacts from strange patterns or distortions. Sophisticated model architectures and loss functions are efficient in penalising such errors and needed for achieving this level of robustness.

2.5.4 Ethical and Legal Considerations

Bias and Fairness: Biases in the training set mean that the learning is amplified by deep learning models. For example, the performance of the different models may get biased due to a particular set where the majority of the images are collected from same demographic conditions. It is not guaranteed that equity and minimising prejudice will occur in certain applications where there is the potential to affect the lives of people, such as autonomous vehicles or medical imaging.

Privacy Concerns: The collection of large datasets present serious privacy issues, especially when personal data is involved. The data must be gathered and handled morally, with the proper consent. Certain privacy concerns would be mitigated if methods such as federated learning, where the models are trained across decentralised devices, were applied.

Misuse of Technology: Different technologies are applied for translating photos from one domain to another by producing deepfake images which can be altered in many different ways. Moral questions are asked about the possibility of fraud, disinformation, and other activities. It is essential to create different policies and procedures for controlling they way these technologies are used and the technological solutions for identifying these issues.

Legal Implications: The image-to-image translation environment is still developing. Complex issues exist, including considering data ownership and intellectual property rights for model errors. Users and developers of these technologies are required to follow all applicable laws and regulations [44–46].

2.6 FUTURE DIRECTIONS

2.6.1 Emerging Trends in Generative Models

As the technology is growing and there are many improvements in designing deep learning architectures, there have been further advancements in the architecture. The following are the some of the improved architectures in existing DL models.

- **Improved GAN Architectures**: Novel architectures aimed at enhancing stability, convergence, and performance are part of the ongoing evolution of generative adversarial networks. New standards in producing realistic, high-quality images are being set by methods such as StyleGAN, BigGAN, and GANs that use attention processes. For example, StyleGAN disentangles the latent space to provide unparalleled control over the style and attributes of generated images [48].
- **Hybrid Models**: Combining several generative models—VAEs and GANs, for example—can help them benefit from each other's advantages. For instance, hybrid models known as VAE-GANs combine the adversarial training of GANs with the explicit likelihood estimates of VAEs to create models that can generate high-quality images while preserving a well-organised latent space.

- **Self-Supervised Learning**: Self-supervised learning is gaining popularity, which entails training models to predict subsets of the data based on other subsets. This method can help generative models become more capable of generalising while also reducing the dependence on labelled data. Self-supervised approaches have the potential to improve the model's robust feature learning from unlabelled images for image-to-image translation.
- **Diffusion Models**: A competitive alternative to GANs is emerging: diffusion models. Diffusion models create images by reversing a steady noise adding process. While avoiding some of the training instabilities linked with GANs, these models offer an alternative approach to generative modelling and have demonstrated potential in generating high-fidelity images.

2.6.2 Potential Improvements in Techniques

Potential improvements in designing deep learning techniques are as follows.

- **Advanced Data Augmentation**: Model robustness can be increased by creating more advanced data augmentation methods. Approaches like automated data augmentation, which makes use of reinforcement learning to identify the optimal augmentation strategies, and adversarial data augmentation, which employs adversarial cases to enhance model performance, are attractive fields of study [49].
- **Better Loss Functions**: Creating loss functions with greater efficiency is essential to raising the calibre of images that are produced. Better visual fidelity and realism can result from adversarial loss designed for a given application and perceptual loss that guides the generation process using data from pretrained networks.
- **Model Interpretability**: Improving generative models' interpretability can reveal more about how these models learn and produce images. Approaches like explainable AI (XAI), attention mechanisms, and feature visualisation can aid in debugging and understanding models, resulting in more dependable and transparent systems.
- **Efficient Training Techniques**: It is crucial to optimise the training process in order to minimise training time and computing needs. Model performance and training efficiency can be greatly increased by using strategies like neural architecture search (NAS), progressive growth, and transfer learning [44–46].

2.6.3 Expanding Applications

When designing new algorithms or applying novel deep learning architectures, there are many new architectures of DL, as follows.

Healthcare: There is a lot of promise for image-to-image translation in the medical imaging field. Applications include creating artificial medical images for training, optimising diagnostic instruments, and raising the quality of MRI or CT scans. Improvements in patient outcomes and more effective healthcare systems may result from these developments.

Autonomous Vehicles: Image-to-image translation has applications in autonomous driving, including creating artificial training data, improving photos in low light or bad weather, and modelling different driving conditions. These applications have the potential to increase autonomous systems' dependability and safety.

Art and Design: Image-to-image translation technologies are useful for creative industries for tasks including content development, graphic design automation, and style transfer. By using these tools to automate tedious activities and experiment with new styles, artists and designers can improve their creative workflows.

Augmented and Virtual Reality (AR/VR): Through realistic texture generation, improved scene reconstruction, and the creation of immersive settings, image-to-image translation can improve AR and VR experiences. More dynamic and interesting training, teaching, and gaming applications may result from these developments [50].

Combining with Natural Language Processing (NLP): Multimodal applications like text-to-image translation—which creates images from written descriptions—and vice versa can be made possible by integrating image-to-image translation with natural language processing. Improvements in domains such as data augmentation, interactive AI systems, and content creation may result from this synergy [43].

Interdisciplinary Research: Research collaborations in computer vision, neurology, psychology, and other fields can help us understand how human perception and creativity are mirrored in generative models. These domains' insights can help create AI systems that are more complex and human-like.

Ethics and Social Sciences: Collaboration between ethicists, legal specialists, and social scientists is necessary to address ethical concerns and comprehend the societal implications of image-to-image translation systems. The development of rules and regulations that guarantee the ethical and responsible use of these technologies can be aided by this cross-disciplinary approach.

Environmental Impact: It is imperative to investigate the effects of training big generative models on the environment. By working together with specialists in energy efficiency and sustainability, greener AI techniques can be developed, which will lower the carbon footprint of developing and implementing deep learning models.

2.7 CONCLUSION

This chapter highlighted notable advancements in image-to-image translation through the use of generative models and deep learning approaches. Notable findings include GANs, where it has been demonstrated that GAN-based super-resolution models provide notable advantages over classical techniques. For instance, superior-quality results and improved texture handling were obtained by employing an enhanced super-resolution GAN rather than a SRGAN. A number of models have been tested for picture inpainting, including VAEs. The evaluation measures demonstrated that the top-performing model, using line masks, obtained a PSNR of 32.143 and an SSIM of 0.949, demonstrating the potency of sophisticated generative models for picture reconstruction. Through the creation of artificial training data and the improvement of images in low-light situations, image-to-image translation has increased the safety and dependability of autonomous driving. The chapter identified several critical implications for both research and practice, including ethical and legal considerations, environmental impact, and efficient training techniques.

REFERENCES

1. Pang, Y., Lin, J., Qin, T., & Chen, Z. (2021). Image-to-image translation: Methods and applications. *IEEE Transactions on Multimedia*, *24*, 3859–3881.
2. Chen, X., & Jia, C. (2021). An overview of image-to-image translation using generative adversarial networks. In *Pattern Recognition. ICPR International Workshops and Challenges: Virtual Event, January 10–15, 2021, Proceedings, Part VI* (pp. 366–380). Springer International Publishing.
3. Jiao, L., & Zhao, J. (2019). A survey on the new generation of deep learning in image processing. *IEEE Access*, *7*, 172231–172263.
4. Cheng, B., Liu, Z., Peng, Y., & Lin, Y. (2023). General image-to-image translation with one-shot image guidance. In *Proceedings of the IEEE/CVF International Conference on Computer Vision* (pp. 22736–22746). IEEE.
5. Senapati, R. K., Satvika, R., Anmandla, A., Ashesh Reddy, G., & Anil Kumar, C. (2023, June). Image-to-image translation using Pix2Pix GAN and cycle GAN. In *International Conference on Data Intelligence and Cognitive Informatics* (pp. 573–586). Singapore: Springer Nature Singapore.
6. Desai, D., Zanjal, S., Kasar, A., Bagade, J., & Dandawate, Y. (2023). Image-to-image translation using generative adversarial networks. In *Generative Adversarial Networks and Deep Learning* (pp. 13–37). Chapman and Hall/CRC.
7. Erdei, T. I., Kapusi, T. P., Hajdu, A., & Husi, G. (2024). Image-to-image translation-based deep learning application for object identification in industrial robot systems. *Robotics*, *13*(6), 88.
8. Cheng, J., Zhu, Y., Zhao, Y., Li, T., Chen, M., Sun, Q., . . . Zhang, X. (2024). Application of an improved U-Net with image-to-image translation and transfer learning in peach orchard segmentation. *International Journal of Applied Earth Observation and Geoinformation*, *130*, 103871.
9. Shi, C., Huang, K., Lu, G. A. N., Liu, H., Zhu, M., Wang, N., & Gao, X. (2024). On the analysis of GAN-based image-to-image translation with gaussian noise injection. In *The Twelfth International Conference on Learning Representations*. Open Review, ICLR.
10. Chakraborty, T., KS, U. R., Naik, S. M., Panja, M., & Manvitha, B. (2024). Ten years of generative adversarial nets (GANs): a survey of the state-of-the-art. *Machine Learning: Science and Technology*, *5*(1), 011001.
11. De Souza, V. L. T., Marques, B. A. D., Batagelo, H. C., & Gois, J. P. (2023). A review on generative adversarial networks for image generation. *Computers & Graphics*, *114*, 13–25.
12. Torbunov, D., Huang, Y., Yu, H., Huang, J., Yoo, S., Lin, M., . . . Ren, Y. (2023). Uvcgan: Unet vision transformer cycle-consistent gan for unpaired image-to-image translation. In *Proceedings of the IEEE/CVF Winter Conference on Applications of Computer Vision* (pp. 702–712). IEEE.

13. Kumari, R., Goel, S., & Das, S. (2023, September). Mathematical modelling of dendritic complexity mechanism in Alzheimer's disease. In *AIP Conference Proceedings* (Vol. 2872, No. 1). AIP Publishing.
14. Kumari, R., Goel, S., & Das, S. (2022, November). A 3D convolutional neural network approach for diagnosing Alzheimer's disease using modified Owl Search Optimization technique. In *TENCON 2022-2022 IEEE Region 10 Conference (TENCON)* (pp. 1–7). IEEE.
15. Samadadiya, K., Das, S., & Kumari, R. (2024, January). Predictive paradigm: AI-driven social media analysis for real estate sales forecasts. In *International Conference on Smart Computing and Communication* (pp. 189–198). Singapore: Springer Nature Singapore.
16. Kumari, R., Goel, S., & Das, S. (2023, April). A patch based 3D CNN approach for diagnosing early stages of Alzheimer's disease by applying OBL-WOA algorithm. In *2023 8th International Conference on Cloud Computing and Big Data Analytics (ICCCBDA)* (pp. 455–459). IEEE.
17. Kumari, R., Das, S., Nigam, A., & Pushkar, S. (2023). Patch-based Siamese 3D convolutional neural network for early Alzheimer's disease using multi-modal approach. *IETE Journal of Research*, 1–19.
18. Kumari, R., Das, S., Singh, R. K., Kohli, A., Sunil, A., & Dadhich, A. (2024). Getting started with computational drug discovery: A comprehensive guide. In *Converging Pharmacy Science and Engineering in Computational Drug Discovery* (pp. 235–258). IGI Global.
19. Kundu, R., Das, S., & Mishra, S. K. (2022, April). A comprehensive review of single and double stage object detection algorithms in self driving cars. In *2022 IEEE 7th International Conference for Convergence in Technology (I2CT)* (pp. 1–8). IEEE.
20. Ahmad, T., Talaan, A., Gola, V., Das, S., & Singh, R. K. (2024, April). Advancing early diagnostic accuracy for Alzheimer's disease through the integration of machine and deep learning paradigms by applying multisource datasets. In *Proceedings of International Conference on Intelligent Systems and New Applications* (Vol. 2, pp. 42–46). Springer.
21. Goodfellow, I., Pouget-Abadie, J., Mirza, M., Xu, B., Warde-Farley, D., Ozair, S., . . . Bengio, Y. (2014). Generative adversarial nets. *Advances in Neural Information Processing Systems, 27*.
22. Huang, X., Liu, M. Y., Belongie, S., & Kautz, J. (2018). Multimodal unsupervised image-to-image translation. In *Proceedings of the European Conference on Computer Vision (ECCV)* (pp. 172–189). Springer.
23. Liang, J., Zeng, H., & Zhang, L. (2021). High-resolution photorealistic image translation in real-time: A laplacian pyramid translation network. In *Proceedings of the IEEE/CVF Conference on Computer Vision and Pattern Recognition* (pp. 9392–9400). IEEE Explore.
24. Atouani, A., Kirchhof, J. C., Kusmenko, E., & Rumpe, B. (2021, October). Artifact and reference models for generative machine learning frameworks and build systems. In *Proceedings of the 20th ACM SIGPLAN International Conference on Generative Programming: Concepts and Experiences* (pp. 55–68). Cornell University.
25. Salehi, P., Chalechale, A., & Taghizadeh, M. (2020). Generative adversarial networks (GANs): An overview of theoretical model, evaluation metrics, and recent developments. *arXiv preprint* arXiv:2005.13178.
26. Li, Q., Li, S., Li, R., Wu, W., Dong, Y., Zhao, J., . . . Aftab, R. (2022). Low-dose computed tomography image reconstruction via a multistage convolutional neural network with autoencoder perceptual loss network. *Quantitative Imaging in Medicine and Surgery, 12*(3), 1929.
27. Henry, J., Natalie, T., & Madsen, D. (2021). Pix2pix gan for image-to-image translation. *Research Gate Publication*, 1–5.

28. Zhu, J. Y., Park, T., Isola, P., & Efros, A. A. (2017). Unpaired image-to-image translation using cycle-consistent adversarial networks. In *Proceedings of the IEEE International Conference on Computer Vision* (pp. 2223–2232). IEEE Explore.
29. Doersch, C. (2016). Tutorial on variational autoencoders. *arXiv preprint* arXiv:1606.05908.
30. Gatys, L., Ecker, A. S., & Bethge, M. (2015). Texture synthesis using convolutional neural networks. *Advances in Neural Information Processing Systems, 28.*
31. Nguyen, N., Milanfar, P., & Golub, G. (2001). A computationally efficient superresolution image reconstruction algorithm. *IEEE Transactions on Image Processing, 10*(4), 573–583.
32. Chen, X., & Jia, C. (2021). An overview of image-to-image translation using generative adversarial networks. In *Pattern Recognition. ICPR International Workshops and Challenges. ICPR 2021. Lecture Notes in Computer Science*. Springer. https://doi.org/10.1007/978-3-030-68780-9_31
33. Hoyez, H., Schockaert, C., Rambach, J., Mirbach, B., & Stricker, D. (2022). Unsupervised image-to-image translation: A review. *Sensors, 22*(21), 8540. https://doi.org/10.3390/s22218540
34. Zhu, Jun-Yan, Park, Taesung, Isola, Phillip, & Efros, Alexei A. (2017). Unpaired image-to-image translation using cycle-consistent adversarial networks. In *Proceedings of the IEEE International Conference on Computer Vision* (pp. 2223–2232). IEEE Explore.
35. Isola, Phillip, Zhu, Jun-Yan, Zhou, Tinghui, & Efros, Alexei A. (2017). Image-to-image translation with conditional adversarial networks. In *Proceedings of the IEEE Conference on Computer Vision and Pattern Recognition* (pp. 1125–1134). IEEE Explore.
36. Choi, Yunjey, Choi, Minje, Kim, Munyoung, Ha, Jung-Woo, Kim, Sung Hun, & Choo, Jaegul. (2018). Stargan: Unified generative adversarial networks for multi-domain image-to-image translation. In *Proceedings of the IEEE Conference on Computer Vision and Pattern Recognition* (pp. 8789–8797). IEEE Explore.
37. Lee, H. Y., Li, Y. H., Lee, T. H., & Aslam, M. S. (2023). Progressively unsupervised generative attentional networks with adaptive layer-instance normalization for image-to-image translation. *MDPI Sensors, 23*(15), 6858.
38. Choi, Yunjey, Choi, Minje, Kim, Munyoung, Ha, Jung-Woo, Kim, Sung Hun, & Choo, Jaegul. (2018). Stargan: Unified generative adversarial networks for multi-domain image-to-image translation. In *Proceedings of the IEEE Conference on Computer Vision and Pattern Recognition* (pp. 8789–8797). IEEE Explore.
39. Richardson, Elad, Alaluf, Yuval, Patashnik, Or, Nitzan, Yotam, Azar, Yaniv, Shapiro, Stav, & Cohen-Or, Daniel. (2020). Encoding in style: A stylegan encoder for image-to-image translation. In *Proceedings of the IEEE/CVF Conference on Computer Vision and Pattern Recognition* (pp. 2287–2296). IEEE Explore.
40. Pang, Y., Lin, J., Qin, T., & Chen, Z. (2021). Image-to-image translation: Methods and applications. *IEEE Transactions on Multimedia, 24*, 3859–3881.
41. Park, Taesung, Efros, Alexei A., Zhang, Richard, & Zhu, Jun-Yan. (2020). Contrastive Learning for unpaired image-to-image translation. In *Computer Vision–ECCV 2020: 16th European Conference, Glasgow, UK, August 23–28, 2020, Proceedings, Part IX 16* (pp. 319–345). Springer International Publishing.
42. Lee, Hsin-Ying, Tseng, Hung-Yu, Huang, Jia-Bin, Singh, Maneesh Kumar, & Yang, Ming-Hsuan. (2018). *Diverse image-to-image translation via disentangled representations*. In *Proceedings of the European Conference on Computer Vision (ECCV)* (pp. 35–51). IEEE Explore.
43. Tang, H., Xu, D., Sebe, N. and Yan, Y., 2019, July. Attention-guided generative adversarial networks for unsupervised image-to-image translation. In *2019 International Joint Conference on Neural Networks (IJCNN)* (pp. 1–8). IEEE.

44. Choi, Yunjey, Choi, Minje, Kim, Munyoung, Ha, Jung-Woo, Kim, Sung Hun, & Choo, Jaegul. (2018). *Stargan: Unified generative adversarial networks for multi-domain image-to-image translation.* In *Proceedings of the IEEE Conference on Computer Vision and Pattern Recognition* (pp. 8789–8797). IEEE Explore.
45. Alotaibi, A. (2020). Deep generative adversarial networks for image-to-image translation: A review. *Symmetry*, *12*(10), 1705. https://doi.org/10.3390/sym12101705
46. Liu, Ming-Yu, Huang, Xun, Mallya, Arun, Karras, Tero, Aila, Timo, Lehtinen, Jaakko, & Kautz, Jan. (2019). *Few-shot unsupervised image-to-image translation.* In *Proceedings of the IEEE/CVF International Conference on Computer Vision* (pp. 10551–10560). IEEE Explore.
47. Nadkarni, P. M., Ohno-Machado, L., & Chapman, W. W. (2011). Natural language processing: An introduction. *Journal of the American Medical Informatics Association*, *18*(5), 544–551.
48. Khamparia, A. (Ed.). (2024). *Microbial Data Intelligence and Computational Techniques for Sustainable Computing* (Vol. 47). Springer Nature.
49. Gupta, D., Gupta, U., & Sarma, H. J. (2024). Functional iterative approach for Universum-based primal twin bounded support vector machine to EEG classification (FUPTBSVM). *Multimedia Tools and Applications*, *83*(8), 22119–22151.
50. Gupta, U., & Jain, V. (2024). Social neuroscience: Inferring mental states in social media. In *Emotional AI and Human-AI Interactions in Social Networking* (pp. 15–39). Elsevier.

3 Generative Models in Medical Imaging

Aarti P. Pimpalkar, Vijaya S. Patil, Nilesh N. Thorat, Mayuresh Gulame, Jayashri D. Palkar, and Poonam Suraj Gham

3.1 INTRODUCTION

With the ability to train two networks in parallel for picture production and discrimination, generative adversarial networks (GANs) are an exceptionally potent family of neural networks. Realistic image production and domain shift handling are among their well-known strengths [1]. Generative adversarial networks produce more instances by utilizing the estimated probability distribution. GANs are very good at creating realistic, detailed images, even if there are alternative deep-learning generative models available. Because GANs are grounded in game theory, as opposed to standard optimization-based generative modeling techniques, they have become increasingly popular in both academia and industry, providing new research opportunities. Through the creation of superior medical images from small datasets, GANs in medical imaging are transforming diagnostic accuracy and image enhancement. In order to assist tasks like resolution augmentation or denoising of medical pictures, pix2pix focuses on image translation, whereas CycleGAN is utilized for domain adaptation [2], translating images in multiple modalities. In the field of medical imaging, UNIT GAN is a noteworthy GAN algorithm that facilitates cross-modal image fusion by identifying a shared latent space between various modalities. Meanwhile, ProGAN facilitates the creation of high-resolution medical images [3], resulting in authentic and detailed images that are essential for diagnostics and healthcare scholarship. With the quality and diversity of medical images being increased by these GAN algorithms, healthcare settings can now perform better analysis and diagnosis. The generator (G) and discriminator (D) neural networks are the two that GANs in medical imaging use. The generator generates random noise-based synthetic medical images in an attempt to mimic real data, while the discriminator assesses and distinguishes between created and real images. The generator contributes to applications such as augmentation, synthesis, classification, detection, reconstruction, and segmentation by improving its output through iterative feedback to provide more realistic data. Healthcare machine learning model development is supported by GANs, which also improve diagnostic picturė quality and handle data limitations. In medical imaging, Figure 3.1 illustrates the fundamental workflow of a GAN. Diagnostic accuracy and image improvement in the field of medical imaging have been transformed by GANs because they can generate high-quality medical

DOI: 10.1201/9781003539483-3

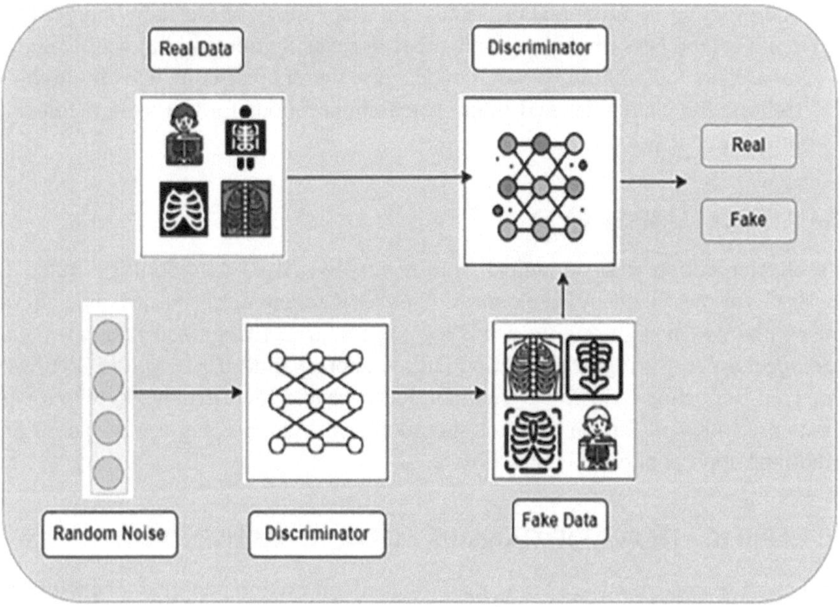

FIGURE 3.1 Workflow of GANs in medical imaging.

images even with sparse datasets. Though they started with the rudimentary adversarial process in 2014, GANs have come a long way over time. However, there are still issues addressing data distribution completely. Image quality was enhanced with the release of DCGAN (Deep Convolutional Generative Adversarial Network) in 2015 [4], and mode stability was addressed with WGAN in 2017 [5]. Without paired training data, CycleGAN allowed image-to-image translation, and PGAN brought a progressive training strategy [6]. Applications of GAN in medical imaging include segmentation, registration, enhancement, detection, classification, and picture synthesis. A comprehensive examination of current advancements that offers insightful information for the field's progress is one of the chapter's main contributions.

In summary, this chapter makes the following contributions:

- A comprehensive examination of the diverse fields in which GANs are applied in medical imaging. This investigation covers a wide range of useful medical imaging applications for GANs and talks about researchers' advancements in this sector.
- Offers a summary of widely used datasets, assessments measures, and data pre-processing methods for the best possible model training in GANs.
- This study examines various GAN models utilized in medical imaging, clarifying their applicability for particular healthcare scenarios and assisting researchers in making well-informed model choices.
- The most recent developments and contributions of GANs by researchers in medical imaging are examined in detail, providing insights into the

cutting-edge experimental outcomes that shape the field's terrain. In order to point researchers toward possible areas of investigation and innovation and to support their future research endeavors, the chapter concludes by highlighting the challenges and future research directions for GANs in medical imaging.

3.2 LITERATURE SURVEY

This chapter adopts a systematic literature review (SLR) methodology based on the paradigm described by Keele et al. [7] and Kitchenham et al. [8]. The survey focuses mainly on high-quality academic papers from recognized databases such as ScienceDirect, SpringerLink, ACM Digital Library, and IEEE Xplore. PRISMA (Preferred Reporting Items for Systematic Reviews and Meta-Analyses) recommendations are followed for the research methodology, guaranteeing a transparent and methodical approach to data collecting.

3.3 APPLICATIONS OF GANS IN MEDICAL IMAGING

Significant advancements are being made in medical imaging applications with generative adversarial networks. Making artificial images that closely resemble actual patient data is one important application, which is essential for enhancing small labeled datasets. Additionally, GANs are excellent at improving medical images by generating high-quality versions from inputs with lower resolution, which increases the accuracy of diagnosis. GANs also enable cross-modal image transformations, which enable the conversion of MRIs to CT scans and vice versa. Healthcare practitioners are able to make more accurate clinical judgments thanks to their ability to produce realistic and diverse medical images, which advances image analysis and segmentation. A few GAN applications for medical imaging are shown in Figure 3.2.

3.3.1 Segmentation

Image segmentation is utilized in medical imaging to provide uncertain estimation, facilitate multi-modal fusion, and improve picture reconstruction. Segmentation-based techniques are used to produce more reliable and accurate medical diagnoses. Table 3.1 highlights a few key applications of medical picture segmentation.

3.3.2 Reconstruction

The technique of reconstructing a picture from imperfect or deteriorated data is known as image reconstruction. It is commonly employed in remote sensing, computer vision, and medical imaging. When referring to generative adversarial networks, picture reconstruction typically means using these networks to create high-fidelity images from noisy or low-resolution input. A generator that learns to produce realistic images from random noise or faulty input is the basis of a GAN. In applications where precise diagnosis and analysis depend on crisp, detailed images, such as super-resolution imaging, denoising, and improving the visual quality of medical

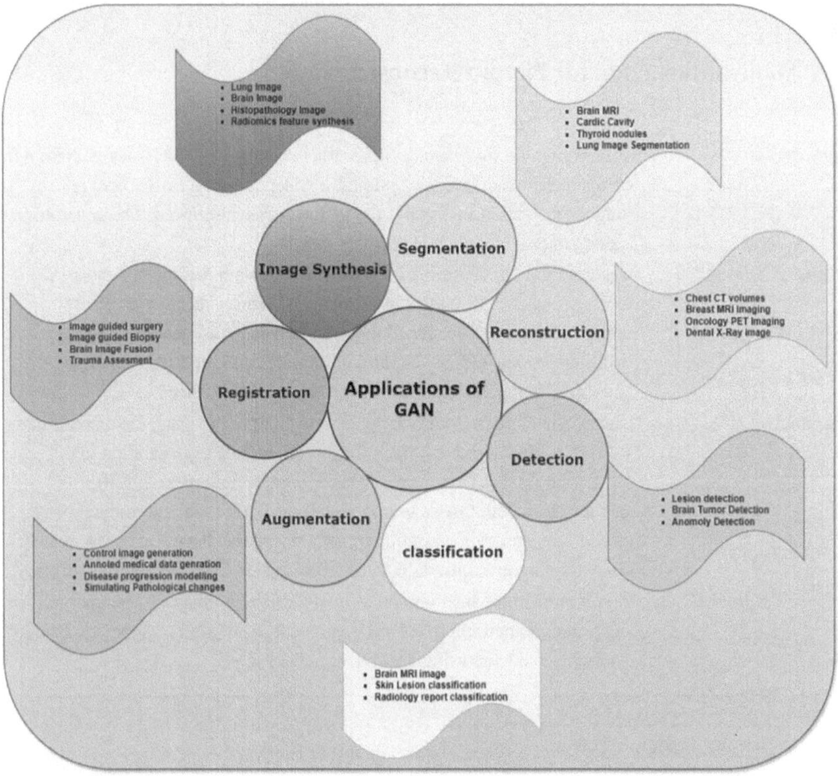

FIGURE 3.2 Applications of GANs in medical imaging.

scans, they are very useful for improving image quality. A few GAN applications for picture reconstruction are displayed in Table 3.2.

The process of creating a new image from damaged or incomplete data is called image reconstruction. It is frequently used in medical imaging, computer vision, and remote sensing. Picture reconstruction, when discussing generative adversarial networks, usually refers to the process of employing these networks to produce high-fidelity images from noisy or low-resolution input. A GAN is essentially a generator that learns to generate realistic images from random noise or flawed input. They are especially beneficial for improving picture quality, particularly in applications like super-resolution imaging, denoising, and enhancing the visual quality of medical scans, where accurate diagnosis and analysis depend on clear, detailed images.

3.3.3 Classification

With the help of data augmentation, domain distribution alignment for robustness, improved image quality for enhanced feature extraction, anomaly detection, and the provision of unlabeled samples for semi-supervised learning, generative adversarial

TABLE 3.1
GAN Applications Used for Picture Reconstruction

Ref	Description
Munawar et al. [9]	Highlighting the significance of accurate chest X-ray (CXR) segmentation for computer-aided diagnostic systems, a generative adversarial network for lung segmentation in chest X-ray pictures was introduced. The generator is trained to provide realistic segment masks.
Zhang et al. [10]	Suggested the segmentation of images to help with medical diagnostics, highlighting the difficulties in using deep learning techniques across different locations because of these variations in distribution. It is suggested that bidirectional GANs, in particular CycleGAN, be used to mitigate this and improve medical picture segmentation performance.
Kunapinum et al. [11]	Using StableSeg GAN with the generator DeeplabV3+ and the discriminator ResNet18, the hybrid approach for thyroid nodule segmentation in ultrasound images is proposed. This approach combines semantic segmentation with GANs to improve performance while introducing closed-loop supervision of output gain loss in the discriminator to reduce GAN training instability. PID control is applied for GAN training stability.
Narayanan et al. [12]	Brain tumors in medical photos were identified by image segmentation; the suggested method improves training and segmentation accuracy by creating synthetic data pairs using generative networks.

TABLE 3.2
GAN Applications for Image Reconstruction

Ref	Description
Du et al. [13]	The suggested T-GANs focus on maintaining texture details and employ deep learning to improve low-resolution medical pictures, especially in low-field MRI.
Wang et al. [14]	Presented TRCT-GAN, a GAN network intended to generate new CT volumes for the chest using biplane images. To improve feature representation and contextual association, it makes use of a transformer network module and a dynamic attention module.
Mishra et al. [15]	An object, number, and character-focused method for creating visual stimuli from EEG data was presented. An attention and auxiliary classifier-based GAN are combined in the suggested design.
Jiang et al. [16]	Proposed a generative adversarial network (PLA-GAN) for low-dose computed tomography (LDCT) reconstruction that is based on the proximal linear ADMM architecture.

TABLE 3.3
Application of GANs in Medical Image Classification

Ref	Description
Mao et al. [17]	Declared the release of pseudo-labeling generative adversarial networks (PLGAN), a novel semi-supervised classification technique for medical imaging. The algorithm uses cyclic consistency loss, self-attention techniques, and MixMatch to enhance classification performance.
Chen et al. [18]	Presented a brand-new method for automatically classifying artery/vein (A/V) retinal images called TW-GAN. Vessel width and topological connection information are integrated into a deep learning framework by TW-GAN.
Tian et al. [19]	Showed how well GANs with an attentional mechanism may be used to augment ultrasound data for the purpose of classifying idiopathic inflammatory myopathics (IIMs).

networks indirectly assist in image classification. In a variety of applications, this improves classifier accuracy and adaptability. Table 3.3 shows image classification

3.3.4 Augmentation

In data and image processing, especially in medical image analysis, image augmentation is often used. To increase the size and diversity of a dataset, it entails applying several transformations, including rotation, scaling, and noise addition. Augmentation becomes vital in medical imaging, where different clinical cases are important yet datasets can be limited. Augmentation enhances the resilience and generalization of machine learning models by creating additional training samples artificially or altering preexisting ones. In the fields of illness detection, classification, and medical image analysis, where a variety of comprehensive datasets are necessary for accurate results and dependable model performance, this aids in the training of models to be more successful.

3.3.5 Registration

In medical imaging, image registration refers to the process of aligning several photographs of the same subject or structure, whether taken with various modalities or at different times, to guarantee spatial congruence. In order to provide thorough diagnoses, it makes multi-modal fusion in healthcare easier by merging information from MRI, CT, and other sources. Time alignment makes it easier to monitor the course of a disease and the effectiveness of treatment. In order to maximize collateral damage reduction and enable precise targeting in image-guided and radiation therapy, image registration is essential. By creating artificial images to aid in the alignment process, GANs are used in image registration to improve registration accuracy in difficult situations. Table 3.4 shows medical picture registration.

TABLE 3.4
GAN Implementation for Medical Picture Registration

Ref.	Description
[20]	Provided an adversarial methods–based unsupervised image registration system for various modalities, tackling multi-modal similarity metrics issues and highlighting modalities' disparities. A geometry-consistent training scheme, a multi-scale registration network with partial sharing, and image-to-image translation are all included in the proposed method, which makes registration easier.
[21]	Suggested using a GAN and a registration network (RegNet) to enhance the quality of synthetic CT (sCT) that is produced using cone-beam computed tomography (CBCT). RegNet was incorporated into GANs, and the results were better than with GANs alone: fewer errors, better picture metrics, and anatomically accurate sCT images.
[22]	Presented the KDE-GAN medical image fusion model, which makes use of a generative adversarial network with dual discriminators and explainable AI that incorporates knowledge distillation.
[23]	Reported on the creation of the U-Patch GAN model, which aims to improve fusion quality and is used for self-supervised fusing of multimodal brain images.
[24]	MGMDcGAN was used to integrate structural and functional information from images of varying resolutions (e.g., MRI-PET, MRI-SPECT, and CT-SPECT) in a novel way for medical image registration. Furthermore, during the fusion process, the suggested method guarantees the greatest possible retention of information from the source pictures.

3.3.6 Image Synthesis

The process of creating artificial medical images that resemble actual patient data is known as medical image synthesis, and it makes use of generative adversarial networks. An adversarial network called the discriminator and a generator work together to create realistic images, with the discriminator's job being to distinguish between genuine and artificial instances. These networks are known as generative adversarial networks. Medical image synthesis plays a critical role in the healthcare industry by producing a variety of privacy-compliant datasets that are needed for the training of reliable machine learning models. It helps ensure the confidentiality of patient data and address difficulties related to data scarcity. It may also be applied to anomaly detection, data augmentation, and medical condition simulation, which improves medical imaging research and diagnostic skills. Table 3.5 displays a few GAN applications for image synthesis.

3.4 DATASETS, EVALUATION METRICS, AND PREPROCESSING METHODS

Popular medical picture datasets, widely used preprocessing techniques, and important evaluation criteria for gauging GAN effectiveness are all covered in this section. Gaining a better understanding of the evaluation criteria, preprocessing methods, and dataset features is the goal of the discussion.

TABLE 3.5
Using GAN for Image Synthesis in Medicine

Ref.	Description
[25]	Noted the potential for contaminated synthetic data and the necessity of defenses against such assaults. Draw attention to the susceptibility of federated GANs (FedGANs) to backdoor attacks in the context of federated learning (FL).
[26]	When it comes to unsupervised brain image synthesis, FedMed-GAN is the standard for translating domains in federated settings. Across paired and unpaired data ratios, FedMed-GAN performs well and handles mode collapse adequately.
[27]	Provided a novel method based on CycleGAN to resolve spatial irregularities in the creation of 3D medical images, specifically when transforming 2D slices of magnetic resonance images into computed tomography images.
[28]	Investigated the creation of synthetic lung pictures using generative adversarial networks with semantic annotations and actual computed tomography scans.

3.4.1 Dataset

The GAN framework thrives on diverse and robust datasets to generate realistic content. The MC dataset, CORN-2, and BraTs2019 exemplify the variety essential for training GANs effectively. With its rich multimedia content, the MC dataset offers a broad spectrum of visual data. BraTs2019, centered on brain tumor images, contributes to medical imaging advancements. These datasets empower GANs to understand and replicate complex patterns across domains, fostering innovation in fields ranging from multimedia generation to medical diagnostics. Their diversity ensures that the GAN model generalizes well and produces authentic outputs across various domains.

3.4.2 Evaluation Metric

Selecting the appropriate model is essential for optimal application performance, but selecting the appropriate assessment metric is equally critical for ensuring optimal results. GANs have various applications, and every industry has developed evaluation standards of its own. However, when deciding on the evaluation criteria for various vocations, researchers have become confused due to the absence of standard measurements.

3.4.3 Preprocessing Methods

Pre-processing is necessary in order to improve training efficiency and generate high-quality images for generative adversarial networks. Image cropping, random flipping, normalization, size correction, contrast enhancement, and other techniques are covered in Table 3.6.

TABLE 3.6
Pre-Processing Techniques for GANs

Pre-Processing Technique	Description	Studies
Picture Crop	As a pre-processing technique, image cropping entails downsizing an image for display or further analysis or deleting a specific portion of the image, usually focusing on a region of interest.	[29–31]
Enhancement of Contrast	By manipulating the brightness and color levels, contrast enhancement—a basic image processing technique—improves the visibility of features, conferring greater distinction upon them.	[29, 32]
Normalization	In machine learning in particular, normalization is a pre-processing technique for data that involves scaling values in a dataset to a predefined range, usually between 0 and 1. This makes analysis more accurate and consistent.	[33, 34]
Coregistration	When many photos of the same area are collected at different times or with different sensors, coregistration is a technique used in image processing and remote sensing to align or integrate them to facilitate data integration and comparative analysis.	[33, 35]
Modification of Size	Reducing the size or quality of an image to meet a particular need is known as size adjustment, for example, changing its size for analysis or presentation.	[34, 36]
Flipping at Random	In machine learning and computer vision, random flipping is often employed and includes randomly mirroring photos either vertically or horizontally in order to increase the variety of training data and strengthen the model's robustness.	[31, 36]
Modifying the Texture	In order to obtain a certain visual or analytical result, artists and analysts frequently employ a variety of image processing techniques to modify the apparent texture of a picture. This process is known as texture transformation.	[37]

3.5 EXPLORING POPULAR GAN VARIANTS

Numerous subcategories of generative adversarial networks in the medical domain are covered in this extensive section on algorithms. The analysis encompasses a range of applications, such as disease progression modeling, image-to-image translation, multimodal GANs, image synthesis, enhancement, regression using time-series data, anomaly detection, registration, segmentation, and augmentation of images, among others. DCGAN, SRGAN, pix2pix, RGAN, SAGAN, and CGAN are a few examples of applications that correspond to particular GAN models.

3.5.1 Data Augmentation and Image Synthesis

A useful framework for creating synthetic images and enhancing data is generative adversarial networks. Through competition between two neural networks, discriminators and generators, GANs can generate realistic synthetic data or visuals. Because GANs generate fresh, varied samples that closely resemble the original data distribution, they enable the augmentation of data sets by extending their limits. GANs are very good at synthesizing realistic, high-quality images, which opens up new possibilities for image editing and other creative uses.

3.5.1.1 Deep Convolutional Generative Adversarial Networks

Radford et al. presented their groundbreaking work developing a convolutional decoder neural network for a generator. In order to maximize its effectiveness in the field of unsupervised learning, this specific technique incorporates some architectural constraints. Using the spatial upsampling capability built into the generator's convolutional decoder operation, a deep convolutional GAN maximizes its potential (G). Through the use of this unique capability, the power of GANs is leveraged to produce images with better resolutions. High-quality image creation and enhanced training stability are the results of improvements made to the original DCGAN design. The primary changes are the replacement of the pooling layers in the generator (G) with fractional-stride convolutions and the usage of stride convolutions in the discriminator (D). Second, the distribution of generated and real samples is centered around a zero by using batch normalization in both the discriminator (D) and the generator (G). Third, by removing related hidden layers, DCGAN chooses a deeper architectural approach. Ultimately, the generator uses Tanh activation for the output layer and ReLU activation for all other layers. Every layer of the discriminator uses LeakyReLU. Distinctly, DCGAN outperforms other subsequently proposed GAN variations in its quantitative production of visually appealing images. One noteworthy shortcoming of DCGAN, meanwhile, is that it is prone to mode collapse. Data augmentation and classification tasks are among the applications of DCGAN, which has been successfully trained on datasets including LSUN and ImageNet. This is the GAN's objective function

$$\underbrace{min}_{G}\ \underbrace{max}_{D}\ V(D,G) = E_{x\sim P_{Data(x)}}\left[\log\left(D(x)\right)\right] + E_{z\sim P_{z(z)}}\left[1-\log\left(D(G(z))\right)\right] \tag{3.1}$$

3.5.1.2 Vanilla Generative Adversarial Networks

The generator and discriminator networks in the generative adversarial network framework participate in a competitive training process. The framework was first suggested by Goodfellow et al. in 2014 [38]. In contrast to the discriminator, which separates real data from created samples, the generator produces data from random noise. Over time, the discriminator attempts to accurately categorize both forms of data, while the generator produces samples that can test the discriminator's accuracy. The discriminator finds it difficult to distinguish between the generator's data, which resembles the training distribution, and this dynamic persists until Nash equilibrium is reached. As a two-player game, GAN training ultimately aims to minimize the value function V(D, G), which represents the trade-off between discriminator and generator performance.

$$\underbrace{min}_{G}\ \underbrace{max}_{D}\ V(D,G) = E_{x\sim P_{Data(x)}}\left[\log\left(D(x)\right)\right] + E_{z\sim P_{z(z)}}\left[1-\log\left(D(G(z))\right)\right] \quad (3.2)$$

While the discriminator discerns between real and created samples, the generator uses random noise to create synthetic images. The generator's ability to generate images and the discriminator's ability to discriminate are both optimized through adversarial training. The generative model that is often produced by this repeated optimization is as follows:

$$G^{*} = \arg \underbrace{min}_{G}\ \underbrace{max}_{D}\ V(D,G) \quad (3.3)$$

Applications for GAN can be found in semi-supervised and unsupervised learning contexts, and it works on the tenets of unsupervised learning. Relying only on backpropagation, it is distinct from Markov chains as a generative model. Backpropagation from the discriminator helps with the generator's parameter updates. By producing more realistic and distinct samples, GAN outperforms other sophisticated models. GAN does, however, have many drawbacks, including a restricted range of generated outputs and training variation that causes mode collapse. The real GAN framework has been the basis for many optimized methods that have been proposed to address these problems. GAN is also not ideal for processing discrete data types such as text because of its ongoing constraints.

3.5.1.3 Auxiliary Classifier Generative Adversarial Networks (The Backup Classifier)

Introduced by Odena et al. [39], the generative adversarial network shares a structure with InfoGAN and cGAN in that it includes an auxiliary classifier. Unlike the previous structures of InfoGAN and cGAN, where these two architectures might apply to various data domains, with the auxiliary classifier generative adversarial network (AC-GAN) framework, the additional information is restricted to the class label. A classifier for classifying samples into different classes is included in the AC-GAN discriminator. Training stability is greatly improved by the addition of a classifier. As the number of labels increases, academic works [40] have noted that although AC-GAN has been shown to provide high-quality images, the model produces images that are often utilized for most classes.

To generate a sample known as Xfake = G(c, z), the generator G in the context of AC-GAN uses inputs of noise Z in conjunction with the corresponding categorical label C sampled from the distribution PC. However, taking into account both the authenticity and the category labels, discriminator D offers the ability to distinguish between real and fake photographs. Optimizing the combined loss Ls + Lc is the main goal of discriminator D training. On the other hand, while the generator G is being trained, the goal is to maximize the difference between losses, which is represented as Ls – Lc. Interestingly, the noise Z representation in the AC-GAN framework is learned independently and is not affected by the class label that corresponds with it.

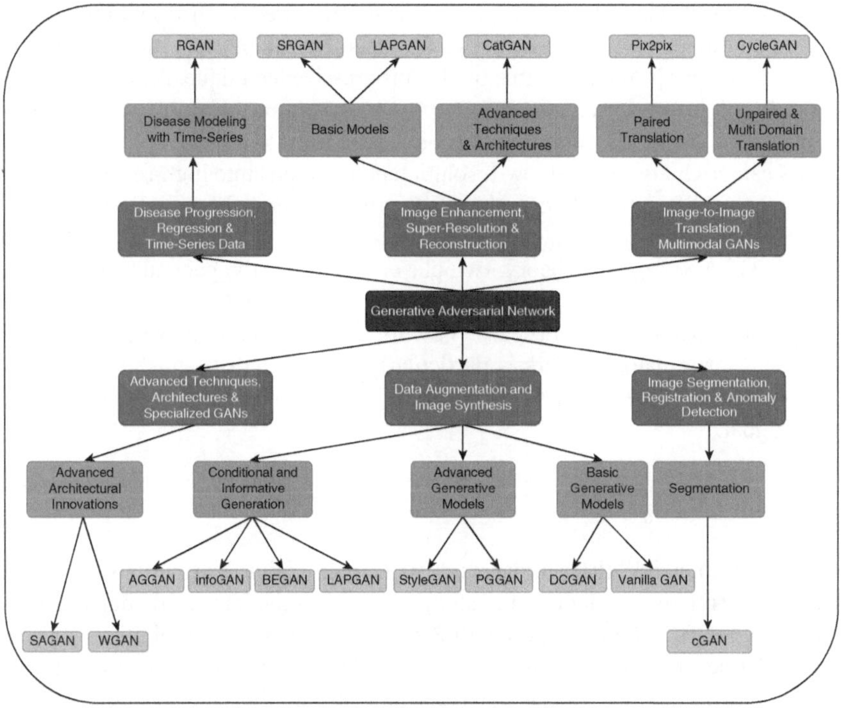

FIGURE 3.3 Taxonomy of generative adversarial networks.

3.5.1.4 Information Maximizing Generative Adversarial Network

Generative Adversarial Networks (GANs) are powerful tools for generating images; however, when specific properties or constraints need to be integrated into the generated images. Chen and colleagues [41] introduced InfoGAN, an unsupervised GAN capable of learning disentangled representations. The information-theoretic approach known as an information maximizing generative adversarial network (InfoGAN) can solve the problem of explaining the hidden variables in GAN. Between the implicit encoding c and the resulting distribution G(z, c), the common information is described by the "info" variable. The variable "info" indicates the information that is shared between the generated distribution G(z, c) and the underlying encoding c. The core GAN objective function is complemented by regular-term constraints, and I(c; G(z, c)) should be maximized in order to close the correlation between x and c. The lower bound on the P(c|x) variation could be ascertained concurrently by defining an auxiliary distribution Q(c|x) to approximate the P(c|x) approximation.

$$\underbrace{min}_{G,Q}\ \underbrace{max}_{C}\ L_1\left(D,G,Q\right)=V\left(D,G\right)-\lambda L_1\left(G,Q\right) \tag{3.4}$$

3.5.1.5 Progressive Growing Generative Adversarial Network

Combining generator and discriminator networks, the progressive growing generative adversarial network (PGGAN) is a well-known GAN version. Owing to

PGGAN's remarkable ability to capture global structures, high-resolution CXR is produced automatically. The learning of tiny features and overall image properties as layers get bigger is made possible by this progressive technique. A notable fade-in method allows lower-resolution layer outputs to have a considerable impact on the high-resolution output. Because it incorporates the knowledge from previous layers, PGGAN can gradually convert low-resolution photographs into high-resolution ones, which makes it distinctive. A formal website utilizing TensorFlow in Python—more precisely, TensorFlow-gpu 1.6.0 and Python 3.4.0—is the gateway to the implementation of PGGAN. In game theory, two players compete: the generator (G) and the discriminator or classifier (C). This is the foundation of PGGAN's training procedure. As the generator network learns how to transfer random noise into the input space, the discriminator network is particularly trained to distinguish between real and artificially produced samples. The loss function is, in theory, determined by the minimax goal.

$$\underbrace{min}_{G}\ \underbrace{max}_{C} + \underbrace{E}_{x\sim P_r}\left[\log C(x)\right] + \underbrace{E}_{x\sim P_g}\left[\log\left(1 - C(\tilde{x})\right)\right] \tag{3.5}$$

Within this framework, the authors work with three major distributions: Pr, which describes how real image data is allocated; Pg, which is the implicit model allocation shaped by x = G(z), where z ~ p(z) with P(z) being a Gaussian distribution; and Px^, which is defined by uniform sampling along linear paths that connect point pairs sampled from Pr and Pg. Because it incorporates a gradient penalty, the progressive growing of GANs technique uses the enhanced Wasserstein GAN loss, also known as the WGAN-GP loss. This method outperforms the original Wasserstein GAN. PGGAN's exceptional training stability—a critical component that makes it possible to synthesize high-resolution images—works in concert with the enhanced Wasserstein GAN loss in this work.

$$L = \underset{\tilde{x}\sim P_R}{E}\left[C(\tilde{x})\right] - \underset{\bar{x}\sim P_R}{E}\left[C(x)\right] + \lambda \underset{\hat{x}\ \sim P_{\hat{x}}}{E}\left[\left(\|\bar{\nabla}_{\hat{x}}\, C(_{\hat{x}})\|_2 - 1\right)^2\right. \tag{3.6}$$

3.5.1.6 Style Generative Adversarial Networks

A style generative adversarial network (StyleGAN) builds on the progressive GAN design, progressively scaling images from poor quality to high resolution. Bi-linear sampling is used for both the generator and discriminator in this version, as opposed to the closest neighbor up/down selection method, and a second-order binomial filter is integrated to increase quality. By creating an intermediate latent vector and incorporating a mapping network into the original, it affects numerous visual aspects. The process involves converting a 512-dimensional latent vector (z) into another 512-dimensional vector (w) by means of an eight-layer MLP-based mapping function and a learned affine operation (A). After being altered, the synthesis network receives this modified w together with the AdaIN module for adaptive instance normalization. As a result, Style GAN represents a significant development in GAN technology. The discriminator's architecture remains consistent with the baseline, but the generator integrates these modifications. As an input, the AdaIN operation requires y = (ys, yb), which is obtained by applying A to w. Its definition can be found in this way:

$$\text{AdaIN}\left(\mathrm{x}_i,\mathrm{y}\right) = y_{s,i}\frac{x_i - \mu\left(x_i\right)}{\sigma\left(x_i\right)} + y_{b,i} \tag{3.7}$$

An indefinitely fine-grained sum is a reasonable explanation for the perceptual path length; in practice, this is implemented by estimating a small subdivision parameter called epsilon (ε). Thus, an average over this approximation is used to calculate the mean perceptual path length in the latent space Z, which includes all possible endpoints:

$$lZ = E\left[\frac{1}{\epsilon^2}d\left(G\left(slerp\left(z1,z2\ ;t\right)\right),G\left(slerp\left(z1,z2\ ;t+\epsilon\right)\right)\right)\right] \tag{3.8}$$

3.5.1.7 Boundary Equilibrium Generative Adversarial Networks

The discriminator auto-encoder architecture, first presented in energy-based GANs by Zhao et al. [42], is incorporated into the boundary equilibrium generative adversarial network (BEGAN). The objective of the auto encoder's training is to improve the reconstruction loss for real and generated images; Berthelot et al. [43] proposed the BEGAN framework. According to this goal, the Wasserstein gap between distributions should be minimized.

3.5.2 Super-Resolution, Reconstruction, and Image Enhancement

In medical imaging, GANs perform well in image enhancement, super-resolution, and reconstruction. Medical image reconstruction can be made more precise and detailed, with higher resolution and better diagnostic accuracy, by utilizing a dual network architecture, where one generator is used to verify authenticity and another to improve image quality.

3.5.2.1 Super-Resolution Generative Adversarial Network

Through the addition of perceptual loss to adversarial loss, the super-resolution GAN enhances the realism of generated images [44]. As a result of the loss of fine, high-frequency features in the recovered images, using mean squared error (MSE) as the loss function during GAN training can produce a high peak signal-to-noise ratio (PSNR). After applying a convolutional neural network to both artificially generated and real images, the feature differences are compared in order to calculate the perceptual loss [45]. SRGAN has been used extensively in investigations to reconstruct high-quality images and restore details from low-quality inputs. For instance, Gu et al. synthesized high-quality pictures from low-quality computed tomography and magnetic resonance images using a GAN-based super-resolution framework. The created photos nonetheless had realistic patterns and textural characteristics because to their technique. Perceptual loss equation:

$$L_{perceptual} = \frac{1}{N}\sum_{i=1}^{n}\left\|\varnothing\left(I^i_{real}\right) - \varnothing\left(I^i_{gen}\right)\right\|_2^2 \tag{3.9}$$

3.5.2.2 Least Squares Generative Adversarial Networks

Fundamentally, a least squares generative adversarial network (LSGAN) uses the least-squares loss function, which was first proposed by Mao et al. [46], in place of the discriminator's cross-entropy loss. With traditional GANs, the discriminator is viewed as a classifier that uses the cross-entropy sigmoid loss. Gradient vanishing issues are caused by this strategy. A fake sample that is identified as a real image does not have an error since it lies on the right side of the decision boundary even though it is obviously not the same as the true samples. Alternatively, data points that are far from the right of the decision border are penalized by the least-squares loss function. Generation of samples more akin to the real data is encouraged by this penalty. More robustness during training and better picture generation than normal GANs are two characteristics that set LSGANs apart. The mode collapse that it experiences, however, has a detrimental effect on the efficacy and diversity of the images that are generated. Equations 3.10 and 3.11 give the expressions for the objective functions of the generator and discriminator.

$$\underbrace{min}_{G} L_G = \frac{1}{2} E_{z\sim} P_z \left[(D(G(z)) - c)^2 \right] \tag{3.10}$$

$$\underbrace{min}_{D} L_{D=} \frac{1}{2} E_{x\sim} P_r \left[\left(D(x) - b \right)^2 \right] + \frac{1}{2} E_{z\sim} P_z \left[\left(D\left(G(z) \right) - a \right)^2 \right] \tag{3.11}$$

3.5.2.3 Category-Based Generative Adversarial Networks

As an alternative to conventional GAN, Springenberg's [47] introduction of category-based generative adversarial networks (CatGANs) employs a distinct methodology. Multiclass classification is used by CatGAN in an unsupervised manner as an alternative to binary classification. Within this framework, all sample data is pre-selected into categories by training the discriminator (D) to discriminate between true and false data. During the process, D assigns classes to the data, even if it doesn't know how the categories are distributed among the samples that the generator (G) creates. Notably, instead of merely replicating samples from a dataset, CatGAN requires G to construct samples linked with particular classes. CatGAN has difficulties efficiently clustering input characteristics, even if it can learn from unlabeled data. H[p(c|x,D)] and H[p(c|D)] maximization and H[p(c|G(z),D)] minimization are the goals of the CatGAN. Applying CatGAN to picture categorization is a remarkable use case, as demonstrated by Reference [48]. Equations 3.12 and 3.13 give the expressions for the objective functions of the generator and discriminator.

$$\text{LD} = \underbrace{max}_{D} \; H_X \left[p(c \mid D) \right] - E_{x\sim X} \left[H \left[p\left(c|x, D \right) \right] \right] + E_{7\sim p(7)} \left[H \left[p\left(c|x, D \right) \right] \right] \tag{3.12}$$

$$LG = \underbrace{min}_{G} - H_G \left[P\left(c|D \right) \right] + E_{z\sim P(z)} \left[H[P(c \mid G\left(z \right), D)] \right] \tag{3.13}$$

H [.] stands for empirical entropy in these equations, whereas X is the data set's distribution.

3.5.3 Image-to-Image Conversion, Multilayer BANANS

Generative adversarial networks in image-to-image translation, which translate images from one domain to another (e.g., CT scan to MRI), use discriminator and generator neural networks. To produce many perspectives or modalities from a single input, for instance, multimodal GANs are used in medical imaging. Through the provision of many viewpoints or features that may be absent from a more thorough medical investigation and explanation, this aids in diagnosis.

3.5.3.1 Pixel-to-Pixel Generative Adversarial Network

Within the area of conditional generative adversarial networks, pix2pix generates an image as a result only if an input (source) image is first generated. The generator and discriminator are the two main parts of the network. An picture's input must be transformed into the desired output image by the generator. The discriminator evaluates how similar the input image is to an unknown image at the same time. This unknown image could be an output image generated by the generator or a target image from the dataset. Determining whether the image was generated by the generator is its aim. To reduce the loss that the discriminator anticipates for the generated images, the generator is continuously adjusted during training. Through an approach where the generator is not explicitly exposed to the training dataset, the training procedure attempts to mitigate the danger of overfitting. The generator is instead controlled by the loss functions as it advances through the training process; dropout layers are used to introduce randomness during both the dataset training and prediction stages. To create the appropriate target image y, which can be represented as x, z → y, the generator in pix2pix learns a mapping that takes as inputs the source image x and a random noise image z. The discriminator's task in the interim is to distinguish between actual target images (y) based on source image x and phone y ones produced by the generator.

3.5.3.2 Cycle Generative Adversarial Networks

The difficulty of switching images between two distinct domains is what Zhu et al. [49] sought to address using a cycle generative adversarial network. This technique creates a cyclic network topology using two complimentary generative adversarial networks. Mapping domain X and domain Y images is the basic objective of CycleGAN. Within this structure, there are two discriminators, Dy and Dx, and two generators, G and F. A domain X image is sent into the generator G, which tries to convert it to a domain Y image. In parallel, the discriminator Dy ascertains if G created a specific image or it is a real image from the domain. Comparably, generator F's job is to transform an image from domain Y into an image from domain X, and discriminator Dx's job is to ascertain if an image was produced by generator F or is part of domain X. The model's resilience is increased by CycleGAN's use of cyclic consistency loss to further improve overall performance. The schematic diagram for CycleGAN is displayed in Figure 3.6.

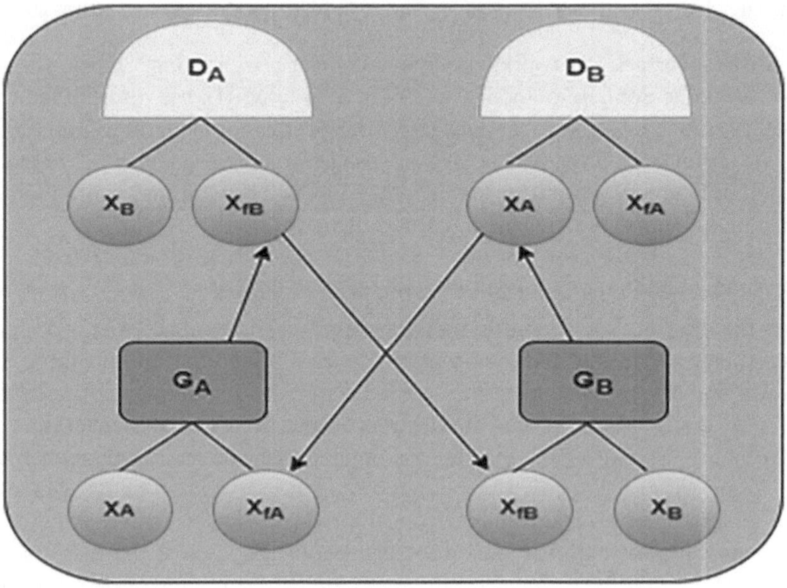

FIGURE 3.4 Schematic diagram of CycleGAN.

3.5.4 *R*-Squared, Time-Series Data, and Disease Progression

Generative adversarial networks produce realistic visuals with time-series medical imaging that show how diseases advance or regress. In order to improve diagnostic and predictive capacities in healthcare, GANs use deep learning to simulate illness histories. This allows for the analysis and forecasting of the advancement or regression of diseases.

3.5.4.1 Relativistic Generative Adversarial Networks

A novel training method to improve GAN performance is introduced by the relativistic GAN. The discriminator of RGAN is designed to determine whether real data is more likely to be genuine than artificial data that is created at random in order to solve the non-convergence problem of traditional GANs. Other training methods have surfaced after RGAN. Song et al. proposed controlling the generator's gradient value to avoid gradient explosion in order to reduce method failure in GANs. This was achieved by including some erroneous samples as real samples during training. With the discriminator constructed as a classifier for positive-unlabeled classification rather than the conventional positive and negative classification, a point cloud upsampling network (PU-GAN) was created to address the training instability inherent in GAN. In line with Goodfellow and associates' research, this approach is based on the core idea of allowing a generative model (G) to be trained with the particular goal of tricking a differentiable discriminator (D). With training, this discriminator learns to distinguish between legitimate images and super-resolved images generated by the generator. This generator will be able to produce results that are almost exactly like real photos if it follows this approach, which will make it difficult for discriminator D to effectively classify the results.

$$\underbrace{max}_{\theta_G}\underbrace{max}_{\theta_D} E_{I^{HR}\sim P_{train}\left(I^{HR}\right)}\left[\log D_{\theta_D}\left(I^{HR}\right)\right]+E_{I^{LR}\sim pG\left(I^{LR}\right)}\left[\log\left(1-D_{\theta_D}\left(G_{\theta_G}\left(I^{LR}\right)\right)\right)\right] \tag{3.14}$$

3.5.5 More Complex Methods, Structures, and Expertise

Modern versions and architectures created specifically for medical imaging are used in GANS advanced methods for generative adversarial networks. Medical research, diagnosis, and treatment planning are aided by the high accuracy and clinical significance of the images produced by these GANs, which are designed with complex optimization procedures.

3.5.5.1 Self-Attention Generative Adversarial Networks

While it generally picks up spatial features, conventional convolutional GAN has trouble learning some classes of images. This second GAN model is better at creating images with certain restrictions, like sky or ocean vistas, but it can't replicate images with intricate geometric patterns. By incorporating a self-monitoring mechanism into a convolutional GAN, Zhang et al. [50] introduced the self-attention generative adversarial network (SAGAN). With this embedding, the model may take into account global long-range dependencies for picture fusion, resulting in a large receptive field without sacrificing computational efficiency. Self-suggestion works by balancing the features from all other regions to determine the response inside a region. The computational cost of computing attention weights is small. To enhance the resilience of training, spectral normalization is utilized for both the generator (G) and discriminator (D) weights. Complex geometric conditions are imposed on the image structure by the discriminator, while the generator creates images with intricate details at various points. In challenges like enhancing human position representation and reaching super resolution, self-attention GAN demonstrates notable advantages over other image generating techniques. An illustration of the self-monitoring mechanism's architecture is provided in Figure 3.5. The key, question, and value are the three sequentially related letters in the figure: g, f, and h. Mapping is represented by the symbol ⊗. The attention map demonstrates long-distance spatial interdependence to better detect anomalies in medical images and provide more accurate and dependable diagnoses by precisely identifying structures, aligning images for particular comparison, and highlighting variations.

3.5.5.2 Wasserstein Generative Adversarial Network

As mentioned [51], the WGAN successfully resolves the unstable GAN problem and facilitates learning. The training instability issue that GANs encounter is resolved by WGAN. As stated in the source, the two primary causes of the issues with the original GAN are (1) the use of impractical difference measurements following equivalent optimization, like the Jensen Shannon (JS) and Kullback Leibler (KL) differences, and (2) the difficulty of achieving overlap between the original randomly initialized generator distribution and the true distribution. The Wasserstein distance

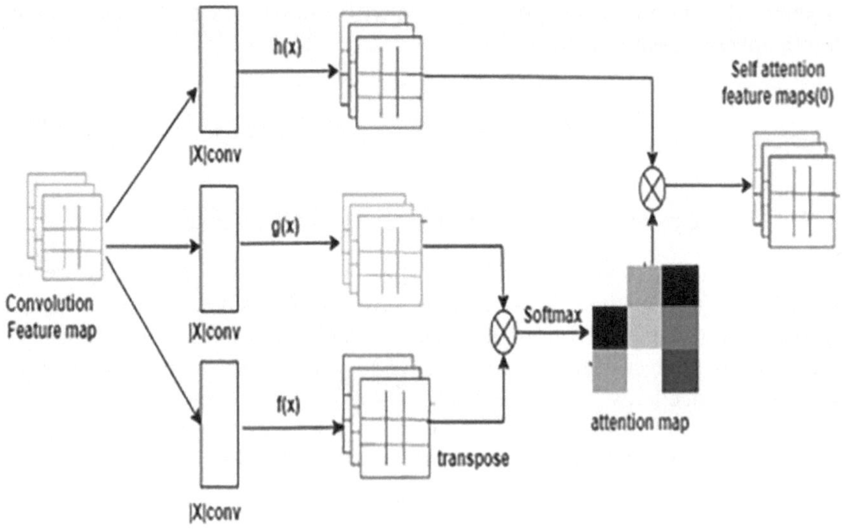

FIGURE 3.5 SAGAN architecture.

is introduced by the WGAN in order to address these problems. When there is no overlapping support between the two distributions, the Wasserstein distance can still be used to measure differences, unlike the KL and JS distributions. Furthermore, compared to the KL and JS differences, the Wasserstein distance offers superior smoothing performance. The gradient vanishing problem is resolved by this advantageous feature, which permits improved harmony between the discriminator and the generator during the learning process. It is possible to maximize the Wasserstein distance mathematically by employing a neural network, represented by the letter D. Then, G is optimized in relation to this roughly ideal D in order to minimize the Wasserstein distance and hence decrease the difference between the generated and real distributions. In the Wasserstein GAN, the generator (G) and discriminator (D) loss functions are defined independently as follows:

$$L_G = -E_{x \in P_g}\left[D_w(x)\right] \tag{3.15}$$

$$L_D = E_{x \in P_g}\left[D_w(x)\right] - E_{x \in P_r}\left[D_w(x)\right] \tag{3.16}$$

where w denotes parameters that have a finite value.

3.5.6 Image Segmentation, Registration, and Anomaly Detection

Medical imaging anomalies can be effectively segmented, registered, and identified using Generative Adversarial Networks (GANs). Studies have shown that Conditional GANs (cGANs) are especially beneficial for image-to-image transformation problems. Its functions include producing photo-realistic images, assisting segmentation tasks, and enabling data augmentation.

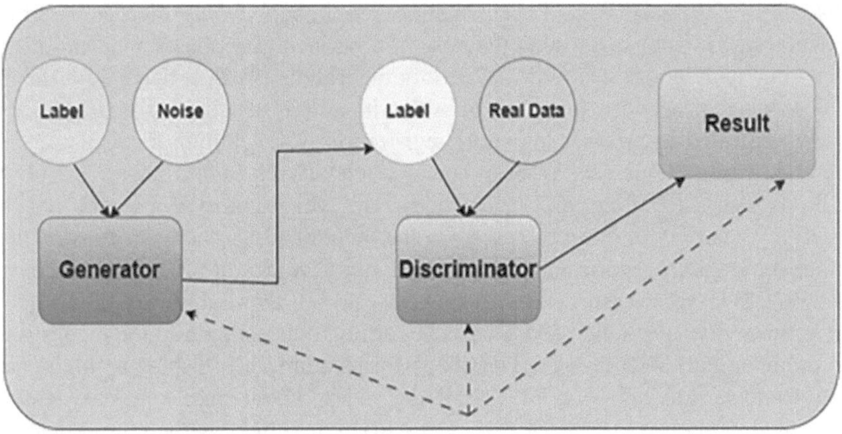

FIGURE 3.6 Schematic diagram of CGAN.

3.5.6.1 Conditional Generative Adversarial Network

The controlled synthesis of generated data is made possible by the cGAN, a conditional model created to add extra information to the generative model. As stated by Mirza et al. [34], this additional data may include class designations or data from several modalities. The cGAN is a GAN framework expansion that requires an extra information vector (c) to be sent as part of the input to the discriminator and generator. This innovation has proved to have improved multi-modal data representation capabilities. Typically, the additional data is encoded as a one-hot vector in the discriminator and generator. It is then mixed with the real data (x) in the discriminator and an encoded noise vector (z) in the generator. It is remarkable, therefore, that the discriminator is unable to generate the class label for the input data on its own. cGANs frequently require pairs of input and output images for training, which may not always be the case in domain adaption circumstances. A multitude of parameters are included in the conditioning part of cGAN, such as characteristics, images, texts, and class labels. cGANs are flexible enough to work with a wide range of data types, including multi-modal datasets like Flickr and unimodal datasets like MNIST [52]. Equation 3.17 displays the loss function related to the cGAN framework.

$$\underbrace{min}_{G} \underbrace{max}_{D} E_{x\sim P_x}\left[\log D(x|c) + E_{z\sim P_z} \log\left(1 - D\left(G(z|c)\right)\right)\right] \qquad [3.17]$$

3.6 RESULT ANALYSIS

Metrics such as SSIM, PSNR, accuracy, AUC, Dice coefficient, MAE, ROC curve, IoU, entropy, and normalization are used in result analysis for GANs in medical imaging. These metrics evaluate the overall performance of the model as well as the segmentation precision, classification accuracy, and image quality. To ensure a thorough assessment of GAN performance in improving medical image synthesis, registration, classification, and segmentation, researchers choose metrics based on particular tasks. Upon examining the table of described GAN-based medical image processing applications, we find that certain algorithms perform better in different medical image processing jobs. MMFGAN, with a high structural similarity index, has demonstrated its prowess in picture registration. The acronym for accuracy and amplitude gain (AG) is acc. When it comes to classifying brain images, ED-GAN excels with an astounding 96.25% accuracy rate, which makes it a useful tool for classifying a variety of brain diseases. On the other hand, the image reconstruction specialist MedGAN reports a comparatively lower accuracy of 62%. When it comes to chest CT image classification, MI-GAN performs admirably, exhibiting good AUC, sensitivity, specificity, and accuracy. Turning our attention to the reconstruction of abdominal MRI images, T-GAN performs admirably, displaying high peak signal-to-noise ratio and structural similarity index. These studies make extensive use of datasets such as OASIS, SRPBS, and ABIDE, highlighting their importance in influencing the field of medical image processing. These datasets have been widely used, which highlights their importance as useful tools that allow researchers to investigate algorithmic skills in a variety of medical imaging studies. To sum up, the complexity of medical imaging necessitates a careful approach to algorithm selection that takes into account the unique requirements of each activity. Even while some algorithms work well for specific applications, performance variation highlights how important it is to make customized decisions when deploying algorithms, which has a big impact on how medical image processing is developing.

3.7 CHALLENGES AND FUTURE RESEARCH DIRECTIONS

GANs have become one of the most potent kinds of machine learning models. Tasks including image synthesis, segmentation, augmentation, classification, registration, reconstruction, denoising, and detection have a lot of potential applications in medical imaging. But there are particular difficulties when using GANs for medical imaging; therefore, more research will be needed to increase productivity. The main issues and prospective research directions for improving GANs in medical imaging will be covered in this section.

3.7.1 Optimization Process

GAN optimization is a complicated process. As a result of the process's nature—which is seen as a mini-max game—achieving the Nash equilibrium, the ideal point in the optimization scenario, is difficult. Several conceptual and numerical factors contribute to the instability of traditional GAN training. This could lead to two convergence issues: mode-hopping and mode collapse. The overall effectiveness of GANs can be increased by looking into more resilient optimization methods and strategies to stabilize the training process, including resolving convergence problems like mode collapse. By reducing the possibility of the generator being overly optimized for a particular discriminator, unrolled GANs reduce mode collapse and improve model stability overall. Potential techniques to improve GAN convergence include punishing discriminator weights and adding noise to discriminator inputs.

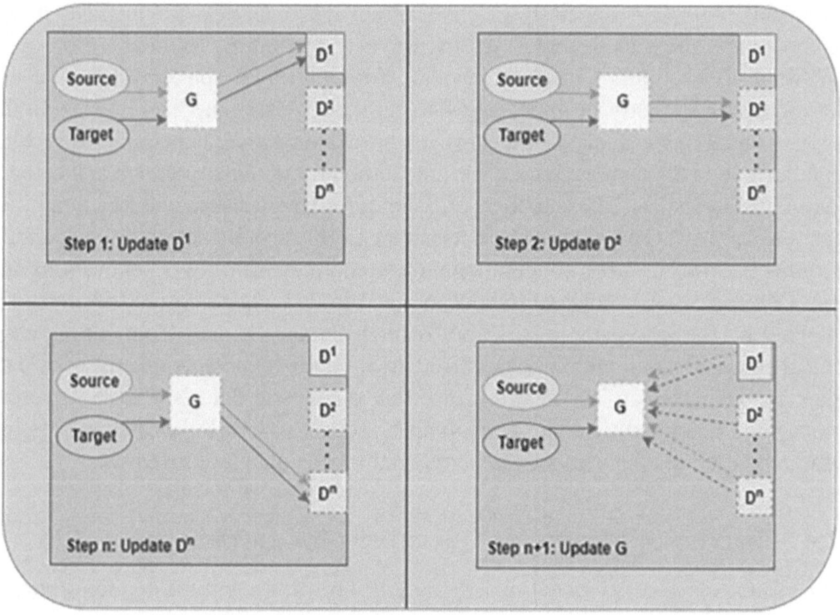

FIGURE 3.7 Optimization process of AsynDGAN.

3.7.2 Privacy Concerns and Trustability of Generated Data

Privacy issues occur in the application and gathering of medical imaging data, especially because such data is sensitive. The asynchronized discriminator GAN (AsynDGAN) framework addresses the crucial need to safeguard patients' sensitive information while facilitating efficient communication and dissemination of GAN-generated medical data in the field of healthcare data privacy. AsynDGAN accomplishes this without requiring the sharing or direct access to sensitive patient information by learning generative distributions from actual medical datasets across many health institutions. One major problem is building trust in medical images that are generated. The reliability of generated data can be improved by utilizing rigorous experiments and physics-based simulations to comprehend GAN convergence in the context of medical imaging. The AsynDGAN optimization process architecture is shown in Figure 3.7.

The brown ellipse represents the real image of the target, while the green ellipse indicates the source mask. Solid arrows represent the forward pass in our iterative updating method, while dotted arrows show the gradient direction during the backward pass. Dotted blocks indicate they stay the same throughout that specific update, while solid blocks indicate ongoing updates.

3.7.3 Limited Integration with Models from Other Domains and Multimodal Medical Image Augmentation

While GANs have been integrated with models from various fields, such as natural language processing, signal graphs, and optimization techniques, their application in medical imaging—especially in creating advanced models for medical image augmentation—remains limited. Absorbing and combining models from other domains, such as attention mechanisms, transformers, and graph convolution, could offer promising avenues for improving GANs for augmented medical images. In the field of medical image analysis, transformers have demonstrated encouraging results, particularly in tasks such as semantic segmentation for the identification and categorization of skin lesions. These models offer unique characteristics and functionalities that could improve GANs' overall performance in this specific situation. It is anticipated that interdisciplinary cooperation will promote the sharing of innovations and ideas. Developing efficient multimodal medical image augmentation techniques is hampered by the increasing availability of multimodal pictures from cutting-edge medical imaging equipment. These difficulties could involve problems with data fusion, model intricacy, and making sure that diagnostic data is preserved across various imaging modalities. The development of GAN-based methods for processing multimodal medical pictures should be the main focus of future research.

3.7.4 Traditional Metrics for Quantitative Evaluation

Medical images' precise visual quality may not be well captured by conventional pixel-wise measurements like MAE, MSE, PSNR, and SSIM. More sophisticated evaluation criteria have been developed and adopted to offer more relevant and human-aligned evaluations of the caliber of generated medical images, such as learning perceptual image path similarity (LPIPS). Prioritizing the complete medical image during the diagnosis procedure is not always evident, though. Medical diagnosis frequently necessitates focusing on narrow, targeted regions of interest. Therefore, developing evaluation metrics that take into account the semantic context and are consistent with both subjective and objective assessments presents a new challenge for the field.

3.7.5 Geometric Correlations and Microscopic Imaging

Strong geometric connections are not always taken into account by current data synthesis approaches, which limits their applicability. Future developments will probably entail refining architectures that address particular geometric properties particular to various medical imaging modalities and workloads in order to get over these restrictions. The challenges of validation and real-time application needs are addressed by this endeavor. The architecture of bidirectional generative adversarial networks (Bi-GANs) offers a viable way to synthesize various microscopic images in various fields. This method considers a number of geometric properties. By effectively tackling certain geometric complexity implicit in certain medical imaging tasks, our approach may significantly expand the field of GAN applications in the medical imaging arena.

3.7.6 Lack of Interpretability and High Training Cost

Deep learning has major problems, particularly in the field of medical image augmentation, due to the interpretability issues in GAN model training and the corresponding high costs. One approach that shows promise for addressing this problem is the combination of deep learning techniques and classical methodologies. For example, improving interpretability could be achieved by creating augmentation methods based on approaches such as temporal-spectral fusion generative adversarial networks (tsf-GANs) and blending generative adversarial networks (blend-GANs). Another problem is that strong GPU hardware is required for the GAN model training process, particularly when training a large amount of picture data. Regretfully, the cost of these systems can be high. Furthermore, it is anticipated that deep network training times will drop noticeably as computer hardware continues to improve, bringing with it greater computational power and efficiency.

3.7.7 Interdisciplinary Collaboration and Semi-Automatic Creation of Medical Image Reports

The semi-automated creation of medical imaging reports has been studied through the use of GANs created especially for text-generation tasks. During report generation, GANs with attention mechanisms can prioritize important disease-related data, hence improving the compilation of diagnostic reports and lessening the strain for doctors. It is obvious that cooperation between medical experts and AI researchers is crucial as we move to the future. Physicians can provide specialized help in feature selection, data tagging, and problem solving due to their clinical experience. The potential of AI in medical imaging must be fully realized through this interdisciplinary partnership. It has the ability to change the way doctors perform their duties by providing targeted advice on feature selection, data tagging, and problem solving, therefore propelling the industry forward [53].

3.7.8 Automatic 3D Image Modality Colorization and 4D Medical Image Augmentation

In the field of medical imaging, automatic colorization of 3D picture modalities constitutes an untapped area. Potential areas for improvement are highlighted by colorizing multi-modal 3D medical data using the generalization powers of GANs and 2D-style exemplars. The goal of this novel strategy is to increase the usefulness of such data. Still, more investigation and improvement are needed in this field. Although the majority of medical imaging research initiatives focus on 2D and 3D images, it is still difficult to harness the power of GANs for 4D-based images. 4D time series prediction using augmented models is a promising avenue for the future. In the future, 4D time series prediction may be enhanced by methods that capitalize on GANs' achievements in 4D imaging.

3.7.9 Class Leakage

Class leakage affects the fidelity of the data when generated images contain properties from another class. To avoid class leakage and guarantee that the generated images accurately reflect the intended class features, it is essential to develop appropriate metrics and constraints in GANs. Researching class leakage is a good avenue to pursue. This may entail creating brand-new loss functions or regularization techniques that mandate class-wise separation throughout training. Furthermore, investigating methods from transfer learning and domain adaptation may provide insightful information on reducing the problem of mixing attributes between classes.

3.7.10 Addressing the Skewed Distribution of Medical Data and Dataset Quality with Availability

Medical data often exhibits a skewed distribution, with a focus on common diseases. To address this imbalance, researchers can combine GANs and attention mechanisms to intentionally generate pathological cases of rare diseases, aiding in research and the diagnosis of less usual conditions. The quality and availability of medical datasets suitable for GANs pose challenges, including sparsity, age, and heterogeneity. Using GAN-based models in biomedical imaging has been severely limited by the lack of a large medical dataset. Efforts should be directed towards creating standardized and diverse medical datasets for GANs. This involves considering specific challenges posed by medical imaging tasks.

3.7.11 Lack of Preservation of Small Abnormalities

When using unpaired data, cross-modality models are not guaranteed to maintain small abnormality zones during the transformation. Biases in pre-trained models such as CycleGAN cause this problem when attempting to match the distribution of the target domain with the generated data. When specific classes are over- or under-represented in the training data, biases may appear. This is true even when there are paired data points. By using techniques like altering the discriminator design and applying penalization based on smaller patches, this bias can be lessened.

3.7.12 Reinforcement Learning

The broad use of reinforcement learning (RL) applied to GANs is hindered by various issues. The intricate design of RL is one of the main obstacles. Minimal changes in the configuration of states, incentives, and actions can result in observably different results, and a great deal of experimentation is needed to identify the ideal hyperparameters. Additional difficulties arise from the low stability and repeatability of RL models, since the same operations may provide different results, especially if the input data source is changed. Future directions for reinforcement learning in GANs applied to medical imaging appear encouraging, notwithstanding these obstacles. Investigating hierarchical reinforcement learning (HRL) is one approach. The goal of HRL is to increase agent productivity by decomposing complicated activities into a hierarchy of smaller jobs. HRL subclasses, including intrinsic motivation, spatio-temporal abstraction, and deep successor RL, have the potential to enhance agent-based pipelines, especially when handling high-dimensional 3D or even 4D image data. Moreover, transfer reinforcement learning and multitasking can improve the flexibility of RL agents. By using transfer learning to make agents capable of doing comparable but distinct tasks, training time can be drastically decreased. Another

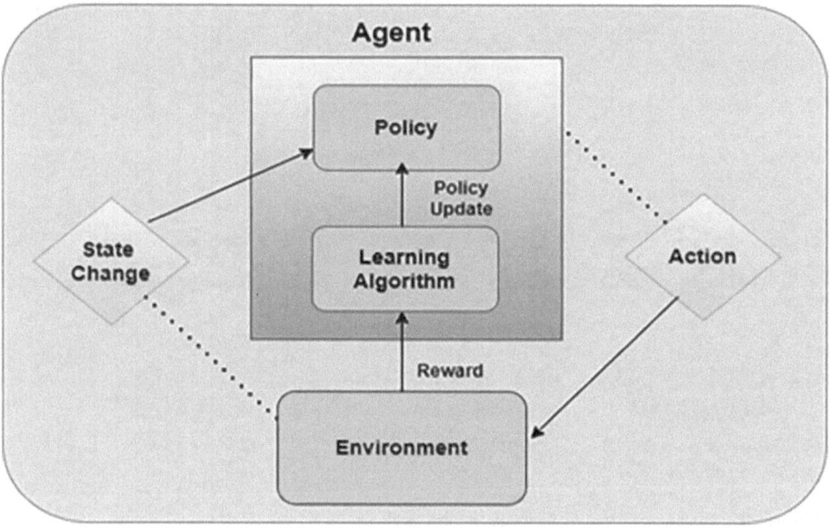

FIGURE 3.8 Framework of reinforcement learning.

fantastic path for the field is presented by active reinforcement learning. Active learning techniques that involve user interaction—especially with doctors—can improve the agent's comprehension of the objectives of the user and maximize performance with the least amount of annotated data. However, because active RL requires human users to be involved, putting it into practice could be difficult. The general reinforcement learning framework is shown in Figure 3.8.

In order to maximize cumulative rewards, an agent interacts with the environment and makes decisions one after the other within the framework of learning. After observing the present state of the environment, the agent decides what to do based on its policy, goes about carrying out these actions, gets feedback in the form of rewards, and changes to a new state. The agent's learning of the best policy to use while making decisions in order to maximize long-term benefits is the aim. This entails using iterative learning procedures to improve the policy.

3.7.13 Federated Learning

Opportunities exist for reducing privacy hazards in generative adversarial networks for medical imaging through federated learning. But it has difficulties. One major challenge in decentralized settings is the requirement for efficient convergence within the limitations of constrained transmission bandwidth. A careful investigation is necessary to strike a compromise between model performance and privacy preservation when integrating federated learning with differential privacy. Collaborative learning is further complicated by the uniqueness and diversity of imaging modalities found in medical datasets. In the future, researchers will focus on improving model robustness, resolving communication bottlenecks, and federated learning's adaptation to the complexities of medical data. Figure 3.9 shows the federated learning process.

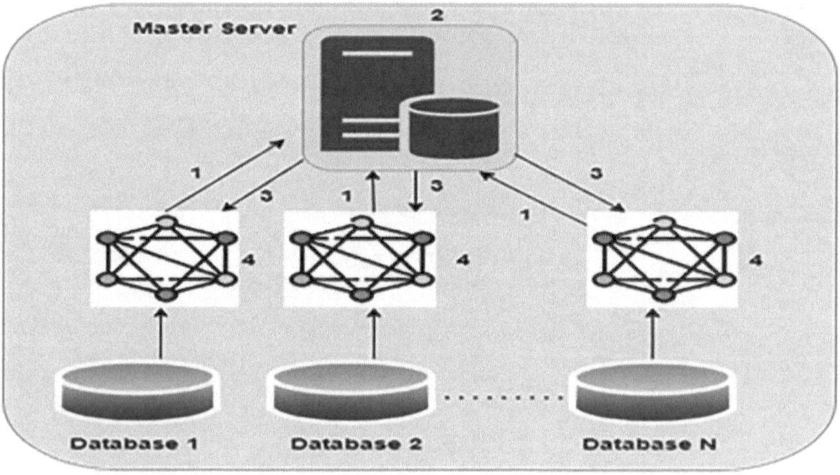

FIGURE 3.9 Federated learning working procedure.

The first stage involves each participant computing the model gradient locally, sending the results to the master server while encrypting the data using methods such homomorphic encryption. The master server must carry out secure aggregation in step two before returning the aggregated results to step three's participants. In step 4, participants modify their model parameters by decrypting the gradients they received. Until the maximum number of iterations is reached or the loss function converges, this iterative procedure is continued. Unlike centralized models on Hadoop, participant data is kept dispersed, protecting anonymity. Federated learning effectively handles growing data volumes without requiring communication bandwidth by enabling any number of databases to cooperatively train the model without moving data to a central place.

3.7.14 Diffusion Models

Diffusion models, an alternative to GANs, are presently being developed. In order to understand the underlying data distribution, these score-based approaches train images by adding noise gradually and according to a Gaussian distribution. The main goal is to represent the complex data distribution rather than explicitly reversing the introduced noise. Diffusion models with steady training and good mode coverage have demonstrated the capacity to produce realistic images. Nonetheless, a significant obstacle is the prolonged sampling duration linked to the diffusion process. Researchers are actively addressing this constraint by improving models for faster sampling, even if this might not be as important in non-real-time applications like medical imaging. Future research in this area will focus on improving diffusion models through sampling time reductions without sacrificing image quality. This entails investigating novel model variations, improving diffusion models' general efficacy and application, particularly in the context of medical imaging, and honing their real-time applicability. The diffusion model procedure is shown in Figure 3.10.

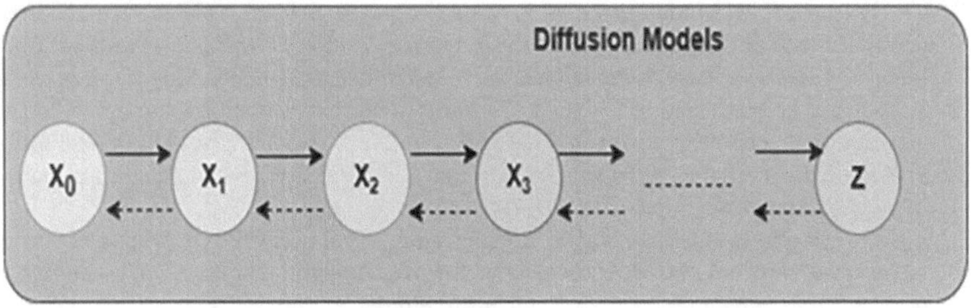

FIGURE 3.10 Diffusion model working procedure.

Both forward and backward diffusion processes are included in diffusion models. A Markov chain is used in the forward diffusion process, which automatically introduces noise into the input data until white noise is reached. This often involves a thousand steps and is not a method that can be learned. Conversely, the goal of the reverse diffusion process is to gradually remove noise in order to recreate the original data, so methodically undoing the forward process. To enable this reversal, a trainable neural network is used.

3.8 CONCLUSION

A generative adversarial network is a particular type of neural network design that trains two networks side by side to generate images and check and evaluate them. In the realm of medical imaging, GANs enhance image quality, produce vital training data, and progress illness identification and diagnosis through the application of cutting-edge image processing techniques. In medical imaging, GANs dramatically raise small datasets, sharpen diagnostic precision, and improve image quality—all of which benefit patient care and the efficacy of research. Nonetheless, research on GANs in medical imaging is lacking. This chapter provides a comprehensive overview of GAN applications in medical imaging across multiple domains, with an emphasis on recent developments. It examines widely used datasets and preprocessing methods, assesses well-known GAN algorithms, and does a thorough current study. Additionally, it outlines the challenges that GANs face in medical imaging and makes recommendations for future directions in study. Because of this, this work is a vital tool for group research, providing informative data to support the development of GANs in medical imaging and supporting scientists and financiers who wish to stay up to date and promote innovation in this area.

REFERENCES

1. D. Saxena and J. Cao, "Generative adversarial networks (GANs) challenges, solutions, and future directions," *ACM Comput. Surv. (CSUR)*, vol. 54, no. 3, pp. 1–42, 2021.
2. A. Almahairi, S. Rajeshwar, A. Sordoni, P. Bachman, and A. Courville, "Augmented cyclegan: Learning many-to-many mappings from unpaired data," in *International Conference on Machine Learning*. PMLR, July 2018, pp. 195–204.

3. J. A. Iglesias, J. M. Monterrubio, M. P. Sesmero, and A. Sanchis, "Generation and evaluation of medical images based on diffusion models," in *2024 IEEE International Conference on Evolving and Adaptive Intelligent Systems (EAIS)*. IEEE, May 2024, pp. 1–8.
4. A. Radford, L. Metz, and S. Chintala, "Unsupervised representation learning with deep convolutional generative adversarial networks," *arXiv preprint* arXiv:1511.06434, 2015.
5. N. Kodali, J. Abernethy, J. Hays, and Z. Kira, "On convergence and stability of gans," *arXiv preprint* arXiv:1705.07215, 2017.
6. F. Kheiri, H. E. Najafabadi, and S. Rahnamayan, "Progressively Growing Generative Adversarial Network Based Auto-encoder for MRI Image Inpainting," *Proceedings of the 37th Canadian Conference on Artificial Intelligence*, May 2024.
7. S. Keele, "Guidelines for performing systematic literature reviews in software engineering," Dept. Comput. Sci., Univ. Durham, Durham, U.K., Tech. Rep. EBSE-2007-01, 2007.
8. B. Kitchenham, "Procedures for performing systematic reviews," Keele Univ., Keele, U.K., Tech. Rep. TR/SE-0401, 2004, vol. 33, pp. 1–26.
9. F. Munawar, S. Azmat, T. Iqbal, C. Grönlund, and H. Ali, "Segmentation of lungs in chest X-ray image using generative adversarial networks," *IEEE Access*, vol. 8, pp. 153535–153545, 2020.
10. L. Zhu, Q. He, Y. Huang, Z. Zhang, J. Zeng, L. Lu, W. Kong, and F. Zhou, "DualMMP-GAN: Dual-scale multi-modality perceptual generative adversarial network for medical image segmentation," *Comput. Biol. Med.*, vol. 144, Art. no. 105387, May 2022.
11. A. Kunapinun, M. N. Dailey, D. Songsaeng, M. Parnichkun, C. Keatmanee, and M. Ekpanyapong, "Improving GAN learning dynamics for thyroid nodule segmentation," *Ultrasound Med. Biol.*, vol. 49, no. 2, pp. 416–430, February 2023.
12. S. J. Narayanan, A. S. Anil, C. Ashtikar, S. Chunduri, and S. Saman, "Automated brain tumor segmentation using GAN augmentation and optimized U-Net," in *Frontiers ICT Healthcare*. Cham, Switzerland: Springer, 2023, pp. 635–646.
13. W. Du and S. Tian, "Transformer and GAN-based super-resolution reconstruction network for medical images," *Tsinghua Sci. Technol.*, vol. 29, no. 1, pp. 197–206, February 2024.
14. Y. Wang, Z.-L. Sun, Z. Zeng, and K.-M. Lam, "TRCT-GAN: CT reconstruction from biplane X-rays using transformer and generative adversarial networks," *Digit. Signal Process.*, vol. 140, Art. no. 104123, August 2023.
15. R. Mishra, K. Sharma, R. R. Jha, and A. Bhavsar, "NeuroGAN: Image reconstruction from EEG signals via an attention-based GAN," *Neural Comput. Appl.*, vol. 35, pp. 9181–9192, December 2022.
16. J. Jiang, Y. Feng, H. Xu, and J. Zheng, "Low-dose CT reconstruction via optimization-inspired GAN," *Proc. IEEE Int. Conf. Acoust. Speech Signal Process (ICASSP)*, pp. 1–5, June 2023.
17. J. Mao, X. Yin, G. Zhang, B. Chen, Y. Chang, W. Chen, J. Yu, and Y. Wang, "Pseudo-labeling generative adversarial networks for medical image classification," *Comput. Biol. Med.*, vol. 147, Art. no. 105729, August 2022.
18. W. Chen, S. Yu, K. Ma, W. Ji, C. Bian, C. Chu, L. Shen, and Y. Zheng, "TW-GAN: Topology and width aware GAN for retinal artery/vein classification," *Med. Image Anal.*, vol. 77, Art. no. 102340, April 2022.
19. R. Zhang, W. Lu, J. Gao, Y. Tian, X. Wei, C. Wang, X. Li, and M. Yu, "RFI-GAN: A reference-guided fuzzy integral network for ultrasound image augmentation," *Inf. Sci.*, vol. 623, pp. 709–728, April 2023.
20. J. Wang, G. Xie, Y. Huang, J. Lyu, F. Zheng, Y. Zheng, and Y. Jin, "FedMed-GAN: Federated domain translation on unsupervised crossmodality brain image synthesis," *Neurocomputing*, vol. 546, Art. no. 126282, August 2023.

21. B. Sun, S. Jia, X. Jiang, and F. Jia, "Double U-Net CycleGAN for 3D MR to CT image synthesis," *Int. J. Comput. Assist. Radiol. Surgery*, vol. 18, no. 1, pp. 149–156, August 2022.
22. J. Mendes, T. Pereira, F. Silva, J. Frade, J. Morgado, C. Freitas, E. Negrão, B. F. de Lima, M. C. da Silva, A. J. Madureira, I. Ramos, J. L. Costa, V. Hespanhol, A. Cunha, and H. P. Oliveira, "Lung CT image synthesis using GANs," *Expert Syst. Appl.*, vol. 215, Art. no. 119350, April 2023.
23. *The Whole Brain Atlas—Med.harvard.edu*. Accessed: 22 October 2023 [Online]. Available: http://www.med.harvard.edu/AANLIB/home.html
24. *CORN: CORneal Nerve Database—Imed.Nimte.Ac.Cn—Imed.Nimte.Ac.Cn*. Accessed: 4 January 2024 [Online]. Available: https://imed.nimte.ac.cn/CORN.html
25. *Polyp—Grand Challenge—Polyp.grand-challenge.org*. Accessed: 22 October 2023 [Online]. Available: https://polyp.grand-challenge.org/CVCClinicDB/
26. P. Porwal, S. Pachade, R. Kamble, M. Kokare, G. Deshmukh, V. Sahasrabuddhe, and F. Meriaudeau, "Indian diabetic retinopathy image dataset (IDRiD): A database for diabetic retinopathy screening research," *Data*, vol. 3, no. 3, p. 25, July 2018.
27. S. G. Mueller, M. W. Weiner, L. J. Thal, R. C. Petersen, C. R. Jack, W. Jagust, J. Q. Trojanowski, A. W. Toga, and L. Beckett, "Ways toward an early diagnosis in Alzheimer's disease: The Alzheimer's disease neuroimaging initiative (ADNI)," Alzheimer's Dementia, vol. 1, no. 1, pp. 55–66, July 2005.
28. *Multimodal Brain Tumor Segmentation Challenge 2019 | CBICA | Perelman School of Medicine at the University of Pennsylvania—Med.upenn.edu*. Accessed: 22 October 2023 [Online]. Available: https://www.med.upenn.edu/cbica/brats-2019/
29. F. Che, X. Zhu, T. Yang, and T.-Y. Yu, "3SGAN: 3D shape embedded generative adversarial networks," *Proc. IEEE/CVF Int. Conf. Comput. Vis. Workshop (ICCVW)*, pp. 3305–3314, October 2019.
30. F. Yu, A. Seff, Y. Zhang, S. Song, T. Funkhouser, and J. Xiao, "LSUN: Construction of a large-scale image dataset using deep learning with humans in the loop," *arXiv preprint* arXiv:1506.03365, 2015.
31. M. Frid-Adar, I. Diamant, E. Klang, M. Amitai, J. Goldberger, and H. Greenspan, "GAN-based synthetic medical image augmentation for increased CNN performance in liver lesion classification," *Neurocomputing*, vol. 321, pp. 321–331, December 2018.
32. A. Madani, M. Moradi, A. Karargyris, and T. Syeda-Mahmood, "Semisupervised learning with generative adversarial networks for chest X-ray classification with ability of data domain adaptation," *Proc. IEEE 15th Int. Symp. Biomed. Imag. (ISBI)*, pp. 1038–1042, April 2018.
33. X. Chen, Y. Duan, R. Houthooft, J. Schulman, I. Sutskever, and P. Abbeel, "InfoGAN: Interpretable representation learning by information maximizing generative adversarial nets," *Proc. Adv. Neural Inf. Process. Syst.*, vol. 29, pp. 1–13, 2016.
34. M. Mirza and S. Osindero, "Conditional generative adversarial nets," *arXiv preprint* arXiv:1411.1784, 2014.
35. Z. Zhuang, W. Shen, A. Damian, and T. D. Tran, "Incorporating knowledge distillation to the training of medical image synthesis," *Proc. Int. Conf. Med. Image Comput. Comput. Assist. Intervent (MICCAI)*, pp. 152–160, 2019.
36. D. Nie, Y. Gao, L. Wang, and D. Shen, "ASDNet: Attention-based semisupervised deep networks for medical image segmentation," *Proc. Int. Conf. Med. Image Comput. Comput. Assist. Intervent (MICCAI)*, pp. 370–378, 2019.
37. S. Ramanathan and M. Ramasundaram, "Low-dose CT image reconstruction using vector quantized convolutional autoencoder with perceptual loss," *Sādhanā*, vol. 48, no. 2, p. 43, March 2023.

38. I. Goodfellow, J. Pouget-Abadie, M. Mirza, B. Xu, D. Warde-Farley, S. Ozair, A. Courville, and Y. Bengio, "Generative adversarial nets," *Proc. Adv. Neural Inf. Process. Syst.*, vol. 27, pp. 1–9, 2014.
39. A. Odena, C. Olah, and J. Shlens, "Conditional image synthesis with auxiliary classifier GANs," *Proc. Int. Conf. Mach. Learn.*, pp. 2642–2651, 2017.
40. T. Miyato and M. Koyama, "CGANs with projection discriminator," *arXiv preprint* arXiv:1802.05637, 2018.
41. C. Chu, A. Zhmoginov, and M. Sandler, "CycleGAN, a master of steganography," *arXiv preprint* arXiv:1712.02950, 2017.
42. J. Zhao, M. Mathieu, and Y. LeCun, "Energy-based generative adversarial network," *arXiv preprint* arXiv:1609.03126, 2016.
43. D. Berthelot, T. Schumm, and L. Metz, "BEGAN: Boundary equilibrium generative adversarial networks," *arXiv preprint* arXiv:1703.10717, 2017.
44. C. Ledig, "Photo-realistic single image super-resolution using a generative adversarial network," *Proc. IEEE Conf. Comput. Vis. Pattern Recognit. (CVPR)*, pp. 4681–4690, July 2017.
45. J. Johnson, A. Alahi, and L. Fei-Fei, "Perceptual losses for real-time style transfer and super-resolution," *Proc. Eur. Conf. Comput. Vis.*, pp. 694–711, 2016.
46. X. Mao, Q. Li, H. Xie, R. Y. K. Lau, Z. Wang, and S. P. Smolley, "Least squares generative adversarial networks," *Proc. IEEE Int. Conf. Comput. Vis. (ICCV)*, pp. 2813–2821, October 2017.
47. J. T. Springenberg, "Unsupervised and semi-supervised learning with categorical generative adversarial networks," *arXiv preprint* arXiv:1511.06390, 2015.
48. X. Yi, E. Walia, and P. Babyn, "Unsupervised and semi-supervised learning with categorical generative adversarial networks assisted by Wasserstein distance for dermoscopy image classification," *arXiv preprint* arXiv:1804.03700, 2018.
49. J.-Y. Zhu, T. Park, P. Isola, and A. A. Efros, "Unpaired image-to-image translation using cycle-consistent adversarial networks," *Proc. ICCV*, pp. 2223–2232, October 2017.
50. H. Zhang, I. Goodfellow, D. Metaxas, and A. Odena, "Self-attention generative adversarial networks," *Proc. Int. Conf. Mach. Learn.*, pp. 7354–7363, 2019.
51. Z. Yang, Y. Chen, Z. Le, F. Fan, and E. Pan, "Multi-source medical image fusion based on wasserstein generative adversarial networks," *IEEE Access*, vol. 7, pp. 175947–175958, 2019.
52. M. Sharma, S. Deswal, U. Gupta, M. Tabassum, and I. Lawal, eds., *Soft Computing Techniques in Connected Healthcare Systems*. CRC Press, 2023.
53. Y. Lecun, L. Bottou, Y. Bengio, and P. Haffner, "Gradient-based learning applied to document recognition," *Proc. IEEE*, vol. 86, no. 11, pp. 2278–2324, January 1998.

4 Revolutionizing Healthcare
The Impact of Generative AI and Large Language Models

Nisha Varghese

4.1 INTRODUCTION

Generative AI, a cutting-edge subset of artificial intelligence, is poised to revolutionize the healthcare industry by enhancing precision, efficiency, and personalization in patient care. By leveraging large language models (LLMs) and advanced algorithms that generate new data from existing datasets, generative AI enables unprecedented capabilities in diagnosing diseases, tailoring treatments, discovering new drugs and more. This technology can analyze complex medical data, simulate various medical scenarios, and predict patient outcomes with remarkable accuracy. As healthcare continues to evolve, generative AI stands at the forefront, offering innovative solutions to some of the industry's most pressing challenges and paving the way for a new era of medical excellence.

This chapter outlines the transformative potential of generative AI and large language models in healthcare, focusing on their applications, possibilities, and the development of domain-specific LLM models. It aims to demonstrate how these technologies can enhance patient care, streamline clinical workflows, support medical research, and address various healthcare challenges. The chapter incorporates a background study with an overview of AI in healthcare and introduction to generative AI. The objectives of this chapter are to describe the role of large language models in the health care sector and the potential of these models to assist the health workers in enhancing patient outcomes by improving clinical efficiency and providing support for medical research and innovation. The potential applications include patient care with personalized medicine, virtual health assistants, and mental health support.

The personalized treatment plans based on individual patient information and predicting patient responses to treatments. The mental health support provides cognitive behavioral therapy and other interventions and also monitors patient mental health through natural language interactions. Clinical operations with documentation and reporting, decision support systems and workflow automation, medical research, drug discovery, clinical trials facilitate the proper identification and monitoring of mental health. Domain-specific LLM models in healthcare and the development data collection and curation, model training and fine-tuning and validation and testing.

DOI: 10.1201/9781003539483-4

The ethical and regulatory considerations discussing data privacy and security, bias and fairness in data and model, and transparency and reliability of the models.

Automating administrative tasks is another application of generative AI and LLM models. Healthcare administrative tasks play a vital role in managing healthcare processes, ensuring adherence to regulations, and enhancing overall administrative efficiency. Some of the tasks are appointment scheduling, documentation and record-keeping, billing and claims processing, data entry and extraction, insurance verification, communication management, regulatory compliance checks, workflow optimization, task prioritization, and more. There are various LLM models in the health sector. Med-PaLM, Clinical-BERT, BioGPT, BioBERT, JSL-BERT, GloVe-Med are the some of the domain-specific models for various applications like clinical note summarization, clinical entity recognition, patient assistance, diagnostic support. All these models are fine-tuned on their foundation models.

There are various advantages while utilizing generative AI and language models in the area of health care such as improved patient outcomes by providing personalized care and enhanced diagnostic accuracy lead to better health outcomes, Increased Efficiency by ensuring the automation of administrative tasks and documentation reduces healthcare providers' workload, allowing more focus on patient care, Accelerated Research by the AI-driven tools expedite research, enabling faster development of new treatments and innovations and Enhanced Patient Engagement with the support of Virtual assistants and personalized education materials improve patient engagement and adherence to treatments. This chapter will include a case study of domain-specific models with covid dataset question answering and concludes with future enhancements in the area of domain-specific models.

4.2 LITERATURE REVIEW/RELATED WORKS

The study [1] introduced a new dataset and proposes a novel model for detecting health misinformation. The online infodemics are bifurcated into two, Central and peripheral levels. The research investigates the four sub classifications of Central and Peripheral Levels such as topic feature (central) and linguistic, sentiment, and user behavioral features (Peripheral) using the Elaboration Likelihood Model (ELM). The model presents 85% accuracy in the testing of the real-world dataset and suggests that in the detection of the misinformation the behavioral features are more informative than linguistic features. The research article [2] proposes a model named as—Domain- and Instance level Transfer Framework for Fake News Detection (DITFEND), which mainly focused on the domain specific fake news detection such as politics and entertainment in English and Chinese. The novelty of the study is the implementation of the cross domain fake news detection. The study [3] assesses the relative effectiveness of social media interventions meant to dispel false information about health through a meta-analysis. The meta-analysis also presents theory-driven moderators that aid in defining the efficacy of interventions on social media. A publication bias could not be ruled out and attempts to correct misinformation on social media had a positive and significant mean effect size.

This research [4] presents a self-ensemble SCIBERT (Scientific BERT) based model that uses domain specific word embeddings for health misinformation detection, specifically in news, which is less explored. The model also uses a custom dataset that contains health articles scraped from the news fact-checking website Snopes.com, along with the already-existing Fake Health dataset. According to classification results, the suggested model yields a weighted F1 score of 0.715. The article examines [5] the three transformer-based language models—Roberta, Distilbert, and BERT from HuggingFace—were refined using training data to create the suggested models, which were then assembled as estimators with majority voting. This paper's main objective is to prevent the spread of false information and raise public awareness of the value of accurate information. It also investigated COVID-19 fake data that was circulated on various social media platforms. The study [6] aims to classify given tweets as either authentic or fraudulent news. The COVID-19 fictitious dataset has been used by the authors to test a number of deep learning models. Finaly, the deep learning models CT-BERT and RoBERTa performed better than BERT, BERTweet, AlBERT, and DistlBERT. Using the multiplicative fusion technique, the proposed ensemble deep learning architecture outperformed CT-BERT and RoBERTa on the COVID-19 fake news dataset. The performance of the suggested model in this method was ascertained by multiplying the final CT-BERT and RoBERTa predictive values. The study [7] employs the language representation model RoBERTa with a binary classification and classification of tweet using BERTweet, which is based on RoBERTa using the pre-trained models are used for both tasks' fine-tuning. The research project [8] has tackled it using a number of Transformer and recurrent models along with a number of contextual words embedding models. Additionally, a different loss function—rather than the traditional Binary cross Entropy loss function—is used to assess the efficacy of the suggested model. One of the downstream tasks of natural language processing is the detection of fake news, which is regarded as a sequence classification task. The highest weighted average F1-score has been observed when using custom loss functions in conjunction with domain-specific language models. For the domain-agnostic multilingual fake news classification, the article [9] suggests an efficient neural model based on the multilingual Bidirectional Encoder Representations from Transformer (BERT). Experiments are carried out in a wide range of settings, including language- and domain-specific ones. In both domain-specific and domain-agnostic experiments, the suggested model outperforms the state-of-the-art models now and achieves high accuracy. We investigate the efficacy of language-agnostic feature transfer between languages using zero-shot settings, and the results are promising. Experiments on cross-domain transfer are also conducted to evaluate the model's language-independent feature transfer. Additionally, we provide a multilingual multidomain fake news detection dataset covering five languages and seven distinct domains, which may prove beneficial for research and development in scenarios with limited resources.

4.3 POTENTIAL APPLICATIONS OF GENERATIVE AI AND LLM IN HEALTHCARE

Generative AI, a rapidly advancing field of artificial intelligence, has the potential to revolutionize various aspects of healthcare and medical research. In patient care, generative AI models can enhance diagnostic speed and accuracy, improving the quality and efficiency of medical services while reducing equipment costs. These models have demonstrated remarkable capabilities in generating and analyzing medical images, as well as assisting in the diagnosis of various conditions. Generative AI assist in the healthcare domain in various ways like Patient Care, Clinical support, Medical Research, Drug Discovery, Clinical Trials, Risk prediction of pandemic preparedness, Generating synthetic medical data, Personalized medicine and many more. Generative AI can also play a crucial role in clinical support, enabling the standardization and optimization of healthcare processes. By supporting and standardizing clinical judgment, these models can help address the challenges of limited access to expert medical practitioners, especially in low- and middle-income countries [10].

Patient Care: Generative AI can significantly enhance patient care by analyzing patient data to predict disease risks, personalize treatment plans, and even provide real-time decision support during clinical interventions. AI models can generate personalized health recommendations based on an individual's unique medical history, lifestyle, and genetic makeup, leading to more tailored and effective care. Moreover, AI-driven chatbots and virtual assistants can provide 24/7 support to patients, answering questions, monitoring symptoms, and ensuring adherence to treatment plans.

Clinical Support: In the realm of clinical support, generative AI can assist healthcare professionals by generating differential diagnoses, suggesting treatment options, and even predicting patient outcomes. By analyzing electronic health records (EHRs) and integrating data from various sources, AI can provide clinicians with evidence-based insights, reducing the likelihood of errors and improving overall patient outcomes. Additionally, AI-powered tools can automate administrative tasks such as documentation and coding, freeing up valuable time for healthcare providers to focus on patient care.

Medical Research: Generative AI is a game-changer in medical research, where it can analyze large datasets, generate hypotheses, and even design experiments. AI can identify patterns and correlations in data that might be missed by human researchers, leading to new insights and discoveries. In genomics, for example, AI can analyze genetic data to identify potential disease-causing mutations or predict how different patients might respond to certain treatments.

Drug Discovery: In drug discovery, generative AI can accelerate the identification of potential drug candidates by simulating chemical interactions and predicting the efficacy and safety of new compounds. AI can generate novel molecular structures with desired properties, significantly speeding up the process of drug development. This capability can reduce the time and cost associated with bringing new drugs to market, ultimately benefiting patients.

Clinical Trials: Finally, generative AI can optimize clinical trials by predicting patient enrollment, identifying suitable candidates, and even generating synthetic data to simulate trial outcomes. This can help in designing more efficient and targeted trials, reducing the time and cost of bringing new treatments to patients. AI can also assist in monitoring trials in real-time, identifying adverse events early, and ensuring that trials are conducted ethically and effectively.

4.3.1 Risk Prediction of Pandemic Preparedness

A pandemic is an epidemic that has swept across a vast geographical area, affecting several countries or continents as well as a sizeable portion of the population. GenAI can identify new diseases early and poses challenges due to the rapid identification of pathogens and the timely acquisition of accurate information. The complexities of vaccine development and distribution present difficulties, particularly in ensuring equitable global distribution, focusing on addressing disparities in low-income nations. Early Detection and Surveillance of these outbreak by Gen AI is possible and which can be process real-time data from diverse sources, including social media, health reports, and environmental data, to identify early signs of emerging infectious diseases. Detecting unusual patterns or clusters can contribute to early warning systems. Gen AI can use historical data and machine learning to predict potential hotspots for disease outbreaks. Analyzing factors such as population density, travel patterns, and environmental conditions can provide insights into areas at higher risk. Gen AI can accelerate drug discovery by analyzing genetic data and predicting potential vaccine candidates. This expedites the development and testing phases, contributing to a faster response to novel pathogens. Supply chain management can be improved by artificial intelligence (AI) through the prediction and reduction of possible interruptions. It can analyze global logistics, monitor inventory levels, and forecast demand, ensuring a more robust and responsive supply chain for medical equipment and pharmaceuticals. Gen AI can analyze public sentiment and identify misinformation trends during a pandemic. By understanding public concerns and sentiments, authorities can tailor communication strategies to address specific issues, manage anxiety, and ensure better compliance. During a pandemic, resource allocation is critical. Gen AI can analyze data on healthcare facility capacities, equipment availability, and workforce distribution to optimize the allocation of resources based on predicted outbreak patterns. Gen AI has the capability to replicate diverse situations by analyzing past data and present circumstances and this assists governmental bodies and healthcare institutions in strategizing and getting ready for a range of potential results, thereby facilitating a proactive and flexible approach.

Generating synthetic medical data: Artificially generated healthcare information that mimics real patient data but is entirely fictional and unrelated to actual individuals. Synthetic medical data is a safe and secure way for researchers and developers to work with realistic data without compromising the privacy of actual patients. It follows all legal and ethical rules governing the use of patient data, protecting against data breaches and reducing the risk of unauthorized access to sensitive medical information. Synthetic data is also helpful for testing and validation, ensuring that health tech works appropriately before it is used in real-world healthcare settings. Generative AI algorithms have the capability to examine pre-existing medical datasets and produce fabricated data that closely resembles authentic patient information. This fabricated data possesses the ability to encompass a broad spectrum of medical conditions, demographics, and scenarios, thereby guaranteeing that the generated datasets are both realistic and reflective of the healthcare environment. Gen AI allows creating synthetic medical data without directly using accurate patient records. This is essential for privacy preservation, as sensitive health information remains confidential. Researchers and developers can work with synthetic datasets without compromising individual privacy, addressing concerns related to data protection regulations. Generative AI models can be fine-tuned to generate synthetic medical data with specific characteristics, allowing researchers to tailor datasets for their needs. This customization ensures that the synthetic data aligns with the requirements of diverse healthcare research and development projects. Synthetic medical data generated by Gen AI provides a safe and controlled environment for testing and validating algorithms, machine learning models, and healthcare systems. This helps researchers ensure the reliability and effectiveness of their technologies before deploying them in real-world healthcare settings. Gen AI plays a vital role in training machine learning models by creating synthetic datasets that replicate the intricacies of real medical data. This method facilitates the development of precise and resilient models without the need for actual patient records, thereby mitigating concerns regarding consent and confidentiality. Using Gen AI-generated synthetic medical data ensures that ethical and legal guidelines are followed when doing medical research. It offers a compliant substitute for utilizing real patient data and effectively addresses the obstacles linked to the regulatory framework and ethical norms concerning health information usage.

Personalized Medicine: Personalized medicine facilitates medical decisions and practices are customized to suit each patient's specific needs. Personalized medicine doctors face challenges in accurately interpreting vast genetic and molecular data. Integrating genetic information into traditional protocols is complex, requiring continuous education to address gaps in genetic training. Effective communication is crucial when explaining complex genetic details to patients, ensuring informed decisions and consent. Limited resources hinder widespread personalized medicine implementation, impacting accessibility. Gen AI can analyze complex genetic and molecular data, assisting healthcare professionals in interpreting information relevant to individualized treatment plans. This helps identify specific genetic markers and understand their implications for personalized care. Gen AI has the capability to offer healthcare professionals with immediate, evidence-driven suggestions for tailored treatment choices, considering the patient's genetic makeup. This significantly improves the decision-making procedure by swiftly and accurately analyzing a vast quantity of data. Gen AI can contribute to educational initiatives by providing continuous updates on advancements in genomics and personalized medicine. This assists healthcare professionals in staying informed about the latest technologies and treatment strategies. Gen AI can support doctors in effectively communicating complex genetic information to patients. It can generate patient-friendly explanations, ensuring individuals understand personalized medicine's benefits and limitations and facilitating informed consent. Gen AI can assist in navigating ethical and legal considerations related to personalized medicine. Ensuring that AI systems adhere to privacy regulations and ethical standards helps build patient trust and maintains compliance with healthcare laws. Gen AI can contribute to optimizing resource allocation by streamlining workflows, automating routine tasks, and enhancing the efficiency of genetic testing processes. This is crucial for overcoming resource limitations and making personalized medicine more accessible. Gen AI can aid in addressing insurance and reimbursement challenges by providing data-driven evidence of the effectiveness of personalized medicine. This supports healthcare professionals in advocating for coverage and reimbursement for genetic testing and personalized treatments. Gen AI can assist in developing and implementing standardized practices for interpreting genetic data and integrating personalized medicine into clinical workflows. Consistent approaches enhance the reliability and quality of personalized care across healthcare institutions. Gen AI has the capability to examine pharmacogenomic data in order to anticipate how individuals will respond to medications. By incorporating pharmacogenomic information, drug prescriptions can be customized according to genetic factors, resulting in improved treatment outcomes and reduced occurrence of adverse effects.

4.4 ROLE OF DOMAIN-SPECIFIC LLM MODELS IN HEALTHCARE

Large language models have emerged as a transformative force in the healthcare industry, revolutionizing various aspects of medical practice and research. The application of these domain-specific large language models, often referred to as Med-LLMs, has yielded significant advancements across a wide range of medical specialties, including cancer care, dermatology, dental care, neurodegenerative disorders, and mental health [10]. One of the key benefits of Med-LLMs is their ability to enhance diagnostic and treatment-related functionalities. By leveraging sophisticated algorithms and deep learning techniques, these models can provide clinicians with more accurate and comprehensive insights, ultimately leading to improved patient outcomes. In the field of cancer care, for instance, Med-LLMs have demonstrated their potential in aiding physicians with early detection and risk assessment, as well as personalized treatment planning [10].

These models can analyze vast amounts of medical data, including patient records, imaging, and genetic information, to identify patterns and anomalies that may indicate the presence of cancer. Moreover, Med-LLMs can assist in the development of personalized treatment strategies by considering various patient-specific factors, such as genetic profiles, comorbidities, and response to previous therapies. Similarly, in the realm of dermatology, Med-LLMs have shown promising results in supporting clinicians in the diagnosis and management of skin conditions.

4.5 ETHICAL AND REGULATORY CONSIDERATIONS

The rapid advancements in generative artificial intelligence have sparked widespread discussion about its potential applications and implications, particularly in the healthcare domain. Generative AI models, such as ChatGPT, have demonstrated remarkable capabilities in synthesizing medical data, generating personalized treatment plans, and assisting clinicians with decision-making. While these technologies hold immense promise, they also raise complex ethical and regulatory concerns that must be carefully addressed. One of the primary concerns is the issue of bias. Generative AI models can potentially perpetuate or amplify existing biases in the data used for training, leading to discriminatory outcomes in healthcare services

[11]. This could exacerbate health disparities and undermine the principle of equitable access to healthcare. The integration of generative AI in healthcare presents both significant opportunities and substantial ethical and regulatory challenges. As these technologies become increasingly sophisticated, the healthcare industry must navigate complex issues surrounding patient safety, privacy, bias, and accountability.

4.5.1 Patient Safety and Efficacy

One of the foremost ethical considerations is ensuring that generative AI systems are safe and effective for medical use. Unlike traditional software, which follows predefined rules, generative AI models can produce novel outputs, including diagnostic suggestions, treatment plans, and even synthetic data for research. This unpredictability raises concerns about the reliability and accuracy of AI-generated content. If a generative AI model produces an incorrect diagnosis or suggests an inappropriate treatment, the consequences for patient health can be severe. Thus, ensuring that AI systems are rigorously tested and validated before deployment is critical. Moreover, ongoing monitoring and post-market surveillance are essential to identify and mitigate any potential risks that emerge after the AI system is in use.

4.5.2 Privacy and Data Security

Generative AI systems often require large datasets for training, many of which contain sensitive patient information. The use of such data raises significant privacy concerns. Protecting patient confidentiality is a cornerstone of medical ethics, and any breach of this confidentiality can erode trust in healthcare systems. Regulatory frameworks like the Health Insurance Portability and Accountability Act (HIPAA) in the United States and the General Data Protection Regulation (GDPR) in Europe impose strict requirements on the handling of personal health data. However, the unique nature of AI, particularly in its capacity to generate data, poses new challenges. For instance, synthetic data generated by AI, while not directly linked to real patients, could still reveal patterns that compromise patient privacy. Therefore, ensuring robust data governance and implementing stringent privacy measures is essential.

4.5.3 Bias and Fairness

AI models are only as good as the data they are trained on. If the training data is biased, the AI system will likely perpetuate or even exacerbate these biases. In healthcare, this can have serious consequences, particularly for marginalized communities. For example, if an AI system is trained predominantly on data from a specific demographic group, it may not perform as well for patients outside that group, leading to disparities in care. Addressing this issue requires a concerted effort to ensure that training datasets are diverse and representative. Additionally, regular audits of AI systems for bias should be conducted, and there should be transparency in how these systems make decisions to allow for external scrutiny.

4.5.4 Accountability and Liability

The deployment of generative AI in healthcare raises complex questions about accountability. If an AI system makes an error, who is responsible? Is it the developers who created the AI, the healthcare providers who used it, or the institutions that integrated it into their practices? Current legal and regulatory frameworks are often ill-equipped to address these questions. Developing clear guidelines that delineate responsibility is essential. Moreover, there may be a need for new legal frameworks that specifically address the unique challenges posed by AI in healthcare.

4.5.5 Regulatory Oversight

Regulatory bodies such as the U.S. Food and Drug Administration (FDA) are beginning to develop frameworks for evaluating AI-based medical devices. However, the fast pace of AI innovation poses a challenge for regulators who must balance the need for rigorous evaluation with the desire to not stifle technological advancement. Continuous collaboration between AI developers, healthcare professionals, ethicists, and regulators is necessary to create flexible yet robust regulatory frameworks that ensure the safe and ethical use of AI in healthcare.

4.6 CASE STUDY OF GENERATIVE AI ON HEALTH CARE

This section incorporates the case study with Machine reading comprehension based on the transformer-based model to extract the relevant information from the reliable sources. With the advent of Transformer-based pre-trained models such as BERT (Bidirectional Encoder Representations from Transformers) and GPT (Generative Pre-training) are outperforming the typical Machine Leaning and Deep Leaning Models in many of the NLP tasks.

Neural machine reading comprehension focuses on developing systems capable of understanding and extracting information from textual sources, much like a human reader. Neural network architectures are used by NMRC systems to analyse and understand textual material, allowing them to do tasks like information extraction, summarization, and question answering based-on passages provided. After the initial pre-processing the MRC goes through the following phases including Encoding and Contextualization, Attention Mechanisms, Answer Prediction and Evaluation and Fine-tuning. The initial stage involves preprocessing textual material and formatting it so that neural network models may use it. Tokenization, which divides the text into words or subwords, is the first step in this process. Word embedding, for example, turns words into dense numerical vectors that represent semantic information.

In this stage, the selection of the appropriate model to fed the pre-processed data. The models of neural network topologies may include transformer models, convolutional neural networks (CNNs), and recurrent neural networks (RNNs). These models capture the connections between words and sentences by encoding the text and contextualising the data. Transformers have become more popular because of how well they can represent long-distance interdependence in text. The next stage is inevitable to give the focus to the weightage for each specific word. NMRC systems

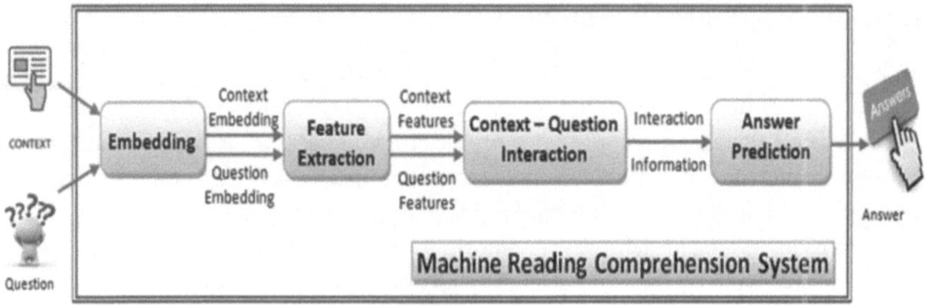

FIGURE 4.1 General Architecture of MRC

frequently use attention mechanisms to concentrate on pertinent textual content while processing. Using these techniques, the model is better able to comprehend context and retrieve pertinent information by dynamically weighing the relevance of certain words or paragraphs. Then, the NMRC system guesses answers to questions or pulls pertinent information from the passage after encoding and contextualising the textual data. In this stage, the model is trained to produce precise answers based on the given task and the input text. The model may provide a single word or phrase, a string of words, or a binary classification denoting the presence or lack of information, depending on the particular job and finally, the metrics Exact Match and F1 score are used to assess the performance of the NMRC system.

A model trained on a dataset of question-answer pairs—each question being linked to a matching answer span within a passage—is usually used for MRC span extraction. The model gains the ability to map a question and passage pair to the appropriate answer span during training. Answer spans for fresh questions and passages can be extracted using the model once it has been trained. The Question-Context Encoding/Embedding, Attention Mechanism, Answer Span Prediction, and Span Selection stages comprise the MRC span extraction method as represented in Figure 4.1.

The technique of identifying and extracting a specific, continuous word sequence, or "span," from a given text passage that answers a question about the passage is known as span extraction in Machine Reading Comprehension (MRC). MRC systems, especially those built for tasks like question answering, require this activity as a basic component. Predicting the beginning and ending locations of the answer span inside the passage is the goal of span extraction. The MRC model is required to determine the range of text in a passage that most effectively addresses a given question, given the material and the query. Span extraction is a crucial component of MRC systems, enabling them to locate specific information within passages and provide accurate answers to questions posed by users or other systems. Transformers have revolutionized natural language processing by introducing a powerful neural network architecture that excels at capturing long-range dependencies in sequential data. Transformers proposed by Ashish Vaswani et al. in 2017 [12] and that transformed the field by introducing attention mechanisms, enabling efficient modeling of long-range dependencies, and achieving state-of-the-art performance on a wide range of NLP tasks. The domain-specific transformer BERT-based models will utilize in this article are SciBERT, BioBERT, and ClinicalBERT.

Transformer is a remarkable advancement in the field of deep learning, created by Ashish Vaswani and colleagues in 2017, represents a significant breakthrough. The most well-known neural network model is called Transformer, and it is excellent at solving tasks like machine translation, phrase classification, and comprehension. The attention mechanism and parallelization are the transformers' primary features. It thus resolves the issues with the RNN and LSTM methods that are currently in use, and it can assist with long-range dependencies without any gradient vanishing or gradient explosion issues. A few additional components are also incorporated into the transformer's architecture: linear layer, positional encoding, SoftMax layers, multi-head attention, and multi-head attention with masking. The encoder executes each entity in the input embedding. It gathers the data from the vector and forwards it to the decoder so that the output can be sent.

The first operation, word embedding, happens at the lowest level of the encoder layer. The process of converting a word into a vector in a vector space is known as word embedding or vectorization. The vector that fills the vector space can capture a significant portion of the words' semantic information with straightforward algebraic operations. Following word embedding, each vector runs parallel to the two encoding layer layers. There are six identical encoders in the transformer, and their weights are not shared. The encoder executes each entity in the input embedding. It gathers the data from the vector and forwards it to the decoder so that the output can be sent. Each encoding layer was composed of two sub-layers: a Position wise feed-forward network layer and a Self-attention (with padding mask) layer. Dependencies exist in the vector flow channel of the self-attention layer. To combat the vanishing gradient issue in deep networks, each of these sub-layers of the encoding layer has a residual dropout followed by the sub-layer input and normalization. LayerNorm(x + Sublayer(x)) is used to determine each sub-layer's output. The FFNN layer has no dependencies, and different vector flow pathways are carried out concurrently. The self-attention layer aids the encoder in emphasizing a particular word and improves the word's encoding. The FFNN layer receives the output from the self-attention layer. The decoder adds an additional Encoder-Decoder Attention layer between the self-attention and FFNN layer that aids in emphasizing the most important aspect of the input context.

4.6.1 Desiderata

The idea of creating the Health News Dataset collection is to create and develop a reading comprehension-based application that can lessen the spread of myths and false information about the COVID-19. Question and Context are inputs to the MRC. As a result, the dataset must be developed with questions and background information from trustworthy sources. To increase the reliability of the dataset, no crowd-sourcing site was used in its creation.

The dataset will therefore be close to 2k bytes in size, however by making use of the prominence of the Transformer models, datasets with less data can still perform with decent accuracy. Due to Health News Dataset's experiment's domain-specific nature, general BERT-based models are inadequate because BERT is pre-trained in general English and does not adhere to any specific domain. As a result, experimentation with the dataset will require specially pre-trained models. Naturally occurring and unrestricted questions and replies are preferred. Additionally, a proper annotation process is sufficient for the dataset's quality assurance.

4.6.2 Scaling Up from the Pilot to Health News Dataset

After the pilot research and desiderata were successfully completed, the Health News dataset is now being introduced. Its development stages included data collecting, an annotation process, and statistical analysis.

4.6.2.1 Data Gathering

Recent days have seen a significant increase in the novel Coronavirus's propagation as well as in the amount of false information being circulated about it. Therefore, gathering information from trustworthy sources is crucial. The World Health Organization (WHO) and the Centers for Disease Control and Prevention (CDC) are two well-known websites from where the data was archived. There are ~ 2000 instances in the dataset. The 4-way annotation is used in the data collation: Context Annotation, Question Annotation, Answer Annotation and Quality Control. This research article extracts the reliable answer for health-related queries using the pre-trained domain-specific Transformer models.

These two websites included policies, recommendations for the general public, technical assistance, responses to false information and myth debunkers regarding the COVID, among other things. About 50 topics are connected to COVID-19, including the following: climate change, mass and public gatherings, masks, contact tracing, herd immunity, lockdown, quarantine, drugs, immunity and antibodies, prevention guidelines, environmental surveillance, food safety, health workers, people with other diseases, vaccines and vaccine safety, virus evolution and mutation, ventilation, and air conditioning.

4.6.2.2 Annotation Protocol

Similar to a human, a machine learning or natural language processing model needs enough training data to grasp certain information. Based on the taught data, the models are able to decide and act. Applications using ML and NLP require correctly categorized and annotated data. The categorizing and labeling of data for a particular use case is known as data annotation. The models that can create and improve ML and NLP applications are facilitated by the high-quality, human- or computer-powered data annotations. An improved method for creating applications like appropriate search engine results, computer vision, personal assistants, chatbots, and speech recognition is to use annotated data.

Context Annotation, Question Annotation, Answer Annotation, and Quality Control are the four types of annotations used in Health News Dataset development. In order to remove noise from the data, the context annotation first generates the context archived from the WHO and CDC Webpages and the context subjected to human-powered annotation. The MRC model will use this updated context as its input context. Second, create a natural form question using the context in the Question annotation. The context may be used to create more than one question. The selection of the topic and context by evaluating the quality of the question and answer, as shown in Figure 2, is the next important annotation.

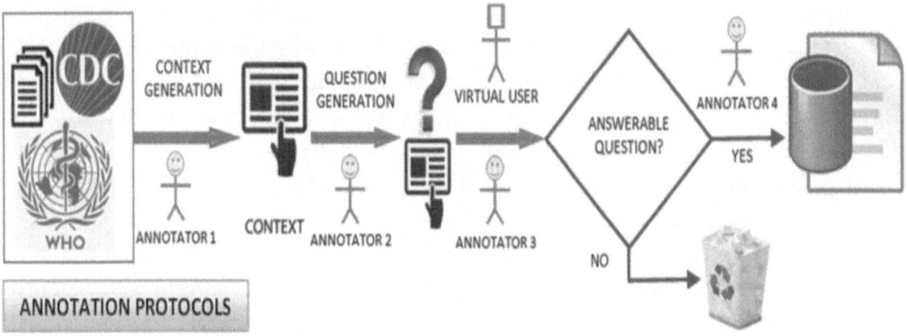

FIGURE 4.2 Annotation Protocols in Data Collection

4.6.2.3 Annotation Protocols for Health News Dataset Generation

For this stage, the right question-context pair is acquired through a human-computer intervention (MRC Model). A virtual user, a software or model for reading comprehension that yields the acceptability score, is then provided with the generated context and question. The procedure will be repeated with a new set of questions and context when any irrelevant, unanswerable, or questions with no answer have been eliminated. The model is derived from the ground truth responses, and by properly annotating the model, it is feasible to determine whether the question can be answered. The high-quality question-context pair will be kept, and the others will be removed from the dataset.

4.6.3 Domain-Specific Models

The general Wikipedia text and the Toronto Book Corpus [15] are used to train BERT with Next Sentence Prediction and Masked Language Modeling. The model created for the English language is therefore inappropriate for use in any other unique corpus or in other types of domain-specific textual documents, such as those found in the academic, clinical, legal, financial, scientific, and biomedical industries. By training BERT with pertinent domain-specific documents from the start, domain-specific models can be developed to circumvent this issue. The newly built model, with its vocabulary and embedding, is better suited for these domain-specific models than the BERT. The current study employs a variety of domain-specific models, including BioBERT, ClinicalBERT, and their combinations.

4.6.3.1 SciBERT

SciBERT [16] is a BERT-based domain-specific model that was trained using scientific articles from Semantic Scholar. According to Ammar et al. [17], the corpus contains 1.14 million full-length articles (not just abstracts), with 82% of the papers coming from the biomedical field and 18% from computer science. The average length of a paper with a corpus size of 3.17 billion tokens is 154 phrases, or approximately 2,769 tokens. The vocabulary is where the BERT and SciBERT differ most noticeably from one another. Rather than using BERT's basevocab vocabulary, SciBERT has its own vocabulary, called scivocab, which was created to best match the training corpus for the particular domain. SciBERT models' cutting-edge performance has demonstrated acceptable results on several NLP tasks in the scientific field. With the exception of being pre-trained on scientific content, SciBERT is comparable to BERT in the architecture domain. By utilizing the SentencePiece library, an unsupervised tokenizer and detokenizer based on neural networks for text processing, the scivocab vocabulary created a new WordPiece vocabulary. The cased and uncased vocabularies in Scivocab and the 30K vocabularies in BERT are of the same size. Just 42% of the tokens in the scivocab and basevocab are shared, indicating a significant difference in token frequency between texts in the general and scientific domains. BASEVOCAB or SCIVOCAB are included with SciBERT in four different configurations: cased or uncased.

4.6.3.2 BioBERT

BioBERT Using massive amounts of textual data, including 18 billion words from two corpora: PubMed and PubMed Central (PMC), [18] is a biomedical domain-specific BERT model that was pre-trained. Pre-trained on PMC full-length articles and PubMed abstracts, BioBERT outperforms the BERT model on the biomedical corpus. The BERT model and BioBERT share the same architecture. Following pre-training, the BioBERT can be modified for a variety of downstream biomedical tasks, including question-answering and named entity recognition.

PubMed: A citation database for biomedical literature, PubMed contains 4.5 billion words and more than 30 million citations from MEDLINE, the journal of the National Library of Medicine, online books and papers, and life science journals. PubMed Central (PMC): PMC is an online database available to the public that is open-source and includes articles published in journals related to the biological and life sciences. 13.5 billion words are in it.

BioBERT uses the WordPiece tokenizer for tokenization. The pre-trained BioBERT combinations are BioBERT + PMC (trained on the PMC corpus), BioBERT + PubMed (trained on the PubMed corpus), and BioBERT + PubMed + PMC (trained on both the PMC and PubMed corpora). The improved BioBERT can also be applied to downstream NLP tasks such as named entity recognition and question answering, in addition to these models. PubMed + BERT BioBERT The models' performance ranking is BioBERT (+ PMC) BioBERT + PubMed + PMC.

4.6.3.3 ClinicalBERT

A clinical domain-specific BERT model for learning deep representations of clinical text, ClinicalBERT [13] was pre-trained on the MIMIC-III (Medical Information Mart for Intensive Care) clinical notes. The vast MIMIC-III database contains information on more than 40,000 patients who were admitted to critical care units. Electronic health records are included in the open-access database, together with 53K other notes on demographics, drugs, diagnoses, procedures, and death. Similar to how we pre-trained the BERT model, ClinicalBERT was trained using masked language modeling and next sentence prediction tasks. The patient's pertinent information is contained in the clinical notes or progress notes, such as the clinical history.

Due to the different styles, grammatical structures, abbreviations, and jargon found in each document, it might be difficult to comprehend clinical notes completely. With the pre-train ClinicalBERT on enormous clinical documents, the relevant information can be extracted and the contextual representation of the clinical corpus can be understood. Understanding different clinical insights, including the clinical summary, the diagnosis details, the therapy measures, and much more, is made easier by clinicalBERT models. ClinicalBERT that has already been trained can be customized for various downstream tasks including readmission forecasts, mortality risk estimation, diagnosis, and a lot more.

4.6.4 Proposed Span Extraction Framework for Health News Dataset

Transfer learning is used by domain-specific transformer models to boost performance. The benefit is that even a tiny dataset can outperform typically pre-trained models in a certain domain. The smaller dataset, which contains just 2,020 cases, led to the selection of the SciBERT, BioBERT, and ClinicalBERT models for the HEALTH NEWS DATASET evaluation. These domain-specific bi-directional models underwent pre-training in fields including science, biomedicine, and medicine. The query and context from the input are used by the pre-trained models to fine-tune for the span extraction tasks before delivering the extracted answer as output. The Health News Dataset includes a variety of examples from different titles, including biomedical, scientific, and clinical information. The collection includes instructions and recommendations for persons with severe illnesses and terrible diseases, as well as the specifics of scientific research and observations related to safety measures, treatments, and drugs. The dataset also contained information on the weather, ecology, preventative recommendations, and much more.

4.7 CONCLUSION AND FUTURE DIRECTIONS

The rise of generative AI and large language models has sparked a transformative paradigm shift in the healthcare industry. These AI-powered technologies have the potential to revolutionize medical education, clinical care, and research, paving the way for a more efficient, accurate, and personalized healthcare system. One of the most promising applications of generative AI in healthcare is in medical image generation and analysis. Generative models have demonstrated the ability to create high-quality synthetic medical images, such as X-rays, CT scans, and MRI scans, which can be used to augment limited training data, improve diagnostic accuracy, and even generate images for rare or difficult-to-visualize conditions. These advancements have the potential to streamline the diagnostic process, reduce wait times, and improve patient outcomes by enabling clinicians to make more informed decisions based on comprehensive and accurate data. Furthermore, large language models, such as GPT-3, have shown remarkable capabilities in natural language processing, allowing for more efficient and effective communication between healthcare providers and patients. These models can be trained to understand and respond to the unique linguistic patterns and nuances of medical terminology, enabling them to assist in tasks like documentation, patient communication, and even medical research.

REFERENCES

1. Zhao Y, Da J, Yan J. Detecting Health Misinformation in Online Health Communities: Incorporating Behavioral Features into Machine Learning Based Approaches. *Information Processing & Management*, 2021, 58.
2. Nan Q, et al. Improving Fake News Detection of Influential Domain via Domain- and Instance-Level Transfer. arXiv:2209.08902v2 [cs.CL], 2022.
3. Walter N, et al. Evaluating the Impact of Attempts to Correct Health Misinformation on Social Media: A Meta Analysis. *Health Communication*, 2021, 36(13):1776–1784.
4. Kumari S, et al. Debunking Health Fake News with Domain Specific Pre-trained Model. *Global Transitions Proceedings*, 2021, 2:267–272.
5. Balouchzahi F, et al. MUCICatCheckThat! 2021: FaDo-Fake News Detection and Domain Identification Using Transformers Ensembling. *CLEF 2021 – Conference and Labs of the Evaluation Forum*, 2021.
6. Mallaa SJ and Alphonse PJA. Fake or Real News About COVID-19? Pretrained Transformer Model to Detect Potential Misleading News. *European Physical Journal Special Topics*, 2022, 231:3347–3356.
7. Ramesh S, et al. BERT Based Transformers Lead the Way in Extraction of Health Information from Social Media. *Proceedings of the Sixth Social Media Mining for Health Workshop*, 2021, pp. 33–38.
8. Hande A, et al. Evaluating Pretrained Transformer-Based Models for COVID-19 Fake News Detection. *5th International Conference on Computing Methodologies and Communication (ICCMC)*, 2021 | 978-1-6654-0360-3.
9. Ciecierski-Holmes T, et al. Artificial Intelligence for Strengthening Healthcare Systems in Low- and Middle-Income Countries: A Systematic Scoping Review. *NPJ Digital Medicine*, 2022, 5:162. doi: 10.1038/s41746-022-00700-y
10. Mumtaz A, Adigun AO, El-Mallakh RS. Frequency of Modification of Pharmacological Treatment is Equivalent for Virtual and in-Person Psychiatric Visits. *Telemedicine Reports*, 2023 Mar 22, 4(1):44–47. doi: 10.1089/tmr.2023.0004. PMID: 36970220; PMCID: PMC10036074.
11. Temsah MH, Jamal A, Aljamaan F, Al-Tawfiq JA, Al-Eyadhy A. ChatGPT-4 and the Global Burden of Disease Study: Advancing Personalized Healthcare Through Artificial Intelligence in Clinical and Translational Medicine. *Cureus*, 2023 May 23, 15(5):e39384. doi: 10.7759/cureus.39384. PMID: 37223340; PMCID: PMC10204616.
12. Vaswani A, Shazeer N, Parmar N, Uszkoreit J, Jones L, Gomez A, Kaiser Ł, Polosukhin I. Attention is All You Need. *Advances in Neural Information Processing Systems*, pp. 5998–6008, 2017.
13. Alsentzer E, Murphy J, Boag W, Weng W-H, Jin D, Naumann T, McDermott M. Publicly Available Clinical BERT Embeddings. *Proceedings of the 2nd Clinical Natural Language Processing Workshop, Association for Computational Linguistics*, pp. 72–78, 2019.
14. Johnson A, Pollard T, Shen L, Lehman L, Feng M, Ghassemi M, Moody B, Szolovits P, Celi LA, Mark R. Data Descriptor: MIMIC-III, a Freely Accessible Critical Care Database. *Scientific Data*, 2016, 3:160035. doi: 10.1038/sdata.2016.35.
15. Zhu Y, Kiros R, Zemel R, Salakhutdinov R, Urtasun R, Torralba A, Fidler S. Aligning Books and Movies: Towards Story-Like Visual Explanations by Watching Movies and Reading Books. arXiv:1506.06724v1 [cs.CV], 2015.
16. Beltagy I, Lo K, Cohan A. SCI BERT: A Pretrained Language Model for Scientific Text. arXiv:1903.10676 [cs.CL], 2019.
17. Ammar W, et al. Construction of the Literature Graph in Semantic Scholar. arXiv: 1805.02262v1 [cs.CL], 2018.
18. Lee J, Yoon W, Kim S, Kim D, Kim S, So CH, Kang J. BioBERT: A Pre-trained Biomedical Language Representation Model for Biomedical Text Mining. *Bioinformatics*, 2019, 1–7, Oxford University Press.

5 Artificial Intelligence in Nanocarrier Design and Drug Delivery via Nanorobotics-Based Personalised Medicine for Cancer Diagnostics and Therapy

Ankit Lodhi, Anshika, Amulya Jindal, Deepak Tomar, Mainuddin, Anoop Kumar, and Kartik Sharma

ABBREVIATIONS

DDS	Drug delivery system
AI	Artificial intelligence
PM	Personalised medicine
NCS	Nanocarriers
SNEDDS	Self-nanoemulsifying drug delivery system
NR	Nanorobots or nanobots
DoC	Disorders of consciousness
ACS	Acute coronary syndrome
CVD	Cardiovascular disease
TME	Tumour microenvironment
TMB	Tumour mutational burden
IBD	Inflammatory bowel diseases
SL	Supervised learning
HRD	Homologous repair deficiency
ML	Machine learning
UL	Unsupervised learning

DOI: 10.1201/9781003539483-5

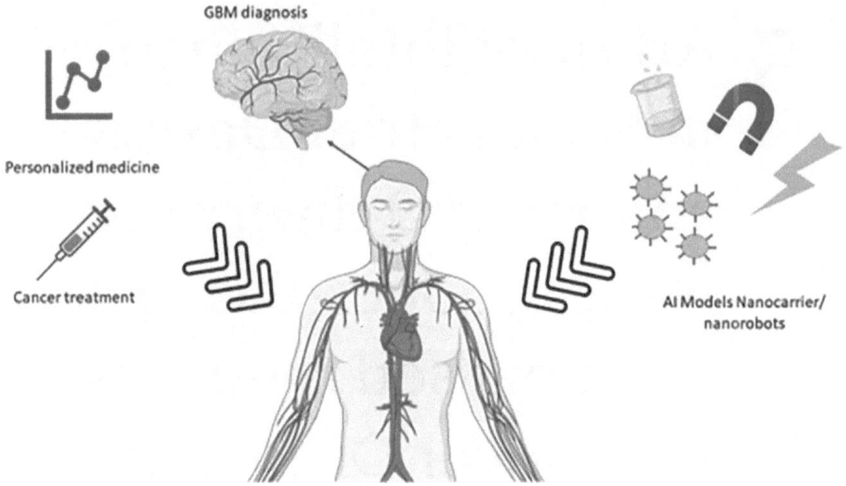

FIGURE 5.1 Graphical abstract.

5.1 INTRODUCTION

Cancer is a complicated and diverse illness that changes throughout time as a result of many different influences. These include molecular modifications, cellular changes, tissue-specific dynamics, genetic mutations, and environmental effects. Cancer development and progression are shaped by various factors, including demographics, population, and socioeconomic status. To address this highly global health challenge, numerous research efforts have been initiated by focusing on new treatment strategies and understanding the disease's biology. While traditional non-precision approaches such as surgery, radiotherapy, chemotherapy, and immunotherapy have shown some success, they remain "one-size-fits-all" solutions that still leave many unresolved challenges. Recurrence, for example, is frequently linked to drug resistance [1], which triggers metastasis of tumours [2] and ultimately leads to cancer [3].

Developing, manufacturing, and modifying materials at the nanoscale is known as nanotechnology [4]. The application of nanotechnology and nanocarriers such as nanorobots/nanobots (NRs) to the mitigation of disease and traumatic injury, as well as the management of pain, is known as nanomedicine [5]. Devices that are capable of sensing, acting, signalling, processing information, and exhibiting intelligence at the nano scale are referred to as NRs [6]. They are made up of different parts that each perform a particular function; the parts are built at the nanoscale size and can have a diameter of 1 – 100nm [7]. Potential uses for NR in medicine include the treatment of cancer [8], surgery, precision medicine [9], dentistry, diabetes and blood monitoring, and drug delivery [4, 5]. Nanomedical robots are widely used in tissue engineering, cardiology, gene delivery systems, drug delivery, invasive brain surgery, vital monitoring, targeted cancer therapy, and diabetes management as well as detection and imaging capabilities and several related applications [7].

The term "personalised medicine" (PM) is a strategy that determines the best course of action and therapeutic agent depending on the particular medical background, genetic makeup, and state of health of each patient. Healthcare professionals can improve the efficacy of treatment by utilising a patient's transcriptome and genetic data. With the use of this method, diseases can be identified with greater accuracy, and drug benefits and side effects can be predicted, resulting in highly successful therapies and treatments. It will also help lower medical expenses and raise the likelihood of developing novel treatments that work, making it one of the fields with the highest hopes for the future [10]. In addition to applying multi-omic investigations of disease pathways, this chapter aims to improve clinical phenotyping in complex conditions by considering the systemic principles of PM (in the broader sense of the 4Ps of medicine, preventive, predictive, participatory, and personalised) [11]. Managing PM has also been found to benefit from proteomics, which involves studying all the proteins inside of a cell or tissue/organism at a particular time. This field mainly focuses on understanding how proteins interact, the modification they undergo after being synthesised, and their specific locations within cells [12]. The basic framework of life, proteins, are essential to the maintenance, structure, and operation of tissues and organs. The proteome is extremely dynamic, in contrast to the comparatively stable genome, which presently predicts roughly 19,773 proteins [13, 14]. Splice variant and post-translational modifications (PTMs) such as methylation, glycosylation, phosphorylation, acetylation, ubiquitination, and farnesylation can sometimes exhibit multiple modifications. These elements alter the function or activity of proteins, as does somatic recombination in some proteins, like immunoglobulins (Igs) and T-cell receptors. Furthermore, not every gene is translated into the RNA and not every RNA into a protein, due to transcriptional and translational constraints on gene expression [15]. These regulatory systems monitor cellular, tissue, or organism changes across time. As a result, proteomics are a valuable tool for researching the underlying-systems biology linked to health, unveiling putative biomarkers and therapeutic targets. Therefore, precision oncology benefits from the combination of proteomics and precision medicine because it increases the likelihood of defining the intricate molecular mechanisms of cancer-causing and diagnostic targets, reveals potential recent biomarkers for imaging and surveillance, and opens up novel methods for assessing the toxicity and efficacy of treatments [16]. Artificial intelligence (AI) solutions may also aid in the analysis of multiple clinical features and their stratification based on shared biological properties to achieve deep phenotyping.

Various clinical studies employing radiomics and radiogenomics techniques in neuroradiology are rising daily, even though AI is still a long way from being commonly used in radiologists' present workflow. In this chapter, we highlight a few AI uses in primary cancer imaging activities and also such AI models which are used by radiologists and helps in their regular therapeutic work [17]. However, accumulating data has demonstrated AI's potent function in oncological neuroimaging using quantitative data extraction from standard radiological exams [18]. The imaging signature is complementary to the molecular signature and, ideally, provides support for the characterisation of the brain tumour. It may also actively direct the design of the most suitable medication and clinical care [19]. Here, AI-based tools serve as a bridge between precision medicines and diagnostics, either independently or in conjunction with techniques based on nanotechnology, such as nanomedicine [20].

5.2 CANCER

5.2.1 Brain Disorders

Neurological illnesses are becoming more widely acknowledged as major global sources of death and disability as populations increase and age [21]. The diverse range of clinical manifestations observed in neurological illnesses can be attributed to the intricate interplay between many hereditary and environmental variables. As a result, individuals with the same illness may exhibit ranges of signs and symptoms in distinct phenotypes. Conversely, various circumstances may occasionally result in the same phenotype. The diagnosis, prognosis, and therapy of several neurological illnesses can now be improved by new developments in neurosciences [22].

5.2.1.1 Degenerative Parkinsonisms

The classic symptoms of Parkinsonian syndrome/disease (PD) are rest tremors, bradykinesia, and extrapyramidal stiffness. It is a typical observation in the elderly, identifying multiple underlying medical diseases, many of which are neurodegenerative [23].

The primary approach to diagnosing PD and other degenerative Parkinsonisms in vivo remains clinical, despite progress in basic sciences and neuroimaging. Misdiagnosis is common, and many patients have their diagnosis change after a few years of observation [24]. Recently, the use of biomarkers has made differentiating PD easier. These biomarkers found in biological samples like cerebrospinal fluid (CSF) and blood indicate whether biological processes are healthy or unhealthy [25].

Applications of biomarkers in PD research include diagnosis, prognosis, illness monitoring, medication response monitoring, and customised treatment [25]. This is a cross-sectional major study that focuses on several aspects:

1. Measuring cerebrospinal fluid biomarkers and characterising clinical and genetic features in both dyskinetic/non-dyskinetic PD patients.
2. Examining how LRRK2 biology with phosphorylation contributes to the signalling cascades triggered by the activation of D1 and glutamate receptors, which are crucial for the synaptic changes associated with levodopa-induced dyskinesias (LIDs).
3. Conducting in vitro tests to investigate the molecular and neuronal modulation associated with LIDs.
4. Determining the synaptic roles (pre and post) of molecular targets that regulate the storage of α-synuclein, which contributes to synaptic alterations.
5. Identifying substances that can either phosphorylate LRRK2 or reduce α-synuclein aggregation and then verifying how these molecules influence PD mice by preventing dyskinetic motor behaviour after levodopa administration.

As per reported clinical studies and pathophysiological models can be modified with the implementation of such strategies (PM) for LIDs in PD.

5.2.1.2 Coma

Coma, also known as acute disorder of consciousness, can result from severe brain damage or systemic disorders (such as infections, vascular diseases, brain hypoxia, and more) [26]. Although misinterpretation is conceivable, behavioural assessments using proven clinical scales [27] can discriminate between such states, which are characterised by reduced awareness and responsiveness. These scales have significant limitations, too, because clinical studies are predicated on studies of motor non-reflex reactions to specific stimuli/commands. Functional neuroimaging studies have suggested evidence of consciousness by demonstrating activity in particular brain regions in patients with chronic disorders of consciousness (DoC) responding to motor commands.

Neurorehabilitation is the primary treatment for such patients and should begin as soon as clinical stability is achieved. Functional outcomes appear to be improved when DoC patients are admitted to specialised neurorehabilitation facilities [28]. Rehabilitative objectives for DoC patients include improving voluntary motor functions and awareness, and various prognostic markers were identified. Most significantly, research has demonstrated that the prognosis deteriorates with time, even if chronic patients have occasionally exhibited signs of improvement [29].

Various methods have been attempted to improve responsiveness and awareness. In addition to traditional neurorehabilitation, pharmacological therapies and invasive and non-invasive brain stimulation have been suggested at DoC diagnosis to promote brain plasticity [30]. Transcranial direct current stimulation (tDCS) and amantadine are two therapies that have, nevertheless, demonstrated some effectiveness in aiding in the regaining of consciousness [31]. Clinical practitioners continue to face several challenges in helping patients regain consciousness. One neurorehabilitation technique that has been tried is sensory stimulation using customised target stimuli to try to help DoC patients become more aware [32].

Due to the wide variation in injuries, rehabilitation medicine cannot be restricted to a single standardised treatment method. Instead, it naturally operates as a model for personalised care. Customising therapy is vital to achieve the best possible clinical results. However, there is a lack of research on functional outcomes and predictive biomarkers specific to this condition. By considering the role of omics, we can better tailor rehabilitation therapies to address the specific needs and experiences per patient [33]. The main challenge in neurorehabilitation is to create a practical method for analysing multiparametric data and multidimensional outcomes, such as the neurobiological response to treatment, within a systems medicine framework. Positron-emission tomography (PET) is utilised to evaluate brain function, while high-density electroencephalography (HD-EEG) can monitor neurophysiological changes before, during, and after personalised stimulation to determine the degree and duration of treatment customisation. This approach is crucial because utilising the patient's familiar emotional pathways can enhance the effectiveness of sensory stimulation. Also, previous research shows that AI and ML algorithms can potentially enhance therapy by analysing clinical and paraclinical symptoms—such as diastolic blood pressure, base deficit, and Glasgow Coma Scale Score—in patients following severe injury resuscitation [34].

5.2.2 Acute Coronary Syndrome–Focused Cardiovascular Diseases

Through examining the interactions between heterogeneous components, omic techniques may aid in understanding the biological processes underlying cardiovascular diseases (CVDs), which are complex conditions resulting from the intersection of environmental factors and individual predisposition [35]. There are various levels at which to investigate the biological complexity of diseases. With a disease like acute coronary syndrome (ACS), these levels move from clinically based approaches, which focus on identifying clinical signs and symptoms, to the basic pharmacological approach, by identifying molecular pathways and biomarkers unique to the disease as well as the molecular effects of various medications [36]. Plaque erosion, plaque without thrombus, and plaque rupture with and without systemic inflammation have all been identified as potential pathogenic routes to ACS to date [37].

The aim of metabolic and lipidomic research is to identify small molecules associated with CVD. Recently, the plasma of participants in a pravastatin study was analysed using a metabolomic platform. When examining the lipid profile, the findings revealed that the metabolomic impact of a PCSK9 loss-of-function variant was similar to that of statin therapy [38]. These results support the therapeutic efficacy of PCSK9-inhibitor drugs and further confirm that reducing levels of plasma LDL lowers CVD risk. The study showed that both PCSK9 inhibitor therapy and statin treatment have similar effects on plasma LDL cholesterol levels [39]. The clinical practice still faces difficulties with ACS prediction. When combined with skilled emergency professionals, AI and ML may be able to anticipate the need for immediate revascularisation in emergency patients [40] and improve clinical outcomes for patients with chest discomfort [41].

5.2.3 Inflammatory Bowel Diseases

One well-known example of a chronic illness with a complicated aetiology is inflammatory bowel disease (IBD). IBD patients are classified into two primary clinical phenotypes (UC or ulcerative colitis and CD/Crohn's disease) according to a clinically based nosographic classification system. For each phenotype, a classification known as the Montreal classification is applied, which is based on endoscopic and radiological data [42]. But there are a lot of drawbacks to this kind of thinking. First, it is increasingly evident that different pathogenic pathways can cause the same clinical sub-phenotype of IBD in different patients. This indicates that IBD does not effectively represent its true clinical heterogeneity and cannot significantly influence patient outcomes [43]. While the precise etiopathogenesis of IBD remains unclear, it is currently widely accepted that these illnesses are multifactorial, resulting from an intricate interplay between environmental stimuli, immune system characteristics, and microbial traits in a genetically predisposed host [44].

Studies have highlighted the potential regulatory importance of a small population of rare cells in immune-mediated disorders, such as inflammatory bowel disease [45]. Single-cell analysis has proved the most effective method in identifying and characterising the functions of these rare cells [46]. This approach could uncover new therapeutic targets and offer a deeper understanding of the pathophysiology of IBD. This strategy may provide a means of clarifying, at least in part, the mechanisms underlying IBD treatment refractoriness and, ideally, provide some indications of the effectiveness of concurrently blocking several inflammatory pathways.

Last, it's important to note the growing significance of gastrointestinal endoscopy in PM. For instance, there has been optimism that AI and ML will be able to address the issues with traditional endoscopic scoring systems, such as poor predictive value and inter-observer variability, in the field of IBD. Also AI-based deep neural network was reported in a study for UC assessment and also predicted the endoscopic as well as histologic remission with >90% accuracy [47].

5.3 IMMUNOTHERAPY

Molecular profiling exhibiting immunogenic traits is widely used to guide immunotherapy, and fresh data in this area is constantly emerging. Tumour mutational burden (TMB), PD-1, and PD-L1 are immunophenotype indicators [48]. In addition to homologous repair-defective and repair-proficient (HRD and HRP, respectively) phenotypes, tumour-infiltrating lymphocytes (TILs) and factors facilitating TME are important markers [49]. When considered together, these factors provide insights into the immunogenicity of cancerous cells, tumour vulnerability to immune system invasion, and the effectiveness of immune cells in executing killing processes.

5.3.1 Tumour Mutational Burden

TMB is a metric used to assess the number of non-synonymous mutations in tumour samples, which helps in evaluating genomic instability and the potential for neoepitope formation on cancer cells [48, 50]. Neoepitopes are proteins that are uniquely expressed on cancer-affected cells and recognisable by the immune system. Although TMB thresholds can vary across different studies, it is typically categorised as high or low, with high TMB generally defined as having more than ten mutations per megabase of DNA [51]. A high TMB indicates an increased number of protein mutations, which could lead to the presence of neoepitopes on the cell surface. This characteristic has been shown in preclinical as well as clinical studies [51, 52], which later acts as reliable indicators of responsiveness to immune checkpoint inhibitor (ICI) therapy in solid tumours. Pembrolizumab (monoclonal antibody PD-1 targeting) has recently been approved in use for tumours with a high TMB (≥10), regardless of tumour type [53]. However, this positive correlation does not consistently apply, as TMB has not reliably predicted responses to immunotherapy in ovarian cancer trials [51]. Ovarian cancer is often classified as a "cold tumour" or TMB low [54]. Despite expectations of high TMB due to insufficient DNA repair, the median and mean TMB in ovarian cancer are 3.6 and 5.3 mutations per megabase, respectively [55].

5.3.2 Homologous Repair Deficiency

HRD is a biomarker used to predict a tumour's response to poly-(ADP ribose) polymerase (PARP)-inhibitors and Pt-based chemotherapy. HRD detects cancers with compromised DNA damage repair mechanisms [56, 57]. Approximately 50% of epithelial ovarian cancers exhibit HRD, and >25% of patients have germline mutations in genes associated with HRD [58]. Additionally, 25.7% of ovarian cancer patients have either somatic or germline BRCA gene mutations, classifying these BRCA mutant cells as HRD positive [59]. Germline BRCA mutations, commonly associated with ovarian and breast cancers, and mismatch repair (MMR) abnormalities, linked to Lynch-syndrome, are two significant familial cancer-related genes connected to homologous repair deficiency. Notably, a hereditary record of cancer is correlated positively with improved outcomes such as objective response rate (ORR), disease control rate (DCR), median time to treatment failure, and median overall survival (OS) following immune checkpoint inhibitor therapy. This suggests that HRD may influence the response to ICIs in hereditary cancers [60]. Additionally, mutations in MMR and other genes in the homologous recombination pathway, such as RAD51, BARD1, and TP53, are associated with reduced DNA repair capacity. Pembrolizumab, a PD-L1 inhibitor, has demonstrated a remarkable response in tumours with MMR [61]. As a result, pembrolizumab was authorised as the initial line of treatment for colorectal tumours lacking MMR [62]. Nevertheless, avelumab and other immunotherapies have not shown any response in BRCA1/2-mutant tumours [63]. Immunocheckpoint inhibitors have had less success in this population than anticipated [64]. Increased carcinogenesis, a rise in tumour mutations, and consequently an increase in the production of tumour neoantigens are among the effects of HRD [65].

5.3.3 Neoantigen Intratumoral Heterogeneity

Intratumoral heterogeneity (ITH) is a difference in neoepitopes expressed by tumour-infiltrating cells. Elevated ITH for neoantigens suggests that the cells in a tumour sample are not homogeneous and have unique neoepitope characteristics. On the other hand, low neoantigen ITH suggests that tumour cells are very homogenous, with the majority of sample cells expressing comparable neoepitope patterns. Subclonal populations of cells survive when neoantigen ITH is high, but the immune system targets the main clonal population. Because fewer T-cells in the tumour can identify the subclonal neoantigen, subclonal populations are not efficiently attacked. According to McGranahan et al., patients with NSCLC and melanoma treated with anti-PD-1 or anti-CTLA-4 antibodies had a favourable outcome when their clonal neoantigen burden was high and their intratumoral heterogeneity was low [66]. In the TME, neoantigen ITH is linked to many indicators. Twenty-five genes showed significantly altered expression in tumours with a high degree of clonal neoantigens (low ITH). The most significantly elevated proteins in the low neoantigen ITH group were PD-L1 and IL-6. Genes related to antigen presentation, immune cell migration, and effector T-cell activity were among the other immunostimulatory genes that were elevated. PD-1 and LAG-3 were among the negatively modulatory genes that were upregulated. Consequently, an inflammatory TME and immune system modulation are linked to low neoantigen ITH or high neoantigen burden along with homogeneity, suggesting a relationship between immunoediting and ITH score.

5.3.4 Tumour-Infiltrating Lymphocytes

TILs are used as a biomarker to assess immune-cell infiltration within the TME and to predict therapeutic responses [49]. Ongoing research has focused more on the roles of T-, NK-, and B-cells within the TME. However, the relationship between TILs and patient prognosis or survival remains unclear. For example, a study on melanoma TME found that higher TIL levels were associated with more aggressive tumours and later disease stages. Interestingly, the same study also identified a link between increased CD69+ levels (lymphocyte activation marker) and longer survival. This suggests that both the quantity and functionality of TILs are essential for accurate prognosis predictions [67]. To predict response, several biomarkers may need to be combined.

5.4 VARIOUS LIMITATIONS OF MOLECULAR-BASED DIAGNOSIS

Though precision medicine has a strong biological foundation, some unfavourable outcomes have brought attention to the strategy's shortcomings with molecularly guided treatment. Patients with solid tumours are randomised into 40 different arms in the NCI-MATCH experiment based on the molecular abnormalities in their tumours. Patients with tumours with FGFR changes, PIK3CA mutations, or ERRB2 amplification were treated with taselisib, FGFR inhibitors, or T-DM1, respectively, in three cohorts from the NCI-MATCH trial. Regretfully, response rates were consistently below 10% for multiple cohorts [68]. In this instance, the existence of populations that were extensively pretreated and concurrent molecular changes may account for the lack of benefit. Furthermore, different outcomes have been found when employing different targets in solid tumours that have the same molecular changes. For example, it is commonly recognised that inhibiting HER2 in breast cancer has been linked to a noteworthy improvement in clinical outcomes [69], even if anti-HER2 medication use in gastric or cancer patients did not have the same effects. The existence of molecular changes that cause primary or acquired resistance is a pertinent drawback of targeted therapy [70]. This tendency in all solid tumours has been extensively researched and documented.

The hyperactivation of intracellular proteins or the amplification of transmembrane receptors within the same pathway targeted by a specific inhibitor can lead to a lack of response to the treatment. Additionally, this resistance can be influenced by other biological processes that support the survival and proliferation of cancer cells [71]. For optimisation and characterisation of context-dependent cancerous mutations and resistance-based mechanisms, a deeper comprehension of cancer biology is required. Preclinical models, like organoids and patient-derived xenografts, may be able to clarify possible codrivers and resistance mechanisms in this case, allowing for the development and testing of sensible combinations to facilitate clinical deployment [72]. Studying circulating tumour DNA can uncover changes linked to how well a treatment works or fails, as shown by the influence of RAS mutations in colorectal cancer patients diagnosed with epidermal growth factor receptor inhibitors.

5.4.1 Personalised Approaches to Overcome Limitations

There is potential for functional precision cancer therapy to supplement existing genomic techniques. The precise validation of precision medicine has been challenging because of the low predictive power of molecular profiling in determining responses to targeted therapies and the limited effectiveness of current animal models used for choosing drugs [73]. The primary goal of functional models is the ability to assess cancer evolution and clonal selection as a result of exposure to anticancer drugs in real time. These models aid in our understanding of potential reasons treatments may fail. In recent years, functional analysis for medication efficacy in solid tumours has been made easier by the use of xenograft models derived from patients and 3-culture, also known as organoids. Models of patient-derived xenografts (PDXs) have helped to apply translational medicine. Tumour cells from patients are transplanted into immunodeficient mice to create these models. Compared to earlier models, it was discovered that these models more closely replicated the original tumour characteristics in vivo. PDXs maintain heterogeneity while retaining the original tumour features. PDXs are a useful tool to enhance personalised treatment plans since they can assist in predicting sensitivity and resistance to drugs in various tumours (Figure 5.1) [74].

The analysis of plasma cell free DNA (cfDNA) by liquid biopsy is another valuable technique that has significantly aided in the dynamic evaluation of solid tumours.

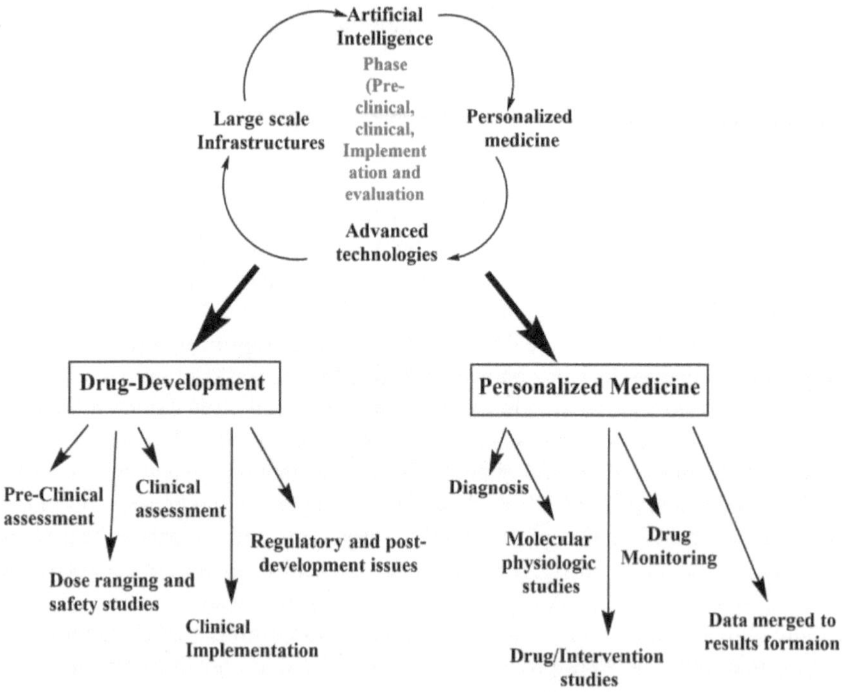

FIGURE 5.2 Various steps for personalised medicine and AI-based modelling in patient care and drug development.

Even when a particular targetable biomarker is found, resistance always emerges. This is why a thorough characterisation of the assessment of tumour heterogeneity and clonal selection as a result of treatment pressure is required. According to several studies, cfDNA may be able to assess tumour heterogeneity by identifying the genetic causes of acquired resistance. This study enables the precise assessment of tumour progression by enabling the examination of genomes and other molecular modifications at a particular point in time. When a patient develops acquired resistance, different tumour sub-clones with separate resistance mechanisms may emerge inside the same lesion, within separate metastatic lesions, or even within the patient [75]. This is due to the evolutionary pressure of therapy. Furthermore, the identification of acquired resistance mechanisms may primarily come from the genomic study of a single biopsy during the disease.

5.4.1.1 Molecular Tumour Microenvironment

A major challenge is the overwhelming amount of genetic tests and information available. Moreover, many pathology and sequencing studies tend to focus primarily on well-known genetic aberrations that can be targeted therapeutically, often overlooking other genetic alterations for which drug access programs or experimental treatments might be available [76]. As new molecular and genetic treatment options are explored, it is increasingly vital to develop and accurately interpret molecular tumour profiles to ensure the most effective cancer treatment. However, careful evaluation is required due to the significant advancements in molecular techniques and the precision attained by these instruments. To convert molecular profiles into clinically useful information, it necessitates talking about the clinical cases and findings from molecular analyses. Optimising patient selection will be made possible by creating molecular tumour boards composed of specialists from several fields [77].

5.4.2 Challenges for Personalised Medicine

There are a lot of chemicals and immunocompetent cells that take part in inflammation and immunity, including different cytokines, and there is currently no clear path forward for PM. Regarding biologics, numerous studies have examined the genetic correlation of therapeutic effects of drugs; nevertheless, no discernible marker genetic alterations or polymorphisms have been discovered. Research looking into genetic biomarkers for TNFα inhibitors has not turned up any indicator signs [78]. A GWAS meta-analysis on rheumatoid arthritis (RA) found that most associated genetic variants are molecular mutations connected to the targets of previous RA-drugs (with pathways). This suggests that meta-analysis could be a valuable tool for developing new medications and identifying novel biomarkers for treating RA [79].

5.5 CURRENT DIRECTIONS WITHIN PERSONALISED IMMUNOTHERAPY/MEDICINE

For immunotherapy to be effective, the TME must stimulate an anti-tumour T-cell response. To do this, a variety of strategies are presently being researched, such as autologous tumour vaccines, combination therapy, and dendritic cells.

5.5.1 Dendritic Cells

Using a tumour peptide to pulse autologous dendritic cells (DCs) is one method [80]. According to a study, the testis' Sertoli cells, the ovary's granulosa cells, and the kidneys all ordinarily express the chosen peptide, Wilms tumour protein-1 (WT1). Nonetheless, in a sample of 100 patients, the prevalence of WT1 protein expression in EOC tissues was reported around 78%, and WT1 was linked to tumours with higher grading ($p = 0.006$) and staging ($p = 0.002$) [81]. A phase I/II clinical trial investigated the function of WT1, a marker for a poor prognosis with a 47% and 5-year survival rate in ovarian cancer. In such patients, along with breast and stomach cancer with WT1 mutation, vaccination with autologous-DCs significantly increased the CD8+ T-cell response against WT1 ($p < 0.05$). Following treatment, seven of the ten patients (70%) had stable disease, with three of the seven indicating tumour decrease on CT scan. Of the ten patients, two (20%) reported a partial response. The diagnosis approach was found to be safe and well tolerated, as the reported adverse effects were of grade 1 or 2 [80]. This study highlights the necessity of tailored immunisations to target particular mutations in patient subgroups, perhaps leading to better results.

5.5.2 Autologous Vaccines

Additionally, autologous vaccinations may play a key role in how immunotherapy is used to treat cancer [82]. Autologous vaccines aim to reduce evasion and enhance immune responses against brain cancer cells. This approach was tested in a pilot study of six patients with advanced metastatic ovarian cancer (OC) who were resistant to chemotherapy. It included surgery, IL-2, ex vivo expended autologous TILs, and nivolumab (an anti PD-1 antibody), in addition to ipilimumab (an anti-CTLA4 antibody). After one year, five patients maintained stable disease, while one showed a partial response. The median progression-free survival was 86 days, ranging from 84 to 342 days. The inclusion of ipilimumab improved the effectiveness of ex-vivo–expended analogous TILs by enhancing CD8+ T-cell activity, compared to previous studies that did not include ipilimumab [83]. Overall, the utilisation of ICIs in combination with autologous vaccinations was emphasised. A potential next step would be to combine ICIs with Vigil, another autologous vaccination previously suggested, which primes T-cells to recognise pertinent clonal tumour neoantigens and boosts peripheral circulating CD3+/CD8+ T-cells. In a Phase I trial, women with relapsed OC were treated with Vigil and atezolizumab. Researchers discovered that administration time affected both safety and effectiveness. Vigil was given before atezolizumab, which improved efficacy and reduced atezolizumab-related side effects [84]. The tiny patient cohort's safety profile and clinical benefit indicate that more research is necessary.

5.5.3 Combination Therapeutic Approaches

It's also crucial to take into account research assessing how well autologous DC vaccination combined with ICIs and chemotherapy works. This study is important because it shows how, if given to the proper patients who have the best chance of responding, the medication may be essential in improving outcomes. Determining the elements that influence a patient's response to treatment is therefore very advantageous and needs to be kept under review. A further significant component of the research centres on the advantages of taking both bevacizumab, cyclophosphamide together, and the autologous DC vaccination. Additional examination of serum reveals that TGF-β was elevated following immunisation and subsequently following cyclophosphamide treatment, indicating the vaccine's responsiveness [85]. Further investigation is necessary to demonstrate the full impact of autologous vaccinations, which may be further beneficial when combined with previously studied, highly effective treatments to give tailored medication.

Additionally, autophagy may be crucial in how the body reacts to immunotherapies [86]. Elevated MHC-II levels are linked to a better prognosis and overall survival in ovarian cancer. One way that cells can produce more neoantigens for MHC-II to present is through autophagy. Autophagy control is multifaceted, with BRCA1/2 being involved in one mechanism. Compared to BRCA1/2 wild type, autophagy is higher in BRCA1/2 mutant cells [86]. Consequently, autophagy inducers in conjunction with immunological treatments such as ICIs and autologous tumour vaccines may be a sensible strategy for BRCA wild-type tumours. Autophagy inhibitors, however, may potentially be utilised to strengthen or resensitise cancers to chemotherapy [87]. Stress, especially chemotherapy, causes an increase in autophagy. According to preclinical research, autophagy inhibitors and chemotherapy can reduce cell viability together [88]. Depending on the situation, autophagy inducers or inhibitors may be used differently.

5.5.4 Affirming Previous Treatment Approaches

A reduced Aβ42/Aβ40 ratio in cerebrospinal fluid indicates the accumulation of Aβ in the brain and can be detected using PET amyloid imaging. Tau buildup is shown by elevated levels of p-tau and tau imaging with PET. Neurodegeneration is assessed in the CSF through markers such as t-tau, neurofilament light chain (NfL), and others (indicative of AD). PET does have many drawbacks, too, including a high cost per scan and few facilities available for use. Moreover, CSF is an extremely intrusive test. The difficulty is that there is a low flow of shared issues between CSF and PET examinations [89]. It is hoped that early practical application of these low-cost, safe, and high-throughput biomarkers would lead to early dementia detection and diagnosis becoming readily available to the general population [90].

5.5.5 Proteomics, the Current Status

Many fascinating advancements in the field of proteomics have occurred since 1994 [91]. As soon as the Human Genome Project was first announced, it became clear that populating the human proteome was crucial for gaining knowledge about pathophysiologic mechanisms, highlighting human health and disorders, and utilising that understanding to design and develop medical diagnostics [92], focusing mainly on cancer. The benefits of chromatographic techniques in automation, sample handling, and recovery have contributed to their increasing popularity. Multidimensional purification enhances proteome analysis by achieving high levels of purification and reducing sample complexity before mass spectrometry (MS) analysis [93]. A straightforward fractionation technique to increase plasma proteome coverage was also developed [94]. Similarly, Ahn et al. used a range of methods to identify biomarkers with altered expression in CRC tissues compared to healthy controls [95].

5.5.6 Major Labelling Strategies

Isobaric tags for relative and absolute quantitation (iTRAQ) enables both relative and absolute quantification of proteins as well as peptides by tagging samples with isotope-encoded reporter ions. This method allows for the detection of variations in target protein expression among samples. Using 8-plex iTRAQ reagents, various proteins can be measured and identified simultaneously at a single trial [96]. iTRAQ-based proteomics is commonly used in cancer research, particularly for complex samples (e.g., plasma) [97]. For example, iTRAQ-based proteomics were utilised to give overview on inflammatory autoimmune disorders. On comparing blood samples (RA patients) both before and after anti-TNF therapy, they identified a novel serum biomarker, leucine-rich α-2 glycoprotein (LRG). It's interesting to note that Crohn's disease (CD) and serum LRG levels were linked [98]. It has been discovered that CRC has a high expression of LRG1, which promotes tumour growth [99]. One major unmet clinical need is the capacity to distinguish between prostate tumours that are likely to develop and those that are indolent.

5.5.7 Targeted Proteomic Approaches

It could facilitate the advancement of sensitive, reproducible, quantitative, and high-throughput assays for identifying and validating potential biomarkers and biomarker panels. Reports indicate that these techniques offer sensitivity levels five to ten times higher than data-dependent analysis (DDA) [100, 101]. Additionally, immune enrichment can further enhance sensitivity. Notably, while immuno-MS specificity is derived from the fragmentation patterns of prototypic peptides, compared to ELISA, there are some less specific requirements for antibodies. The growing popularity of targeted proteomics is highlighted by a recent review that underscored its clinical potential [102].

5.5.8 Label-Free Approaches

Label-free techniques offer several advantages. Unlike labelled methods, which generally require samples to be physically homogenised and measured in a single run for direct comparison, label-free methods allow for direct comparison between any samples. Additionally, label-free techniques provide extensive proteome coverage due to their broad dynamic range, enabling the analysis of low-abundance proteins [103]. For example, label-free proteomics were used to identify a novel immune escape mechanism in HCC cells. They found that lysyl oxidase-like 4 (LOXL4) primarily suppresses macrophage immunity through PD-L1 activation. The correlation between elevated LOXL4 levels and poor survival in HCC patients highlights the role of LOXL4 in HCC progression and suggests new avenues for therapeutic intervention [104].

5.5.9 Proteogenomics

Proteogenomics investigates the relationship between proteomics and genomics [105]. Bridging the gap between the genome and the proteome requires integrating proteomics with other omics platforms, such as lipidomics, transcriptomics, metabolomics, glycomics, and microbiomics. This comprehensive approach enhances our understanding of disease mechanisms, identifies potential biomarkers for detecting and monitoring diseases, and supports both basic as well as clinical research in precision oncology. Through significant financial investments in proteogenomics, CPTAC has accelerated the speed of proteogenomic research and precision oncology, leading to a greater knowledge of the molecular causes of cancer and numerous publications covering a variety of cancer types. Primary breast cancer samples were examined using a combination of next generation DNA and RNA sequencing with TMT-based proteomics, including phosphoproteome and acetylproteome profile. This comprehensive analysis provided insight into metabolic abnormalities, tumour immunogenicity, cell cycle progression and the diversity of therapeutic targets. These findings challenged the traditional methods of diagnosing breast cancer and offered fresh perspectives on precision and customised treatment. Proteogenomic characterisation was employed in a different investigation to discover differentially expressed proteins that show potential for usage in both therapeutic and diagnostic contexts. Additionally, the study revealed therapeutic weaknesses in lung cancer treatment [106].

5.5.10 Bioinformatics

Bioinformatics is a key element of HUPO resources and is vital for managing the higher volumes of proteomics data being generated currently. Numerous online tools and platforms have been created as analytical techniques [107], including those specifically designed for cancer research, such as Perseus [108] and the Cancer Genome Atlas (TCGA) [109].

5.6 NANOROBOTS AND NANOCARRIERS IN MEDICAL DIAGNOSIS

Nanocarriers loaded with lipids or other surfactants generally developed a novel drug delivery system (DDS) which is helpful in enhancing the bioavailability of drug or carriers and also modulated its targeting efficacy with respect to its development form. Also, it can be designed as a PM and loaded with advanced nanotechnology called nanorobots/nanobots. When it comes to sensing detection, detoxification, and purification, NRs are extremely useful. The controlled driving properties of nanorobots allow them to actively seek and target materials for cleaning, enhancing the efficiency of detection and removal. Their ability to accurately detect proteins, cells, bacterial toxins, metal ions, and other substances enables NRs to offer valuable pre-treatment analysis for various diseases. To safeguard human health, it is possible to avoid high ion concentrations by accurately detecting metal ions in the blood [110]. Furthermore, NRs have enormous potential in intelligent sensing and drive systems like biosensors.

Relying on individuals or in groups to monitor is a crucial clinical use of medical NRs. Their potential for medical imaging cannot be overlooked because they are easily detected and guided and can even deliver signals to promote trigger release [111]. Iacovacci et al. [112] proposed a magnetically driven nanorobot developed from thermally responsive double-layer hydrogels. This NR integrates radioactive elements and magnetic nanoparticles into its hydrogel structure, enabling remote control and shape modifications of the micro-device while also serving as imaging agents. The imaging agents facilitate the tracking of the NR throughout the body. A single PET scan confirmed the presence of the NR in the mouse abdomen after imaging mouse epithelial tissues. This work paved the door for single-robot closed-loop control by demonstrating that hydrogel structures as small as 100 μm may be employed for imaging individual NRs. Additionally, the NR was successfully monitored in both superficial tissues and deep organs using magnetic resonance imaging (MRI) and autologous fluorescence (AF). MRI revealed the NR in mouse stomachs after subcutaneous and abdominal injections [113]. In conclusion, the NR has a broad range of potential applications in targeted therapy due to its strong propulsion, precise guidance, and adjustable loading and release properties.

5.6.1 Drug Carriers

For designing and developing the DDS, there are various types of drugs selected majorly, which are classified as per the BCS classification. If the conventional DDS shows good results already but designed with slight modifications in their dosage form to avoid the chances of patient adherence and drug abuse sometimes, which also leads to toxicity and adverse effects. It is anticipated that the toxicity issue brought on by excessive drug use will be resolved by the precise delivery potential of NRs at the targeted site [114]. The average size of the magnesium particles used to make a drug-loaded NR for the diagnosis of stomach bacterial infection is about 20 μm. It can propel itself efficiently; in vitro, it was examined at an average velocity of about 120 μm/s in gastric juice (pH = 1.3) [115]. Because the NR can be accurately manoeuvred to the desired position, and the ultrasonic focus can selectively release the medicine or advanced designed BCS drugs loaded contained in it, ultrasound-mediated therapy can lessen the drug's negative effects [116].

5.6.2 Surgery Tools

Traditional surgical instruments are unable to operate at cellular or at micro-level, and to overcome such limitations, the micro/nanoscale surgical instruments were deployed. The employment of tiny NRs as surgical instruments will undoubtedly lower the danger of infection, speed up healing, and enhance surgical precision and control. NRs can directly find the focus to treat disease by using the properties of the material itself as well as the external physical field. By concentrating magnetic fields to specifically target and eliminate pathogens, Chen et al. controlled magnetic bacteria NRs [117]. To target and connect to *Staphylococcus aureus*, first the magnetotactic bacteria NR was guided in a microfluidic chip. Targeted thermal therapy is feasible through the use of in vitro cell lines. This method of killing cancer cells minimises harm to the body. When combined with AI-based technology, NR has proved an excellent way to target cancer using NCS, and this approach can effectively combat chronic diseases like cancer (Figure 5.3) [118].

5.7 ARTIFICIAL INTELLIGENCE–BASED DIAGNOSIS

AI refers to a technique which copies human cognitive processes, such as learning, thinking, and problem solving. Initially a subfield of computer science, modern AI has grown into a broad, multidisciplinary domain that incorporates insights from informatics, statistics, physics, and other fields, as seen in Figure 5.4, and various AI-based tools are also discussed (Table 5.1).

5.7.1 Radiomics

This new method is based on the concept that radiological images should be interpreted not just as visual images but as sources of numerical data. This approach provides more detailed information than a radiologist's qualitative assessment.

The radiomic paradigm aims to quantify and reproducibly extract data from diagnostic images, particularly complex patterns that are visually not possible to recognise/measure. The integration of AI into biomedical imaging is expected to advance precision medicine by modulating the accuracy and utility of imaging data [119].

5.7.1.1 Radiogenomics

Radiogenomics is a subfield of radiomics that seeks to connect biological information with imaging data. It also performs identification of patterns in proteomics and genomics based on features obtained from imaging data [120].

5.7.1.2 Radiomics-Workflow

A sophisticated procedure known as "radiomics workflow" is used to create and validate AI-based tools that are intended to extract diagnostic and/or prognostic data from biological pictures [121]. The radiomic paradigm involves several established techniques, including segmentation, feature extraction and harmonisation, data mining or model building, data collection, and post-processing or reconstruction. The final step is to effectively extract crucial information from imaging data using ML algorithms, which must be trained, validated, and accessed to ensure the reliability and clinical relevance [122].

5.7.1.3 Machine-Learning

ML is a branch of AI dedicated to identifying meaningful patterns in a dataset, supporting data mining techniques [123]. In radiology, it can be utilised to derive valuable insight from imaging data [124]. ML models are categorised as either supervised or unsupervised, depending on their training methods. Initial data preparation is

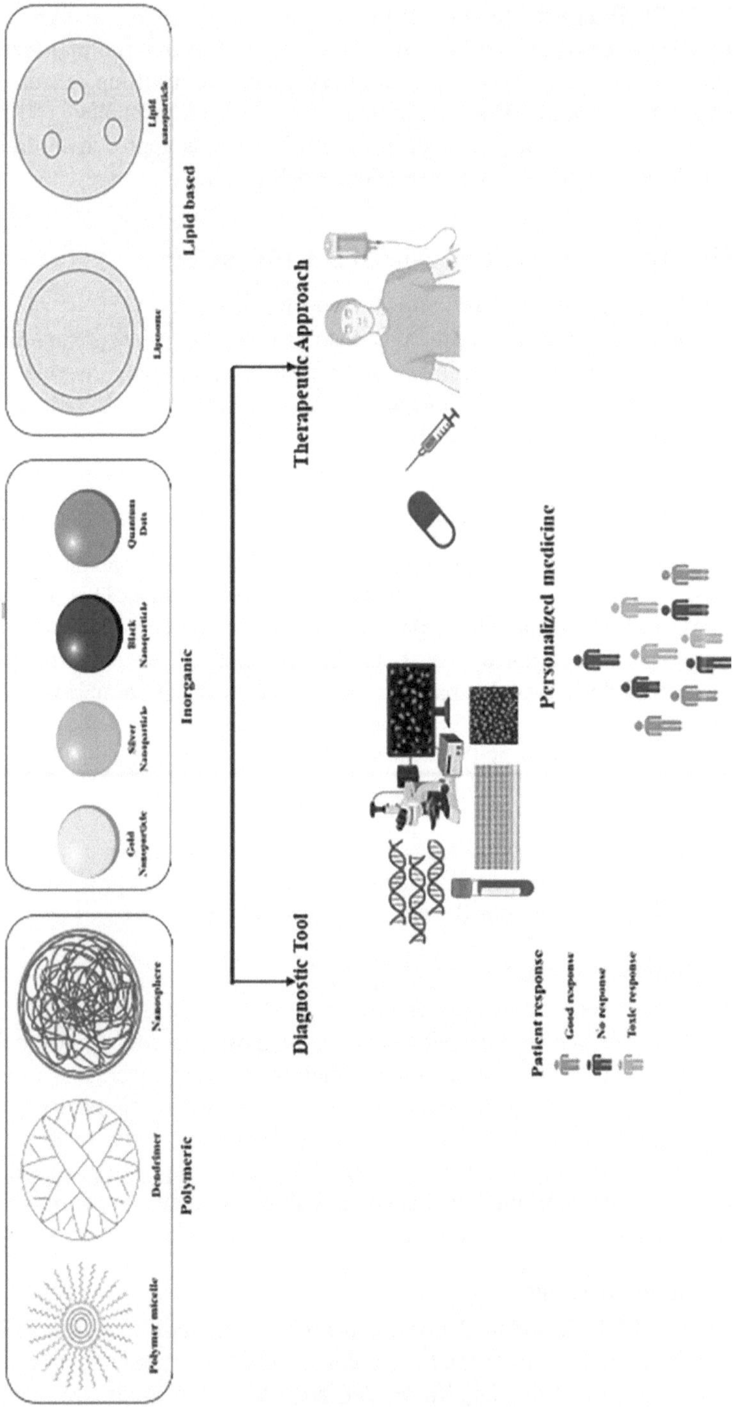

FIGURE 5.3 Nanocarrier- and nanotechnology-based therapeutic approaches for diagnosis of chronic diseases in combination with PM.

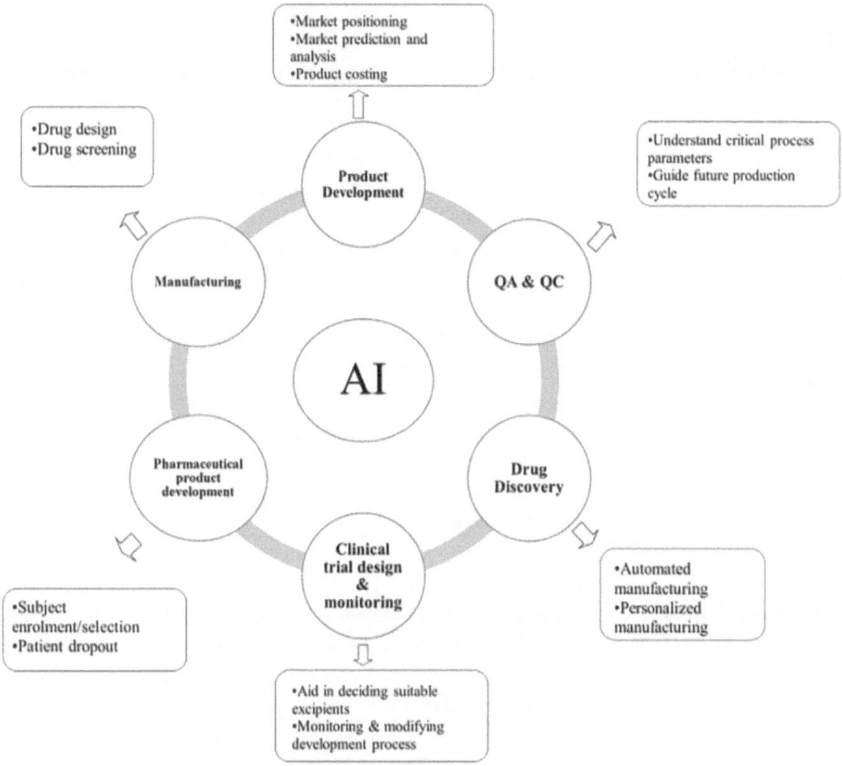

FIGURE 5.4 Implementation of AI in drug development and design of DDSs with patient-related approaches.

necessary to train these algorithms for medical imaging tasks. Subsequently, modern computing power automates these processes either fully or partially, aiming to enhance human decision making. The four main types of ML are discussed in the following [125].

5.7.1.3.1 Supervised Learning

The most fundamental ML method is called SL, which requires some level of human supervision to be educated. Algorithms in SL mimic the cognitive process of "learning by example" in humans. For highly generic classification problems, where fresh components need to be labelled according to a set of predetermined categories, this type of machine learning is suitable. To train these algorithms, a dataset containing input–output pairs (x, y) is necessary, where (x) represents the input data and (y) the corresponding labels. Human experts annotate the input data with labels (e.g., categorising a brain mass as "tumour/non-tumour") to make these labelled data points. The goal of the algorithm is to identify the interrelationship between input and output. Unlike traditional programming, which involves executing a predefined operation to achieve a result, the algorithm is trained to evaluate various hypotheses to

TABLE 5.1
Different AI-Based Tools Utilised in Design and Development of DDSs

Tool	Application in Drug Discovery
Reinforcement learning	Implemented to maximise intended results and optimise medicine combinations and dosages by taking into account a number of interaction variables.
DeepChem	Deep learning chemistry resource and open-source drug discovery.
DeepTox	Open-source framework for DL developed specifically for assessing and predicting toxic characteristics.
PotentialNet	Ligand-binding affinity predicted by using a graph convolutional neural network (CNN)
Predictive ADME/tax modelling	Tools that use machine learning approaches to simulate and forecast drug candidates' absorption, distribution, metabolism, excretion, and possible toxicity
Natural language processing tools	Aid in the extraction and analysis of data from patents, clinical trial data, and scholarly literature.
Cheminformatics tools	The investigation and modification of chemical structures and characteristics are made possible by tools.
QSAR/QSPR modelling	Establishes a relationship between biological activities or characteristics and molecular structures to forecast the behaviour of compounds.
Deep learning	Used for projects such as De-Novo drug design, virtual screening, and drug property prediction.
Machine learning	Assists in biological activity analysis, drug–target interaction prediction, and lead compound optimisation.

discover patterns or correlations (x → y) in the data. This approach mirrors how an experienced human annotator might classify visual features based on their knowledge [126, 127].

5.7.1.3.2 Unsupervised Learning

Self-organising algorithms that uncover hidden patterns in data use only the inherent structure of unlabelled, unclassified, or uncategorised data [127]. In this approach, the algorithm is provided with a raw dataset and tasked with extracting meaningful insights. These algorithms are typically used for clustering, which groups data based on specific criteria, and association, which identifies rules connecting different data points.

5.7.1.3.3 Semi-Supervised Learning

A ML paradigm known as semi-supervised learning operates mainly on unlabelled data with a minor quantity of labelled data, placing it between unsupervised and supervised learning [127].

5.7.1.3.4 Self-Supervised Learning

Self-supervised learning is a ML approach where the system generates its own labels to complete tasks rather than relying on external labels [127]. Although it shares similarities with unsupervised learning due to the absence of provided labels, it aims to tackle problems typically addressed by supervised learning. This approach leverages large amounts of readily available unlabelled data to overcome the challenge of limited labelled data, making it useful when it's impractical to label all the necessary data for comprehensive training. Autoencoders, a neural type of network, are commonly used as a tool for self-supervised learning.

5.7.1.3.5 ML Models

This is a system designed to adjust data according to theoretical assumptions about potential relationships within a dataset. Models generally fall into two major categories: those based on statistical methods and artificial neural networks. Statistical models are especially valuable because they are computationally feasible, meaning they can be readily converted into code for automated analysis. Automated techniques allow for the evaluation of a model's ability to infer relationships within a dataset and the comparison of various models' performances. In machine learning, predictions can be made about specific outcomes based on predefined factors, such as the relationship between an image and a radiologist's label. To determine the effectiveness of the model's proposed mappings, it is important to compare the results from the training phase with those from the validation and testing phases, assessing how well the model performs with new, unseen data [127, 128].

5.7.1.3.5.1 Features Generally, there is a distinction between manually crafted features and those automatically extracted, often through DL algorithms. First-level features, such as shape, volume, and intensity measurements, are fundamental and easily interpreted qualitatively. In contrast, second-order features, which are either derived from combinations of first-level features or automatically generated by DL networks, may be less clinically informative for radiologists [129]. However, it is precisely from these advanced characteristics that AI-powered instruments derive their promise, enabling them to catch information that radiologists are unable to. Because features serve as the foundation for training and validating AI models, they are a required step in the radionics workflow. Thus, in the radiomic procedure, selecting strong and repeatable characteristics is crucial (Table 5.2) [130, 131].

5.7.2 Artificial Neural Networks

ANNs are learning models derived from the neural network of the human brain. ANN consists of nodes and layers, each serving as a distinct computational unit. Each node processes input in a specific way and transmits its output to the following nodes through connections. While these nodes are simpler and less connected than biological neurons, the overall network can exhibit complex and emergent properties. This complexity arises from the collective action of many simple units, each of which combines inputs (often with different weights) and transmits the result to the next node once a certain threshold is met. ANNs learn by adjusting their computational properties rather than by testing statistical hypotheses to find data correlations [132].

TABLE 5.2
Various Applications, Significances, and Cancer-Targeting Approaches via AI in DDS Development

Application	Significance	Hypothesised for Cancer Targeting
Drug design	• Predicting 3D structures of target protein. • De-Novo drug design. • Determination of drug activity. • Predicting drug–protein interactions.	Advanced DDSs designed and can be optimised for cancer targeting at various sites of action via different approaches for a number of drugs.
Chemical synthesis	• Designing bio-specific drug molecules. • Designing multitarget drug molecules.	Chemically modified the drug structure and designed new diagnostic approach against cancer or tumour.
Poly-pharmacology	• Prediction of reaction yield. • Prediction of retrosynthesis pathways. • Gaining knowledge about how reactions work. • Designing synthetic routes.	Advanced reactions give chances of new approaches for cancer treatment.
Drug screening	• Predicting 3D structures of target protein.	Enhance the chances of cancer treatment via designing targeted DDS.
Repurposing	• Predicting 3D structures of target protein.	Proteomics can be delivered for cancer targeting, specifically brain cancer.

5.7.3 Deep Learning

DL is a major area within artificial intelligence that utilises advanced neural networks, such as convolutional neural networks, to uncover complex patterns in data [133]. CNNs are particularly useful for extraction of automated radiomics feature because they can detect deep features automatically, identify subtle information in detailed manner, and efficiently handle large volumes of data [134]. These models are based on the structure of the mammalian brain's visual cortex, whose layers are arranged hierarchically and process progressively complex intermediate visual elements, like forms, edges, and lines, before returning to the meaning of the full visual object. The "black box phenomenon" refers to the difficulty in understanding how the processing of the intermediate layers adds up to the final result; it makes analysing the output of AI tools more difficult [135].

DL models improve image recognition by understanding how local features relate to the overall image. Popular CNNs used for medical image classification include AlexNet [136], VGG [137], and GoogLeNet [138]. In DL-based radiomics, various network designs, such as CNNs and autoencoders, or combinations of linear and nonlinear functions help to identify important features in radiological images [139].

5.7.4 Lesion Detection and Differential Diagnosis

Neuroradiologists can benefit from AI-powered systems in diagnosing brain lesions. Although experienced neuroradiologists can usually identify large, symptomatic gliomas with ease, detecting small brain metastases (BMs) early in cancer patients can be challenging. This difficulty arises because MRI sensitivity can vary, and different MRI acquisition techniques can affect the results [140]. Early detection of even small metastases is crucial, as it influences treatment decisions and stereotactic radiosurgery procedures, significantly impacting patient outcomes. Consequently, many computer-aided detection (CAD) methods in neuro-oncology focus on automatically identifying brain metastases.

5.8 DISCUSSION

Artificial intelligence is increasingly capturing the interest of healthcare professionals and industry leaders due to its transformative potential in diagnostics and preventive care [141]. Personalised precision medicine (PPM) seeks to maximise AI's impact by guiding the selection of optimal treatment strategies for individual patients. Specifically, tools like QPOP and CURATE are designed to determine personalised medication regimens and initial dosages. Additionally, AI creates adaptable patient profiles to ensure precise dosing throughout the treatment process. QPOP and CURATE are mechanism-independent techniques. AI can work even with a lack of pharmacokinetic and drug–drug interaction data, and it can even produce new knowledge particular to a certain system. When PPM is fully implemented clinically, a patient will have QPOP applied to a sample taken from their blood or a tumour that has been removed, and they will have discovered an effective and customised combination—CURATE—after that. The dose modulation in the same person will be guided by AI. As a result, every aspect of the patient's care will be customised, from choosing the medications and their starting dosages to controlling the dosage along the course of therapy. This is a very likely outcome as soon as the two methods are independently verified for every individual signal. ACCURATE.AI's ability to modify combination therapy for individuals has been clinically proven in a prospective pilot trial for mCRPC [142].

Nanostructured DDS also act as targeting DDSs such as nanostructured lipid carriers (NLCs) [143], self-nano-emulsifying DDSs [144], and sometimes modified formulations for targeting a particular effect in a NCS-based system [145], which may be implemented as a PM. It also found in some nanoparticles that AI-based DDS was proved to be effective as a targeted DDS against cancer or any severe disease. Additionally, such DDS enhanced the bioavailability, half-life, and potential of the drug [146–148]. Nowadays, cancer is the most tremendous disorder and the cure is still not developed. So, such AI-based approaches are under trial stage for management of such diseases.

The treatment of various chronic diseases such as cancer, neurological disorders (Alzheimer's, Parkinson's), and cardiovascular diseases which can be fatal are possible or can be controlled at initial stage of detection. Additionally, there are a number of traditional DDS available for the prevention and control of these diseases; however, they have certain drawbacks, either in terms of system bioavailability or their safety and efficacy profile. To overcome these drawbacks, PM has been shown to be successful, and when combined with AI-based techniques, this has developed a safe and effective DDS for the diagnosis of cancer as well as a therapeutic approach [149]. The discussed AI models may be utilised to design PMs loaded with NCS by taking algorithms set with the help of the patient's family and previous disease profile and can be helpful in avoiding the chances of adverse effects as well as ensuring the safety of the developed medicine or DDS [150].

5.9 CONCLUSION

In conclusion, artificial intelligence has emerged as an effective and versatile tool in the realm of diagnosis and therapeutic activity against hereditary disease or cancer. There are various conventional DDS used previously but have some limitations, which was replaced by nanotechnology-based DDS with various nanocarriers loaded with drugs and active components and found effective and have targeted efficacy against such diseases, which makes them a suitable candidate for PM. PM deals with the genetic codes and genomics of patients, which is very effective against neurodegenerative disorders, cardiovascular system diseases, and gastrointestinal tract disorders, as reported by previous researchers. These PMs are designed and developed based on the patient's complete profile and hereditary information, which can be used as an input in various AI models by which the AI-based PM loaded with NCS or modern nanotechnology approaches such as nanoemulsion, self-nano emulsifying systems, and lipid nanoparticles showed advancement in cancer therapeutics, drug delivery, and diagnostics. Also, NRs have been reported effective against cancer cells and have also been used as a PM approach, and NRs have drawn attention for complicated surgeries. This chapter mainly focuses on combining all these approaches. It presents AI-based models with NCS as a PM that can be an effective treatment available for cancer or another fatal disease. Apart from the pharmaceutical and healthcare point of view, AI-based tools will emerge as a major future therapy outcome with the least adverse effects and greater efficacy over conventional DDSs.

5.10 FUTURE PERSPECTIVES

Prospects for this field's future include combining PM and NCS methodologies with intelligent AI-based technology. The field of disease/gene-targeted drug delivery will continue to change with the introduction of combination medicines, continuous manufacturing technologies, and multifunctional nanoformulations. Lipid-based nanoformulations have the approach and efficacy to administer drugs by providing a precise care, which also has good patient compliance, provided research continues to uncover new possibilities and overcome barriers.

REFERENCES

1. Middleton, J.D., Stover, D.G. and Hai, T., 2018. Chemotherapy-exacerbated breast cancer metastasis: A paradox explainable by dysregulated adaptive-response. *International Journal of Molecular Sciences*, *19*(11), p. 3333.
2. Karagiannis, G.S., Pastoriza, J.M., Wang, Y., Harney, A.S., Entenberg, D., Pignatelli, J., Sharma, V.P., Xue, E.A., Cheng, E., D'Alfonso, T.M. and Jones, J.G., 2017. Neoadjuvant chemotherapy induces breast cancer metastasis through a TMEM-mediated mechanism. *Science Translational Medicine*, *9*(397), p. eaan0026.

3. Ren, Y., Zhou, X., Yang, J.J., Liu, X., Zhao, X.H., Wang, Q.X., Han, L., Song, X., Zhu, Z.Y., Tian, W.P. and Zhang, L., 2015. AC1MMYR2 impairs high dose paclitaxel-induced tumor metastasis by targeting miR-21/CDK5 axis. *Cancer Letters*, *362*(2), pp. 174–182.
4. Nice, E.C., 2021. The separation sciences, the front end to proteomics: An historical perspective. *Biomedical Chromatography*, *35*(1), p. e4995.
5. Omenn, G.S., Lane, L., Overall, C.M., Cristea, I.M., Corrales, F.J., Lindskog, C., Paik, Y.K., Van Eyk, J.E., Liu, S., Pennington, S.R. and Snyder, M.P., 2020. Research on the human proteome reaches a major milestone: > 90% of predicted human proteins now credibly detected, according to the HUPO human proteome project. *Journal of Proteome Research*, *19*(12), pp. 4735–4746.
6. Kolch, W., Mischak, H. and Pitt, A.R., 2005. The molecular make-up of a tumour: Proteomics in cancer research. *Clinical Science*, *108*(5), pp. 369–383.
7. Ponomarenko, E.A., Poverennaya, E.V., Ilgisonis, E.V., Pyatnitskiy, M.A., Kopylov, A.T., Zgoda, V.G., Lisitsa, A.V. and Archakov, A.I., 2016. The size of the human proteome: The width and depth. *International Journal of Analytical Chemistry*, *2016*(1), p. 7436849.
8. Ali, M.R., Wu, Y., Han, T., Zang, X., Xiao, H., Tang, Y., Wu, R., Fernández, F.M. and El-Sayed, M.A., 2016. Simultaneous time-dependent surface-enhanced Raman spectroscopy, metabolomics, and proteomics reveal cancer cell death mechanisms associated with gold nanorod photothermal therapy. *Journal of the American Chemical Society*, *138*(47), pp. 15434–15442.
9. Abdel Razek, A.A.K., Alksas, A., Shehata, M., AbdelKhalek, A., Abdel Baky, K., El-Baz, A. and Helmy, E., 2021. Clinical applications of artificial intelligence and radiomics in neuro-oncology imaging. *Insights into Imaging*, *12*, pp. 1–17.
10. Singh, G., Manjila, S., Sakla, N., True, A., Wardeh, A.H., Beig, N., Vaysberg, A., Matthews, J., Prasanna, P. and Spektor, V., 2021. Radiomics and radiogenomics in gliomas: A contemporary update. *British Journal of Cancer*, *125*(5), pp. 641–657.
11. Vagvala, S., Guenette, J.P., Jaimes, C. and Huang, R.Y., 2022. Imaging diagnosis and treatment selection for brain tumors in the era of molecular therapeutics. *Cancer Imaging*, *22*(1), p. 19.
12. Rudie, J.D., Rauschecker, A.M., Bryan, R.N., Davatzikos, C. and Mohan, S., 2019. Emerging applications of artificial intelligence in neuro-oncology. *Radiology*, *290*(3), pp. 607–618.
13. Thangavel, K., Balamurugan, A., Elango, M., Subiramaniyam, P. and Senrayan, M., 2014. A survey on nano-robotics in nano-medicine. *Nanotechnology*, *8*(9), pp. 525–528.
14. Al-Sharif, M., Awen, B. and Molvi, K., 2010. Nanotechnology in cancer therapy: A review. *Journal of Chemical and Pharmaceutical Research*, *2*(5), pp. 161–168.
15. Rahul, V.A., 2017. A brief review on nanorobots. *SSRG-IJME*, *4*, pp. 15–21.
16. Neto, A.M.J.C., Lopes, I.A. and Pirota, K.R., 2010. A review on nanorobotics. *Journal of Computational and Theoretical Nanoscience*, *7*(10), pp. 1870–1877.
17. Schmidt, C.K., Medina-Sánchez, M., Edmondson, R.J. and Schmidt, O.G., 2020. Engineering microrobots for targeted cancer therapies from a medical perspective. *Nature Communications*, *11*(1), p. 5618.
18. Soto, F., Wang, J., Ahmed, R. and Demirci, U., 2020. Medical micro/nanorobots in precision medicine. *Advanced Science*, *7*(21), p. 2002203.
19. Yamamoto, Y., Kanayama, N., Nakayama, Y. and Matsushima, N., 2022. Current status, issues and future prospects of personalized medicine for each disease. *Journal of Personalized Medicine*, *12*(3), p. 444.
20. Hood, L., Balling, R. and Auffray, C., 2012. Revolutionizing medicine in the 21st century through systems approaches. *Biotechnology Journal*, *7*(8), pp. 992–1001.
21. Neurology Collaborators GBD, 2019. Global, regional, and national burden of neurological disorders, 1990–2016: A systematic analysis for the global burden of disease study 2016. *The Lancet. Neurology*, *18*, pp. 459–480.

22. Tan, L., Jiang, T., Tan, L. and Yu, J.T., 2016. Toward precision medicine in neurological diseases. *Annals of Translational Medicine*, *4*(6).
23. Williams, D.R. and Litvan, I., 2013. Parkinsonian syndromes. *Continuum: Lifelong Learning in Neurology*, *19*(5), pp. 1189–1212.
24. Caslake, R., Moore, J.N., Gordon, J.C., Harris, C.E. and Counsell, C., 2008. Changes in diagnosis with follow-up in an incident cohort of patients with parkinsonism. *Journal of Neurology, Neurosurgery & Psychiatry*, *79*(11), pp. 1202–1207.
25. Parnetti, L., Gaetani, L., Eusebi, P., Paciotti, S., Hansson, O., El-Agnaf, O., Mollenhauer, B., Blennow, K. and Calabresi, P., 2019. CSF and blood biomarkers for Parkinson's disease. *The Lancet Neurology*, *18*(6), pp. 573–586.
26. Davis, T. and Ings, A., 2015. Head injury: Triage, assessment, investigation and early management of head injury in children, young people and adults (NICE guideline CG 176). *Archives of Disease in Childhood-Education and Practice*, *100*(2), pp. 97–100.
27. Gerrard, P., Zafonte, R. and Giacino, J.T., 2014. Coma recovery scale–revised: Evidentiary support for hierarchical grading of level of consciousness. *Archives of Physical Medicine and Rehabilitation*, *95*(12), pp. 2335–2341.
28. Phillips, C.L., Bruno, M.A., Maquet, P., Boly, M., Noirhomme, Q., Schnakers, C., Vanhaudenhuyse, A., Bonjean, M., Hustinx, R., Moonen, G. and Luxen, A., 2011. "Relevance vector machine" consciousness classifier applied to cerebral metabolism of vegetative and locked-in patients. *Neuroimage*, *56*(2), pp. 797–808.
29. Katz, D.I., Polyak, M., Coughlan, D., Nichols, M. and Roche, A., 2009. Natural history of recovery from brain injury after prolonged disorders of consciousness: Outcome of patients admitted to inpatient rehabilitation with 1–4 year follow-up. *Progress in Brain Research*, *177*, pp. 73–88.
30. Nardone, R., Sebastianelli, L., Versace, V., Brigo, F., Golaszewski, S., Manganotti, P., Saltuari, L. and Trinka, E., 2020. Repetitive transcranial magnetic stimulation in traumatic brain injury: Evidence from animal and human studies. *Brain Research Bulletin*, *159*, pp. 44–52.
31. Giacino, J.T., Whyte, J., Bagiella, E., Kalmar, K., Childs, N., Khademi, A., Eifert, B., Long, D., Katz, D.I., Cho, S. and Yablon, S.A., 2012. Placebo-controlled trial of amantadine for severe traumatic brain injury. *New England Journal of Medicine*, *366*(9), pp. 819–826.
32. Padua, L., Cuccagna, C. and Pazzaglia, C., 2019. Novel sensory paradigms for neuromodulation in disorders of consciousness in traumatic brain injury. *Current Opinion in Neurology*, *32*(6), pp. 844–849.
33. Wagner, A.K. and Kumar, R.G., 2019. TBI rehabilomics research: Conceptualizing a humoral triad for designing effective rehabilitation interventions. *Neuropharmacology*, *145*, pp. 133–144.
34. Paydar, S., Parva, E., Ghahramani, Z., Pourahmad, S., Shayan, L., Mohammadkarimi, V. and Sabetian, G., 2021. Do clinical and paraclinical findings have the power to predict critical conditions of injured patients after traumatic injury resuscitation? Using data mining artificial intelligence. *Chinese Journal of Traumatology*, *24*(01), pp. 48–52.
35. Barwari, T., Joshi, A. and Mayr, M., 2016. MicroRNAs in cardiovascular disease. *Journal of the American College of Cardiology*, *68*(23), pp. 2577–2584.
36. Joshi, A., Rienks, M., Theofilatos, K. and Mayr, M., 2021. Systems biology in cardiovascular disease: A multiomics approach. *Nature Reviews Cardiology*, *18*(5), pp. 313–330.
37. Crea, F. and Liuzzo, G., 2013. Pathogenesis of acute coronary syndromes. *Journal of the American College of Cardiology*, *61*(1), pp. 1–11.
38. Sliz, E., Kettunen, J., Holmes, M.V., Williams, C.O., Boachie, C., Wang, Q., Maennikkoe, M., Sebert, S., Walters, R., Lin, K. and Millwood, I.Y., 2018. Metabolomic consequences of genetic inhibition of PCSK9 compared with statin treatment. *Circulation*, *138*(22), pp. 2499–2512.

39. Karatasakis, A., Danek, B.A., Karacsonyi, J., Rangan, B.V., Roesle, M.K., Knickelbine, T., Miedema, M.D., Khalili, H., Ahmad, Z., Abdullah, S. and Banerjee, S., 2017. Effect of PCSK9 inhibitors on clinical outcomes in patients with hypercholesterolemia: A meta-analysis of 35 randomized controlled trials. *Journal of the American Heart Association*, *6*(12), p. e006910.
40. Al-Zaiti, S., Besomi, L., Bouzid, Z., Faramand, Z., Frisch, S., Martin-Gill, C., Gregg, R., Saba, S., Callaway, C. and Sejdić, E., 2020. Machine learning-based prediction of acute coronary syndrome using only the pre-hospital 12-lead electrocardiogram. *Nature Communications*, *11*(1), p. 3966.
41. Goto, S., Kimura, M., Katsumata, Y., Goto, S., Kamatani, T., Ichihara, G., Ko, S., Sasaki, J., Fukuda, K. and Sano, M., 2019. Artificial intelligence to predict needs for urgent revascularization from 12-leads electrocardiography in emergency patients. *PLoS One*, *14*(1), p. e0210103.
42. Maaser, C., Sturm, A., Vavricka, S.R., Kucharzik, T., Fiorino, G., Annese, V., Calabrese, E., Baumgart, D.C., Bettenworth, D., Borralho Nunes, P. and Burisch, J., 2019. ECCO-ESGAR guideline for diagnostic assessment in IBD Part 1: Initial diagnosis, monitoring of known IBD, detection of complications. *Journal of Crohn's and Colitis*, *13*(2), pp. 144–164.
43. Sturm, A., Maaser, C., Calabrese, E., Annese, V., Fiorino, G., Kucharzik, T., Vavricka, S.R., Verstockt, B., van Rheenen, P., Tolan, D. and Taylor, S.A., 2019. ECCO-ESGAR guideline for diagnostic assessment in IBD Part 2: IBD scores and general principles and technical aspects. *Journal of Crohn's and Colitis*, *13*(3), pp. 273–284.
44. Neurath, M.F., 2020. Host–microbiota interactions in inflammatory bowel disease. *Nature Reviews Gastroenterology & Hepatology*, *17*(2), pp. 76–77.
45. Alivernini, S., MacDonald, L., Elmesmari, A., Finlay, S., Tolusso, B., Gigante, M.R., Petricca, L., Di Mario, C., Bui, L., Perniola, S. and Attar, M., 2020. Distinct synovial tissue macrophage subsets regulate inflammation and remission in rheumatoid arthritis. *Nature Medicine*, *26*(8), pp. 1295–1306.
46. Privitera, G., Onali, S., Pugliese, D., Renna, S., Savarino, E., Viola, A., Ribaldone, D.G., Buda, A., Bezzio, C., Fiorino, G. and Fantini, M.C., 2021. Dual targeted therapy: A possible option for the management of refractory inflammatory bowel disease. *Journal of Crohn's and Colitis*, *15*(2), pp. 335–339.
47. Takenaka, K., Ohtsuka, K., Fujii, T., Negi, M., Suzuki, K., Shimizu, H., Oshima, S., Akiyama, S., Motobayashi, M., Nagahori, M. and Saito, E., 2020. Development and validation of a deep neural network for accurate evaluation of endoscopic images from patients with ulcerative colitis. *Gastroenterology*, *158*(8), pp. 2150–2157.
48. Keenan, T.E., Burke, K.P. and Van Allen, E.M., 2019. Genomic correlates of response to immune checkpoint blockade. *Nature Medicine*, *25*(3), pp. 389–402.
49. Plesca, I., Tunger, A., Müller, L., Wehner, R., Lai, X., Grimm, M.O., Rutella, S., Bachmann, M. and Schmitz, M., 2020. Characteristics of tumor-infiltrating lymphocytes prior to and during immune checkpoint inhibitor therapy. *Frontiers in Immunology*, *11*, p. 364.
50. Meléndez, B., Van Campenhout, C., Rorive, S., Remmelink, M., Salmon, I. and D'Haene, N., 2018. Methods of measurement for tumor mutational burden in tumor tissue. *Translational Lung Cancer Research*, *7*(6), p. 661.
51. Choucair, K., Morand, S., Stanbery, L., Edelman, G., Dworkin, L. and Nemunaitis, J., 2020. TMB: A promising immune-response biomarker, and potential spearhead in advancing targeted therapy trials. *Cancer Gene Therapy*, *27*(12), pp. 841–853.
52. Fan, S., Gao, X., Qin, Q., Li, H., Yuan, Z. and Zhao, S., 2020. Association between tumor mutation burden and immune infiltration in ovarian cancer. *International Immunopharmacology*, *89*, p. 107126.

53. Chung, H.C., Lopez-Martin, J.A., Kao, S.C.H., Miller, W.H., Ros, W., Gao, B., Marabelle, A., Gottfried, M., Zer, A., Delord, J.P. and Penel, N., 2018. Phase 2 study of pembrolizumab in advanced small-cell lung cancer (SCLC): KEYNOTE-158. *Journal of Clinical Oncology*, *36*, p. 8506.
54. Park, J., Lee, J.Y. and Kim, S., 2019. How to use immune checkpoint inhibitor in ovarian cancer?. *Journal of Gynecologic Oncology*, *30*(5).
55. Morse, C.B., Elvin, J.A., Gay, L.M. and Liao, J.B., 2017. Elevated tumor mutational burden and prolonged clinical response to anti-PD-L1 antibody in platinum-resistant recurrent ovarian cancer. *Gynecologic Oncology Reports*, *21*, pp. 78–80.
56. Hoppe, M.M., Sundar, R., Tan, D.S. and Jeyasekharan, A.D., 2018. Biomarkers for homologous recombination deficiency in cancer. *JNCI: Journal of the National Cancer Institute*, *110*(7), pp. 704–713.
57. Keung, M.Y.T., Wu, Y. and Vadgama, J.V., 2019. PARP inhibitors as a therapeutic agent for homologous recombination deficiency in breast cancers. *Journal of Clinical Medicine*, *8*(4), p. 435.
58. Moschetta, M., George, A., Kaye, S.B. and Banerjee, S., 2016. BRCA somatic mutations and epigenetic BRCA modifications in serous ovarian cancer. *Annals of Oncology*, *27*(8), pp. 1449–1455.
59. Manchana, T., Phoolcharoen, N. and Tantbirojn, P., 2019. BRCA mutation in high grade epithelial ovarian cancers. *Gynecologic Oncology Reports*, *29*, pp. 102–105.
60. Cortellini, A., Bersanelli, M., Buti, S., Gambale, E., Atzori, F., Zoratto, F., Parisi, A., Brocco, D., Pireddu, A., Cannita, K. and Iacono, D., 2018. Family history of cancer as surrogate predictor for immunotherapy with anti-PD1/PD-L1 agents: Preliminary report of the FAMI-L1 study. *Immunotherapy*, *10*(8), pp. 643–655.
61. Le, D.T., Durham, J.N., Smith, K.N., Wang, H., Bartlett, B.R., Aulakh, L.K., Lu, S., Kemberling, H., Wilt, C., Luber, B.S. and Wong, F., 2017. Mismatch repair deficiency predicts response of solid tumors to PD-1 blockade. *Science*, *357*(6349), pp. 409–413.
62. Marabelle, A., Le, D.T., Ascierto, P.A., Di Giacomo, A.M., De Jesus-Acosta, A., Delord, J.P., Geva, R., Gottfried, M., Penel, N., Hansen, A.R. and Piha-Paul, S.A., 2020. Efficacy of pembrolizumab in patients with noncolorectal high microsatellite instability/mismatch repair–deficient cancer: Results from the phase II KEYNOTE-158 study. *Journal of Clinical Oncology*, *38*(1), pp. 1–10.
63. Disis, M.L., Patel, M., Pant, S., Hamilton, E.P., Lockhart, A.C., Kelly, K., Thaddeus-Beck, J., Gordon, M., Weiss, G.J., Ejadi, S. and Taylor, M.H., 2015. 2749 Avelumab (MSB0010718C), an anti-PD-L1 antibody, in patients with recurrent or refractory ovarian cancer: A phase Ib trial reporting safety and clinical activity. *European Journal of Cancer*, *3*(51), pp. S546–S547.
64. Coleman, R.L., Brady, M.F., Herzog, T.J., Sabbatini, P., Armstrong, D.K., Walker, J.L., Kim, B.G., Fujiwara, K., Tewari, K.S., O'Malley, D.M. and Davidson, S.A., 2017. Bevacizumab and paclitaxel–carboplatin chemotherapy and secondary cytoreduction in recurrent, platinum-sensitive ovarian cancer (NRG Oncology/Gynecologic Oncology Group study GOG-0213): a multicentre, open-label, randomised, phase 3 trial. *The Lancet Oncology*, *18*(6), pp. 779–791.
65. Solinas, C., Marcoux, D., Garaud, S., Vitória, J.R., Van den Eynden, G., de Wind, A., De Silva, P., Boisson, A., Craciun, L., Larsimont, D. and Piccart-Gebhart, M., 2019. BRCA gene mutations do not shape the extent and organization of tumor infiltrating lymphocytes in triple negative breast cancer. *Cancer Letters*, *450*, pp. 88–97.
66. Riaz, N., Havel, J.J., Makarov, V., Desrichard, A., Urba, W.J., Sims, J.S., Hodi, F.S., Martín-Algarra, S., Mandal, R., Sharfman, W.H. and Bhatia, S., 2017. Tumor and microenvironment evolution during immunotherapy with nivolumab. *Cell*, *171*(4), pp. 934–949.

67. Hillen, F., Baeten, C.I., van de Winkel, A., Creytens, D., van der Schaft, D.W., Winnepenninckx, V. and Griffioen, A.W., 2008. Leukocyte infiltration and tumor cell plasticity are parameters of aggressiveness in primary cutaneous melanoma. *Cancer Immunology, Immunotherapy*, *57*, pp. 97–106.
68. Eckhardt, S.G. and Lieu, C., 2019. Is precision medicine an oxymoron?. *JAMA Oncology*, *5*(2), pp. 142–143.
69. Verma, S., Miles, D., Gianni, L., Krop, I.E., Welslau, M., Baselga, J., Pegram, M., Oh, D.Y., Diéras, V., Guardino, E. and Fang, L., 2012. Trastuzumab emtansine for HER2-positive advanced breast cancer. *New England Journal of Medicine*, *367*(19), pp. 1783–1791.
70. Gambardella, V., Fleitas, T., Tarazona, N., Cejalvo, J.M., Gimeno-Valiente, F., Martinez-Ciarpaglini, C., Huerta, M., Roselló, S., Castillo, J., Roda, D. and Cervantes, A., 2019. Towards precision oncology for HER2 blockade in gastroesophageal adenocarcinoma. *Annals of Oncology*, *30*(8), pp. 1254–1264.
71. Birkbak, N.J. and McGranahan, N., 2020. Cancer genome evolutionary trajectories in metastasis. *Cancer Cell*, *37*(1), pp. 8–19.
72. Clevers, H., 2016. Modeling development and disease with organoids. *Cell*, *165*(7), pp. 1586–1597.
73. Letai, A., 2017. Functional precision cancer medicine—moving beyond pure genomics. *Nature Medicine*, *23*(9), pp. 1028–1035.
74. Okada, S., Vaeteewoottacharn, K. and Kariya, R., 2018. Establishment of a patient-derived tumor xenograft model and application for precision cancer medicine. *Chemical and Pharmaceutical Bulletin*, *66*(3), pp. 225–230.
75. Gerlinger, M., Rowan, A.J., Horswell, S., Larkin, J., Endesfelder, D., Gronroos, E., Martinez, P., Matthews, N., Stewart, A., Tarpey, P. and Varela, I., 2012. Intratumor heterogeneity and branched evolution revealed by multiregion sequencing. *New England Journal of Medicine*, *366*(10), pp. 883–892.
76. Van der Velden, D.L., Van Herpen, C.M.L., Van Laarhoven, H.W.M., Smit, E.F., Groen, H.J.M., Willems, S.M., Nederlof, P.M., Langenberg, M.H.G., Cuppen, E., Sleijfer, S. and Steeghs, N., 2017. Molecular tumor boards: Current practice and future needs. *Annals of Oncology*, *28*(12), pp. 3070–3075.
77. van de Haar, J., Hoes, L. and Voest, E., 2019. Advancing molecular tumour boards: Highly needed to maximise the impact of precision medicine. *Esmo Open*, *4*(2).
78. Mirkov, M.U., Janss, L., Vermeulen, S.H., van de Laar, M.A., van Riel, P.L., Guchelaar, H.J., Brunner, H.G., Albers, C.A. and Coenen, M.J., 2015. Estimation of heritability of different outcomes for genetic studies of TNFi response in patients with rheumatoid arthritis. *Annals of the Rheumatic Diseases*, *74*(12), pp. 2183–2187.
79. Okada, Y., Wu, D., Trynka, G., Raj, T., Terao, C., Ikari, K., Kochi, Y., Ohmura, K., Suzuki, A., Yoshida, S. and Graham, R.R., 2014. Genetics of rheumatoid arthritis contributes to biology and drug discovery. *Nature*, *506*(7488), pp. 376–381.
80. Zhang, W., Lu, X., Cui, P., Piao, C., Xiao, M., Liu, X., Wang, Y., Wu, X., Liu, J. and Yang, L., 2019. Phase I/II clinical trial of a Wilms' tumor 1-targeted dendritic cell vaccination-based immunotherapy in patients with advanced cancer. *Cancer Immunology, Immunotherapy*, *68*, pp. 121–130.
81. Salvatorelli, L., Parenti, R., Leone, G., Musumeci, G., Vasquez, E. and Magro, G., 2015. Wilms tumor 1 (WT1) protein: Diagnostic utility in pediatric tumors. *Acta Histochemica*, *117*(4–5), pp. 367–378.
82. Thomas, S. and Prendergast, G.C., 2016. Cancer vaccines: A brief overview. *Vaccine Design: Methods and Protocols: Volume 1: Vaccines for Human Diseases*, pp. 755–761.
83. Kverneland, A.H., Pedersen, M., Westergaard, M.C.W., Nielsen, M., Borch, T.H., Olsen, L.R., Aasbjerg, G., Santegoets, S.J., van der Burg, S.H., Milne, K. and Nelson, B.H., 2020. Adoptive cell therapy in combination with checkpoint inhibitors in ovarian cancer. *Oncotarget*, *11*(22), p. 2092.

84. Rocconi, R.P., Stevens, E.E., Bottsford-Miller, J.N., Ghamande, S.A., Aaron, P., Wallraven, G., Bognar, E., Manley, M., Horvath, S., Manning, L. and Nemunaitis, J.J., 2020. A phase I combination study of vigil and atezolizumab in recurrent/refractory advanced-stage ovarian cancer: Efficacy assessment in BRCA1/2-wt patients. *Journal of Clinical Oncology, 38.*
85. Tanyi, J.L., Bobisse, S., Ophir, E., Tuyaerts, S., Roberti, A., Genolet, R., Baumgartner, P., Stevenson, B.J., Iseli, C., Dangaj, D. and Czerniecki, B., 2018. Personalized cancer vaccine effectively mobilizes antitumor T cell immunity in ovarian cancer. *Science Translational Medicine*, *10*(436), p. eaao5931.
86. Morand, S., Stanbery, L., Walter, A., Rocconi, R.P. and Nemunaitis, J., 2020. BRCA1/2 mutation status impact on autophagy and immune response: Unheralded target. *JNCI Cancer Spectrum*, *4*(6), p. pkaa077.
87. Zhan, L., Zhang, Y., Wang, W., Song, E., Fan, Y., Li, J. and Wei, B., 2016. Autophagy as an emerging therapy target for ovarian carcinoma. *Oncotarget*, *7*(50), p. 83476.
88. Chung, Y.C., Lu, L.C., Tsai, M.H., Chen, Y.J., Chen, Y.Y., Yao, S.P. and Hsu, C.P., 2013. The inhibitory effect of ellagic acid on cell growth of ovarian carcinoma cells. *Evidence-Based Complementary and Alternative Medicine*, *2013*(1), p. 306705.
89. Kaneko, N., Nakamura, A., Washimi, Y., Kato, T., Sakurai, T., Arahata, Y., Bundo, M., Takeda, A., Niida, S., Ito, K. and Toba, K., 2014. Novel plasma biomarker surrogating cerebral amyloid deposition. *Proceedings of the Japan Academy, Series B*, *90*(9), pp. 353–364.
90. Blennow, K. and Zetterberg, H., 2018. Biomarkers for Alzheimer's disease: Current status and prospects for the future. *Journal of Internal Medicine*, *284*(6), pp. 643–663.
91. Wasinger, V.C., Cordwell, S.J., Cerpa-Poljak, A., Yan, J.X., Gooley, A.A., Wilkins, M.R., Duncan, M.W., Harris, R., Williams, K.L. and Humphery-Smith, I., 1995. Progress with gene-product mapping of the Mollicutes: Mycoplasma genitalium. *Electrophoresis*, *16*(1), pp. 1090–1094.
92. The Financial Times, 2021. Proteomics: Searching for the real stuff of life. *The Financial Times*, *14*, p. 20.
93. Kota, U. and Stolowitz, M.L., 2016. Improving proteome coverage by reducing sample complexity via chromatography. In *Modern Proteomics–Sample Preparation, Analysis and Practical Applications*, pp. 83–143. Springer.
94. Kaur, G., Poljak, A., Ali, S.A., Zhong, L., Raftery, M.J. and Sachdev, P., 2021. Extending the depth of human plasma proteome coverage using simple fractionation techniques. *Journal of Proteome Research*, *20*(2), pp. 1261–1279.
95. Ahn, S.B., Sharma, S., Mohamedali, A., Mahboob, S., Redmond, W.J., Pascovici, D., Wu, J.X., Zaw, T., Adhikari, S., Vaibhav, V. and Nice, E.C., 2019. Potential early clinical stage colorectal cancer diagnosis using a proteomics blood test panel. *Clinical Proteomics*, *16*, pp. 1–20.
96. Prudova, A., Gocheva, V., Auf dem Keller, U., Eckhard, U., Olson, O.C., Akkari, L., Butler, G.S., Fortelny, N., Lange, P.F., Mark, J.C. and Joyce, J.A., 2016. TAILS N-terminomics and proteomics show protein degradation dominates over proteolytic processing by cathepsins in pancreatic tumors. *Cell Reports*, *16*(6), pp. 1762–1773.
97. Jain, M., Howe, G.R., Harrison, L. and Miller, A.B., 1989. A study of repeatability of dietary data over a seven-year period. *American Journal of Epidemiology*, *129*(2), pp. 422–429.
98. Serada, S., Fujimoto, M., Ogata, A., Terabe, F., Hirano, T., Iijima, H., Shinzaki, S., Nishikawa, T., Ohkawara, T., Iwahori, K. and Ohguro, N., 2010. iTRAQ-based proteomic identification of leucine-rich α-2 glycoprotein as a novel inflammatory biomarker in autoimmune diseases. *Annals of the Rheumatic Diseases*, *69*(4), pp. 770–774.
99. Zhang, Q., Huang, R., Tang, Q., Yu, Y., Huang, Q., Chen, Y., Wang, G. and Wang, X., 2018. Leucine-rich alpha-2-glycoprotein-1 is up-regulated in colorectal cancer and is a tumor promoter. *OncoTargets and Therapy*, pp. 2745–2752.

100. Bauer, M., Ahrné, E., Baron, A.P., Glatter, T., Fava, L.L., Santamaria, A., Nigg, E.A. and Schmidt, A., 2014. Evaluation of data-dependent and-independent mass spectrometric workflows for sensitive quantification of proteins and phosphorylation sites. *Journal of Proteome Research*, *13*(12), pp. 5973–5988.
101. Whiteaker, J.R., Zhao, L., Yan, P., Ivey, R.G., Voytovich, U.J., Moore, H.D., Lin, C. and Paulovich, A.G., 2015. Peptide immunoaffinity enrichment and targeted mass spectrometry enables multiplex, quantitative pharmacodynamic studies of phospho-signaling. *Molecular & Cellular Proteomics*, *14*(8), pp. 2261–2273.
102. Zhang, B., Whiteaker, J.R., Hoofnagle, A.N., Baird, G.S., Rodland, K.D. and Paulovich, A.G., 2019. Clinical potential of mass spectrometry-based proteogenomics. *Nature Reviews Clinical Oncology*, *16*(4), pp. 256–268.
103. Patel, V.J., Thalassinos, K., Slade, S.E., Connolly, J.B., Crombie, A., Murrell, J.C. and Scrivens, J.H., 2009. A comparison of labeling and label-free mass spectrometry-based proteomics approaches. *Journal of Proteome Research*, *8*(7), pp. 3752–3759.
104. Tan, H.Y., Wang, N., Zhang, C., Chan, Y.T., Yuen, M.F. and Feng, Y., 2021. Lysyl oxidase-like 4 fosters an immunosuppressive microenvironment during hepatocarcinogenesis. *Hepatology*, *73*(6), pp. 2326–2341.
105. Nesvizhskii, A.I., 2014. Proteogenomics: Concepts, applications and computational strategies. *Nature Methods*, *11*(11), pp. 1114–1125.
106. Gillette, M.A., Satpathy, S., Cao, S., Dhanasekaran, S.M., Vasaikar, S.V., Krug, K., Petralia, F., Li, Y., Liang, W.W., Reva, B. and Krek, A., 2020. Proteogenomic characterization reveals therapeutic vulnerabilities in lung adenocarcinoma. *Cell*, *182*(1), pp. 200–225.
107. Das, T., Andrieux, G., Ahmed, M. and Chakraborty, S., 2020. Integration of online omics-data resources for cancer research. *Frontiers in Genetics*, *11*, p. 578345.
108. Tyanova, S. and Cox, J., 2018. Perseus: A bioinformatics platform for integrative analysis of proteomics data in cancer research. *Cancer Systems Biology: Methods and Protocols*, pp. 133–148.
109. Weinstein, J.N., Collisson, E.A., Mills, G.B., Shaw, K.R., Ozenberger, B.A., Ellrott, K., Shmulevich, I., Sander, C. and Stuart, J.M., 2013. The cancer genome atlas pan-cancer analysis project. *Nature Genetics*, *45*(10), pp. 1113–1120.
110. Molinero-Fernández, Á., Moreno-Guzmán, M., Arruza, L., López, M.Á. and Escarpa, A., 2020. Polymer-based micromotor fluorescence immunoassay for on-the-move sensitive procalcitonin determination in very low birth weight infants' plasma. *ACS Sensors*, *5*(5), pp. 1336–1344.
111. Li, D., Dong, D., Lam, W., Xing, L., Wei, T. and Sun, D., 2019. Automated in vivo navigation of magnetic-driven microrobots using OCT imaging feedback. *IEEE Transactions on Biomedical Engineering*, *67*(8), pp. 2349–2358.
112. Iacovacci, V., Blanc, A., Huang, H., Ricotti, L., Schibli, R., Menciassi, A., Behe, M., Pané, S. and Nelson, B.J., 2019. High-resolution SPECT imaging of stimuli-responsive soft microrobots. *Small*, *15*(34), p. 1900709.
113. Yan, X., Zhou, Q., Vincent, M., Deng, Y., Yu, J., Xu, J., Xu, T., Tang, T., Bian, L., Wang, Y.X.J. and Kostarelos, K., 2017. Multifunctional biohybrid magnetite microrobots for imaging-guided therapy. *Science Robotics*, *2*(12), p. eaaq1155.
114. Singh, A.V., Ansari, M.H.D., Laux, P. and Luch, A., 2019. Micro-nanorobots: Important considerations when developing novel drug delivery platforms. *Expert Opinion on Drug Delivery*, *16*(11), pp. 1259–1275.
115. de Ávila, B.E.F., Angsantikul, P., Li, J., Angel Lopez-Ramirez, M., Ramírez-Herrera, D.E., Thamphiwatana, S., Chen, C., Delezuk, J., Samakapiruk, R., Ramez, V. and Obonyo, M., 2017. Micromotor-enabled active drug delivery for in vivo treatment of stomach infection. *Nature Communications*, *8*(1), p. 272.

116. Park, J., Kim, J.Y., Pane, S., Nelson, B.J. and Choi, H., 2021. Acoustically mediated controlled drug release and targeted therapy with degradable 3D porous magnetic microrobots. *Advanced Healthcare Materials*, *10*(2), p. 2001096.
117. Chen, C., Chen, L., Wang, P., Wu, L.F. and Song, T., 2019. Steering of magnetotactic bacterial microrobots by focusing magnetic field for targeted pathogen killing. *Journal of Magnetism and Magnetic Materials*, *479*, pp. 74–83.
118. Jindal, A., Mainuddin, Kumar, A., Ratnesh, R.K. and Singh, J., 2024. Nanotechnology driven lipid and metalloid based formulations targeting blood–brain barrier (3B) for brain tumor. *Indian Journal of Microbiology*, pp. 1–28.
119. Soda, P., D'Amico, N.C., Tessadori, J., Valbusa, G., Guarrasi, V., Bortolotto, C., Akbar, M.U., Sicilia, R., Cordelli, E., Fazzini, D. and Cellina, M., 2021. AIforCOVID: Predicting the clinical outcomes in patients with COVID-19 applying AI to chest-X-rays. An Italian multicentre study. *Medical Image Analysis*, *74*, p. 102216.
120. Shui, L., Ren, H., Yang, X., Li, J., Chen, Z., Yi, C., Zhu, H. and Shui, P., 2021. The era of radiogenomics in precision medicine: An emerging approach to support diagnosis, treatment decisions, and prognostication in oncology. *Frontiers in Oncology*, *10*, p. 570465.
121. Avery, E., Sanelli, P.C., Aboian, M. and Payabvash, S., 2022, April. Radiomics: A primer on processing workflow and analysis. In *Seminars in Ultrasound, CT and MRI*, Vol. 43, No. 2, pp. 142–146. WB Saunders.
122. Cellina, M., Pirovano, M., Ciocca, M., Gibelli, D., Floridi, C. and Oliva, G., 2021. Radiomic analysis of the optic nerve at the first episode of acute optic neuritis: An indicator of optic nerve pathology and a predictor of visual recovery?. *La radiologia Medica*, *126*, pp. 698–706.
123. Tan, P.-N., Steinbach, M., Karpatne, A. and Kumar, V., 2018. *Introduction to Data Mining*, 2nd ed.; What's New in Computer Science; Pearson: London, UK.
124. Vicini, S., Bortolotto, C., Rengo, M., Ballerini, D., Bellini, D., Carbone, I., Preda, L., Laghi, A., Coppola, F. and Faggioni, L., 2022. A narrative review on current imaging applications of artificial intelligence and radiomics in oncology: Focus on the three most common cancers. *La radiologia Medica*, *127*(8), pp. 819–836.
125. Cellina, M., Cè, M., Irmici, G., Ascenti, V., Caloro, E., Bianchi, L., Pellegrino, G., D'Amico, N., Papa, S. and Carrafiello, G., 2022. Artificial intelligence in emergency radiology: Where are we going?. *Diagnostics*, *12*(12), p. 3223.
126. Yasmin, G. Gupta, U., 2024, March 25. An improved supervised machine learning model for gold price prediction. *InAIP Conference Proceedings*, Vol. 2919, No. 1. AIP Publishing.
127. Müller, A.C. and Guido, S., 2016. *Introduction to Machine Learning with Python: A Guide for Data Scientists*. O'Reilly Media, Inc.
128. Pal, S., Roy, S., Banerjee, A., Majumdar, K., Gupta, U., Rana, S. and Shetty, S., 2023, November. A unified approach for identification and analysis of the sources of uncertainty in machine learning techniques. In *International Conference on Computing and Communication Networks*, pp. 443–453. Singapore: Springer Nature Singapore.
129. Sansone, M., Fusco, R., Grassi, F., Gatta, G., Belfiore, M.P., Angelone, F., Ricciardi, C., Ponsiglione, A.M., Amato, F., Galdiero, R. and Grassi, R., 2023. Machine learning approaches with textural features to calculate breast density on mammography. *Current Oncology*, *30*(1), pp. 839–853.
130. Fusco, R., Di Bernardo, E., Piccirillo, A., Rubulotta, M.R., Petrosino, T., Barretta, M.L., Mattace Raso, M., Vallone, P., Raiano, C., Di Giacomo, R. and Siani, C., 2022. Radiomic and artificial intelligence analysis with textural metrics extracted by contrast-enhanced mammography and dynamic contrast magnetic resonance imaging to detect breast malignant lesions. *Current Oncology*, *29*(3), pp. 1947–1966.

131. Gupta, U., Pranav, A., Kohli, A., Ghosh, S. and Singh, D., 2024. The contribution of artificial intelligence to drug discovery: Current progress and prospects for the future. *Microbial Data Intelligence and Computational Techniques for Sustainable Computing*, pp. 1–23.
132. Agatonovic-Kustrin, S. and Beresford, R., 2000. Basic concepts of artificial neural network (ANN) modeling and its application in pharmaceutical research. *Journal of Pharmaceutical and Biomedical Analysis, 22*(5), pp. 717–727.
133. Santosh, K.C., Das, N. and Ghosh, S., 2021. Deep learning models for medical imaging. In *Deep Learning Models for Medical Imaging*, pp. i–iii. Amsterdam, The Netherlands: Elsevier.
134. Abd-Ellah, M.K., Awad, A.I., Khalaf, A.A. and Hamed, H.F., 2019. A review on brain tumor diagnosis from MRI images: Practical implications, key achievements, and lessons learned. *Magnetic Resonance Imaging, 61*, pp. 300–318.
135. Parekh, V.S. and Jacobs, M.A., 2019. Deep learning and radiomics in precision medicine. *Expert Review of Precision Medicine and Drug Development, 4*(2), pp. 59–72.
136. Krizhevsky, A., Sutskever, I. and Hinton, G.E., 2012. Imagenet classification with deep convolutional neural networks. *Advances in Neural Information Processing Systems, 25*.
137. Simonyan, K., 2014. Very deep convolutional networks for large-scale image recognition. *arXiv preprint* arXiv:1409.1556.
138. Szegedy, C., Liu, W., Jia, Y., Sermanet, P., Reed, S., Anguelov, D., Erhan, D., Vanhoucke, V. and Rabinovich, A., 2015. Going deeper with convolutions. In *Proceedings of the IEEE Conference on Computer Vision and Pattern Recognition*, pp. 1–9. IEEE.
139. Abiwinanda, N., Hanif, M., Hesaputra, S.T., Handayani, A. and Mengko, T.R., 2019. *Brain Tumor Classification Using Convolutional Neural Network.* Singapore: Springer.
140. Pope, W.B., 2018. Brain metastases: Neuroimaging. *Handbook of Clinical Neurology, 149*, pp. 89–112.
141. Gupta, U., Trivedi, G. and Singh, D., 2024. Human AI: Social network analysis. In *Emotional AI and Human-AI Interactions in Social Networking*, pp. 213–235. Academic Press.
142. Blasiak, A., Khong, J. and Kee, T., 2020. CURATE. AI: optimizing personalized medicine with artificial intelligence. *SLAS Technology: Translating Life Sciences Innovation, 25*(2), pp. 95–105.
143. Mainuddin, Kumar, A., Ratnesh, R.K., Singh, J., Dumoga, S., Sharma, N. and Jindal, A., 2024. Physical characterization and bioavailability assessment of 5-fluorouracil-based nanostructured lipid carrier (NLC): In vitro drug release, hemolysis, and permeability modulation. *Medical Oncology, 41*(5), p. 95.
144. Kumar, A., Jindal, A. and Singh Arya, P.K., 2023. Cytotoxicity and bioavailability assessment from thiamin-phospholipid complexation loaded Ajwain oil based self nano-emulsifying system. *Journal of Dispersion Science and Technology*, pp. 1–17.
145. Jindal, A. and Kumar, A., 2022. Physical characterization of clove oil based self Nano-emulsifying formulations of cefpodoxime proxetil: Assessment of dissolution rate, antioxidant & antibacterial activity. *OpenNano, 8*, p. 100087.
146. Kumar, A. and Jindal, A., 2024. Cytotoxicity and bioavailability assessment from micellar system based Thiamine-Phospholipid complexes. *Journal of Molecular Liquids*, p. 125177.
147. Kumar, A., Singh Arya, P.K. and Jindal, A., 2024. Modulation of intestinal permeability of 5-fluorouracil via phospholipid interaction based lipophilic complex designing and pharmacokinetic assessment. *Journal of Dispersion Science and Technology*, pp. 1–13.

148. Kumar, A., Shipam, K. and Kumar, S., 2024. Raspberry ketone loaded self nanoemulsifying system of cardamom oil: Assessment of phase behavior, dissolution rate and anti-hyperlipidemic activity. *Journal of Drug Delivery Science and Technology*, *99*, p. 105937.
149. Khan, J., Jindal, A., Kumar, A. and Sharma, N., 2025. Tuning stimuli-triggered mesoporous silica nanoparticles in novel way of brain cancer therapy. *Bio Nano Science*, *15*(1), pp. 1–16.
150. Gulati, G., Jain, R., Jha, H.A., Sharma, M., Gupta, D. and Gupta, U., 2023, September. Face mask detection using CNN model and transfer learning. In *2023 3rd International Conference on Innovative Sustainable Computational Technologies (CISCT)*, pp. 1–6. IEEE.

6 Large Language Models in Healthcare Information Systems

Overcoming Challenges to Achieve Personalized Care

Sreenivasan M and Abhay Narayan

6.1 INTRODUCTION

The healthcare landscape is undergoing a profound transformation, driven by rapid advancements in artificial intelligence (AI) and the emergence of large language models (LLMs) such as GPT-4 [1]. These technologies have captured global attention due to their impressive capabilities, igniting widespread discussions about their potential to revolutionize various sectors, particularly healthcare. The remarkable success of conversational AI tools like ChatGPT, which attracted over 100 million users within just two months of its November 2022 launch, as shown in Figure 6.2 [2], underscores the transformative power and broad appeal of these innovations. This swift adoption reflects a growing interest in leveraging AI to address persistent challenges in healthcare delivery and provides the potential to enhance efficiency, accuracy, and personalization. It also helps address long-standing issues such as excessive paperwork, diagnostic mistakes, and inefficient treatment processes. Implementing AI in healthcare systems presents a promising opportunity to improve patient outcomes and streamline operations. The technology can transform how healthcare services are delivered and managed by enhancing the speed and accuracy of diagnoses, personalizing treatment plans, and improving overall patient care. The evolving capabilities of these technologies promise to address and manage healthcare challenges more effectively.

The advanced capabilities of LLM models are well suited to facilitate the transformation of healthcare due to their proficiency in processing and analyzing vast amounts of unstructured data. These technologies excel at interpreting patient records, analyzing extensive medical literature, and utilizing real-time clinical information [3–6]. They generate actionable insights that represent a significant advancement in medical practice, enabling them to assist in diagnosing conditions, recommending treatment options, and predicting patient outcomes based on historical data. Their clinical applications are complemented by their growing role

DOI: 10.1201/9781003539483-6

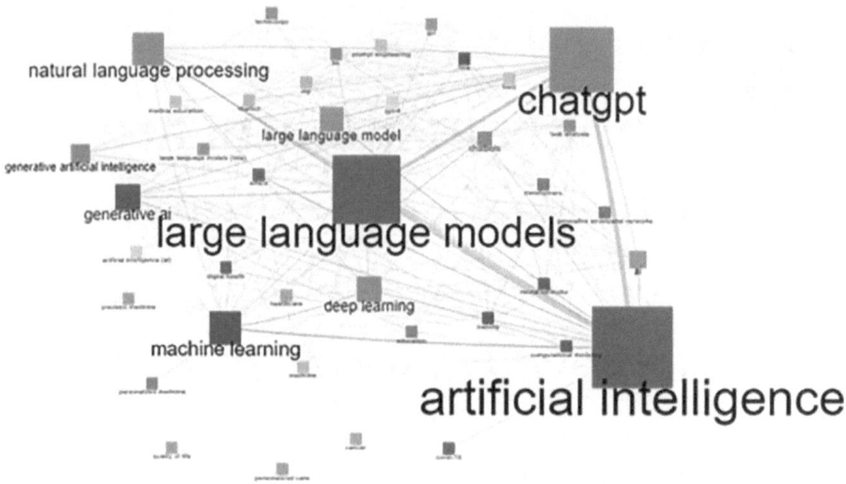

FIGURE 6.1 Common keywords.

in automating administrative tasks within healthcare settings. These models can manage appointment scheduling, patient record management, and communication between patients and providers, which helps reduce healthcare costs and enhance operational efficiency [7, 8]. Automation eases the administrative burden on healthcare professionals, allowing them to focus more on direct patient care. This shift is expected to significantly enhance the overall quality of care. The advancement in the AI technologies are anticipated to further refine personalized medicine, enabling the development of treatment plans tailored to each patient's unique genetic and lifestyle factors. Such personalized approaches helps to contribute more precise and effective healthcare. These evolving capabilities of AI offer the potential for a more efficient and individualized healthcare system (Figure 6.1 shows common terminology).

A major challenge in modern healthcare is the fragmentation of healthcare information systems (HISs), which often results in incomplete and decentralized patient data [9, 10]. This fragmentation complicates healthcare providers' efforts to obtain a comprehensive view of patient information, leading to delays in diagnosis, inappropriate treatments, and redundant tests [11, 12]. Integrating disparate HIS systems is crucial to overcoming these challenges and improving care delivery. Technologies such as Health Level Seven (HL7) and Fast Healthcare Interoperability Resources (FHIR) play a key role in this integration process by facilitating seamless data exchange and bridging gaps between isolated systems [13]. Enhancing interoperability through these technologies supports more coordinated and efficient care, which is essential for improving the accuracy and effectiveness of treatments. Utilizing these integration technologies is fundamental to advancing the healthcare system and ensuring that patients receive timely, comprehensive care based on unified and accurate information [14–17].

This chapter embarks on a comprehensive exploration of the integration of large language models within healthcare information systems, with a particular focus on

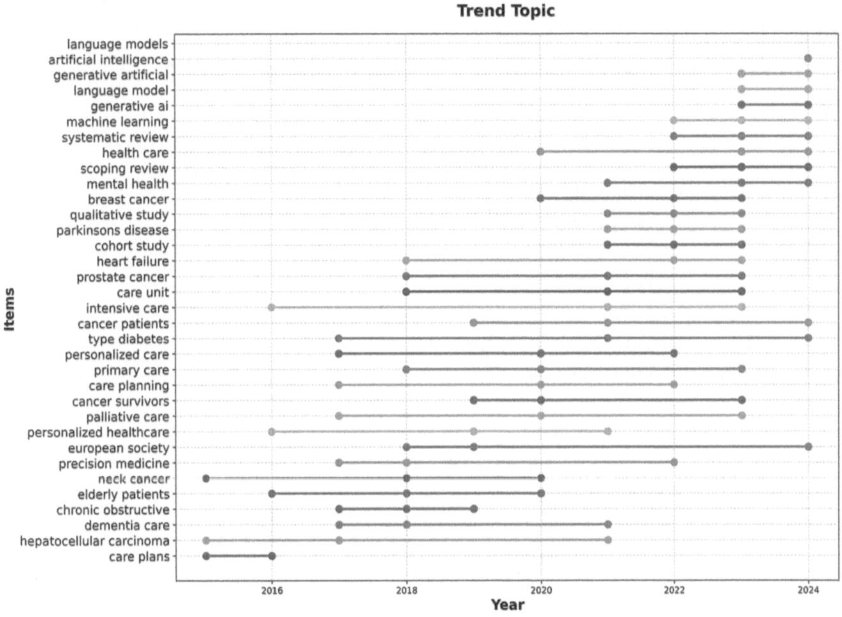

FIGURE 6.2 Trends.

advancing personalized care. It examines how LLMs can address the limitations of traditional HIS by improving communication between disparate systems and enabling a more comprehensive view of patient health. Additionally, the chapter delves into the technical, ethical, and practical considerations of deploying these models in clinical settings. Strategies to mitigate potential risks and ensure the ethical use of LLMs are also discussed. Providing a roadmap for harnessing the full potential of LLMs, the chapter contributes to the development of a new standard of personalized care in healthcare. Improving patient outcomes and advancing public health are central goals of this exploration. The integration of LLMs represents a significant step forward in achieving these objectives. This examination highlights the transformative potential of LLMs in creating a more connected and patient-centered healthcare system.

6.2 INTEGRATION OF HIS AND PERSONALIZED CARE

The integration of healthcare information systems plays a crucial role in advancing personalized care by enabling seamless communication between various healthcare systems. This integration allows healthcare providers to access comprehensive patient data, which leads to more accurate diagnoses and the development of tailored treatment plans, ultimately improving patient outcomes [18]. Moreover, it enhances care coordination and supports the delivery of personalized interventions by leveraging data from multiple sources. The successful implementation of HIS integration is supported by technologies such as interoperability standards

TABLE 6.1
Survey of the Integration of Health Information Systems and Personalized Care

Aspect	Description	Impact Level	Reference
Data Integration	Combining data from various HIS sources (e.g., EHRs, lab results) to create comprehensive patient profiles.	High	[23–25]
	Ensuring seamless data exchange between different HIS to support personalized care.	High	[24, 25]
Clinical Decision Support Systems	Integrating CDSSs with HISs to provide real-time, personalized recommendations during patient care.	High	[26, 27]
	Leveraging HIS data to enhance the accuracy and relevance of CDSS outputs.	Medium	[28]
Patient Engagement and Portal Access	Utilizing patient portals within HIS to offer personalized health insights and care plans.	Medium	[29]
	Enabling patients to interact with their health data, enhancing engagement and self-management.	High	[30, 31]
Privacy and Security	Ensuring that integrated HIS systems comply with privacy regulations while providing personalized care.	High	[32–34]
	Implementing robust security measures to protect sensitive patient data in a personalized care context.	High	[34, 35]
Interoperability	Enhancing interoperability between HIS components to facilitate the integration of personalized care models.	High	[36]
	Standardizing data formats and communication protocols across HISs to support personalized care.	High	[36, 37]

and application programing interface (APIs), which facilitate data exchange and system compatibility. Real-world examples demonstrate how integrated HISs can streamline healthcare workflows, reduce errors, and promote patient-centered care [19–22].

The integration of healthcare information systems provides several critical benefits that enhance personalized care, as shown in Table 6.1. Data integration merges information from various HIS sources, such as electronic health records (EHRs) and laboratory results, to create comprehensive patient profiles and ensure seamless data exchange between systems, which significantly supports personalized care. Clinical decision support systems (CDSSs), when integrated with HISs, offer real-time, personalized recommendations that improve decision-making accuracy. Patient engagement is bolstered through portals that provide personalized health insights and care plans, promoting greater patient involvement and self-management. Privacy and security are crucial, requiring robust measures to protect sensitive data and ensure compliance with regulations. Finally, improvements in interoperability and the standardization of data formats and communication protocols are essential for effectively integrating personalized care models. Collectively, these aspects demonstrate how HIS integration can transform patient care by enhancing data accessibility, decision-making, engagement, and security.

6.2.1 Benefits of Integrating HISs

6.2.1.1 Comprehensive Patient Data Access

The integration of healthcare information systems provides healthcare providers with access to complete and unified patient histories, encompassing critical details such as past treatments, allergies, and test results. Having a comprehensive view of a patient's medical history supports more informed clinical decisions, allowing physicians to consider all relevant factors when making treatment choices. This access to detailed information significantly reduces the likelihood of medical errors, ensuring that treatments are both safe and appropriate. Additionally, it helps avoid unnecessary and repetitive tests, leading to time and resource savings. The ability to review a holistic set of patient data contributes to a more accurate and efficient diagnosis. Healthcare providers can make better decisions about care plans when they have a full understanding of the patient's medical background. Enhanced data access improves coordination among different care providers, fostering a more collaborative approach to treatment. This thorough knowledge of a patient's health status ultimately leads to higher quality care and more effective management of health conditions. Integrating comprehensive data into patient care workflows supports better patient outcomes and resource utilization [32, 38–40, 41].

6.2.1.2 Improved Care Coordination

The integration of health information systems enhances communication and collaboration among healthcare providers by ensuring that all members of a patient's care team have access to the same up-to-date information. This seamless data sharing is crucial for managing patients with complex or chronic conditions, where multiple specialists are often involved. Improved coordination helps maintain continuity of care, as each provider is kept informed of the others' actions and decisions. This collaborative approach enables the development of multidisciplinary treatment plans that are cohesive and aligned with the patient's overall health needs. Effective care coordination reduces the risk of duplication and errors by facilitating timely information exchange. An integrated HIS also supports better tracking of patient progress and treatment responses across different care settings. Enhanced communication among care team members fosters a more holistic approach to patient management, addressing all aspects of a patient's health. This leads to more informed decision-making and tailored treatment strategies. With improved care coordination, healthcare teams work more effectively together, optimizing patient care and resource utilization. Better alignment among providers often results in improved patient outcomes and more efficient care delivery [29, 41, 42].

6.2.1.3 Tailored Treatment Plans

Access to comprehensive and detailed patient data through integrated health information systems enables healthcare providers to create personalized treatment plans that cater to the unique needs and preferences of each patient. These systems facilitate the development of customized care strategies by providing a thorough view of a patient's medical history, current health status, and other relevant factors. Predictive analytics further enhance these plans by analyzing data to forecast potential health issues and suggest preemptive interventions. Decision support tools embedded within HISs can analyze patient data in real time, recommending specific treatments, medications, or lifestyle changes based on the latest evidence and clinical guidelines. This approach ensures that treatment plans are not only effective but also tailored to the individual's specific conditions and preferences. Adapting care plans dynamically based on ongoing data contributes to more precise and responsive health care. Personalized treatment plans align with patient-centered care models, emphasizing the importance of addressing each patient's unique circumstances. Integrating these advanced tools supports a more individualized approach to medicine, making treatments as unique as the patients themselves. This personalized approach can lead to better adherence to treatment protocols and improved health outcomes. Furthermore, it enhances the overall patient experience by making healthcare more relevant and specific to their needs. The result is a more effective and patient-centric healthcare delivery system [24, 25, 41].

6.2.1.4 Enhanced Patient Engagement

Integrated health information systems enable patients to engage more actively in their healthcare through accessible patient portals that offer personalized health information and management tools. These portals enable patients to view their medical records, track their health metrics, and take part in the decision-making process regarding their care. Providing direct access to their health information empowers patients to manage chronic conditions more effectively, adhere to treatment plans, and make informed decisions about their health. This increased level of engagement is linked to improved health outcomes, as patients who are more involved in their care often demonstrate better adherence to treatments and adopt healthier lifestyles. Enhanced patient engagement also strengthens the patient-provider relationship, which is essential for effective healthcare delivery. Additionally, patients who actively use these portals can more easily communicate with their healthcare providers, ask questions, and report issues. Ongoing communication helps address concerns promptly and ensures that care plans are adjusted as needed. The interactive nature of patient portals supports proactive health management and preventive care. Overall, integrated HISs contribute to a more collaborative and patient-centered approach to healthcare. Fostering greater involvement and communication helps enhance the overall quality of care [43].

6.2.1.5 Efficient Healthcare Workflows

Integrating health information systems into healthcare settings can significantly enhance efficiency by automating various administrative tasks, such as scheduling, billing, and documentation. Traditionally, these tasks consume a considerable amount of time for healthcare providers, but automation through an HIS alleviates this burden. As a result, healthcare professionals can focus more on direct patient care, improving the quality of interactions and treatment. Integrated systems also streamline workflows by eliminating redundant processes, leading to a smoother and more efficient operation within healthcare facilities. This increased efficiency not only shortens patient wait times but also enhances the overall service delivery experience. Moreover, automating administrative functions helps reduce operational costs, making healthcare facilities more financially sustainable. The optimization of resources through HISs contributes to better productivity and more effective use of staff time. Integrating these systems enables healthcare organizations to achieve a higher level of operational performance and resource management. Improved workflow efficiency fosters a more responsive and patient-centered approach to care. The combination of reduced administrative workload and enhanced operational efficiency ultimately benefits both patients and healthcare providers [44].

6.2.2 Technological Enablers

6.2.2.1 Interoperability Standards

Interoperability standards like Health Level Seven and Fast Healthcare Interoperability Resources are crucial for ensuring that different healthcare information systems can communicate effectively with one another. These standards define how data is structured and transmitted between systems, ensuring that information remains consistent and accurate across various platforms. Adhering to these standards enables healthcare providers to integrate disparate systems, facilitating seamless data exchange and collaboration. This is particularly important in environments where multiple systems from different vendors are used, as it ensures that all systems can work together harmoniously. The result is a more connected healthcare ecosystem, where information flows freely and supports coordinated care [25, 29, 40].

6.2.2.2 APIs and Integration Platforms

Application programming interfaces and integration platforms are essential tools for enabling different software applications to communicate and share data within an integrated HIS. APIs act as bridges between systems, allowing them to interact and exchange information seamlessly, regardless of their underlying technology. This facilitates the integration of new tools and technologies into existing HISs, enabling healthcare providers to adopt innovative solutions without overhauling their entire IT infrastructure. Integration platforms further enhance this capability by managing data flow between systems, ensuring that information is synchronized and up to date across the board. These technologies are key enablers of a flexible, scalable, and responsive healthcare IT environment that can adapt to the evolving needs of patient care [22, 39, 40, 45–47].

6.2.2.3 Data Security and Privacy

Data security and privacy are critical considerations in the integration of HISs, particularly as the exchange of sensitive patient information increases. Secure data exchange protocols, such as encryption, ensure that patient information is protected during transmission and storage, preventing unauthorized access or breaches. Compliance with regulations like the Health Insurance Portability and Accountability Act (HIPAA) is also essential to maintaining patient trust and ensuring that healthcare organizations are accountable for protecting patient privacy. Robust security measures, including access controls and audit trails, are necessary to safeguard data within integrated systems. Prioritizing data security and privacy enables healthcare providers to build a trusted and secure HIS environment that supports personalized care while protecting patient rights [32, 34, 48].

6.3 ROLE OF LARGE LANGUAGE MODELS IN HEALTHCARE

Large language models like ChatGPT represent a significant advancement in artificial intelligence, particularly in the domain of natural language processing (NLP) [2, 49]. Their ability to generate human-like text and perform various language tasks has led to transformative changes across various industries [50]. In healthcare, LLMs offer innovative applications that enhance patient care and medical practice [3, 4]. Leveraging advanced algorithms and extensive datasets, these models contribute to multiple aspects of healthcare delivery. The integration of LLMs into healthcare systems presents both opportunities and challenges, necessitating careful consideration of their impact on patient outcomes, clinical decision-making, and overall healthcare efficiency [7, 8, 51].

6.3.1 Patient Engagement through Conversational AI

LLMs enhance patient engagement by providing real-time, interactive communication through digital health platforms. These models enable patients to ask questions about their health, treatment options, and care processes, receiving immediate and contextually relevant responses. This real-time interaction improves accessibility to healthcare information, making it available 24/7 and reducing the need for direct provider contact for routine queries. Enhanced patient engagement through conversational AI also aids in reducing patient anxiety and improving understanding of medical conditions. Moreover, LLMs can assist in managing appointments, sending medication reminders, and guiding patients through follow-up care. The ability of LLMs to converse naturally helps patients feel more connected to their healthcare providers. This increased connectivity supports patient adherence to treatment plans and fosters a more patient-centered approach. Additionally, conversational AI can provide educational resources and answer questions in a manner that is easy for patients to understand. Integrating LLMs in patient engagement ultimately contributes to improved health outcomes and greater patient satisfaction [52, 53].

6.3.2 Supporting Clinical Decision-Making

In clinical decision support systems, LLMs assist healthcare providers by analyzing patient data to offer evidence-based recommendations. These models process diverse data sources, including electronic health records, lab results, and medical histories, to support accurate diagnosis and treatment planning. Providing real-time insights and suggestions helps streamline the decision-making process, reducing the cognitive load on clinicians. This assistance is particularly valuable in complex cases where integrating information from various sources is crucial for effective decision-making. LLMs can also cross-reference patient data with the latest medical research and clinical guidelines, ensuring that recommendations reflect current best practices. Offering targeted advice based on comprehensive data analysis contributes to reducing diagnostic errors and improving treatment outcomes. Additionally, LLMs help identify potential drug interactions and contraindications, enhancing patient safety. Integrating LLMs into CDSSs promotes a more data-driven approach to clinical decision-making. While LLMs improve clinical efficiency, they must be used with caution, ensuring that recommendations are validated by healthcare professionals. The continued evolution of LLMs promises further enhancements in clinical decision support and patient care [49, 54].

6.3.3 Automating Medical History Collection

LLMs facilitate the automation of medical history collection, which enhances both the accuracy and efficiency of gathering patient information. These models interact with patients through structured dialogues, prompting them to provide detailed information about their medical histories, symptoms, and lifestyle factors. Automating this process reduces the time and effort required from healthcare professionals to collect and document patient histories manually. This method also minimizes the risk of human error and ensures that all relevant data is systematically captured. Automated systems help maintain consistency across different healthcare settings and improve the completeness of the collected data. Accurate medical histories are essential for effective diagnosis and treatment planning, as they provide a comprehensive view of the patient's health. Furthermore, LLMs can adapt their questioning based on patient responses, allowing for a more personalized data collection experience. The efficiency gained through automation allows healthcare providers to focus more on patient care rather than administrative tasks. Despite these advantages, it is crucial to regularly review and validate automated data collection processes to ensure they meet high standards of accuracy and reliability. Overall, LLMs contribute to more efficient and precise medical history collection, supporting better patient outcomes [5, 51].

6.3.4 Enhancing Research and Clinical Trials

LLMs significantly enhance the efficiency of research and clinical trials by improving patient recruitment and matching. These models can analyze large and complex databases to identify patients who meet the criteria for specific clinical trials, thereby accelerating the recruitment process. By efficiently processing and cross-referencing patient data with trial protocols, LLMs ensure that the right participants are selected for each study. This targeted approach helps in maintaining the integrity and relevance of research findings, as trials are populated with appropriate candidates. LLMs also assist in managing patient engagement throughout the trial, providing updates, answering questions, and ensuring compliance with study protocols. This improved alignment between patients and trials leads to more accurate and reliable research outcomes. Additionally, LLMs can streamline the data collection process during trials, reducing administrative burdens and enhancing data accuracy. The use of LLMs in research also facilitates the identification of trends and patterns across trials, contributing to the advancement of medical knowledge. Despite these benefits, it is important to address potential challenges such as data privacy and bias in the model's recommendations. Future advancements in LLMs promise to further enhance the efficiency and effectiveness of clinical research [55, 56].

6.3.5 Medical Education and Training

In medical education, LLMs provide valuable tools for simulation-based training and realistic case scenarios. These models generate complex and diverse patient cases, offering learners the opportunity to practice clinical reasoning and decision-making in a risk-free environment. Simulation-based training helps medical students and professionals develop critical thinking skills and apply theoretical knowledge to practical situations. LLMs can create scenarios that mimic real-world medical challenges, allowing for a more immersive and effective learning experience. Additionally, these models offer instant feedback on learners' decisions, highlighting areas for improvement and reinforcing best practices. This feedback loop accelerates the learning process and enhances the quality of education. LLMs also help in keeping medical professionals updated with the latest research and clinical guidelines, ensuring their knowledge remains current. By integrating LLMs into educational programs, healthcare training becomes more adaptable and responsive to the needs of learners. Overall, LLMs contribute to more effective and comprehensive medical education, preparing students and professionals for high-quality patient care [57–62].

6.3.6 Language Translation and Accessibility

LLMs play a pivotal role in addressing language barriers in healthcare, enabling real-time translation services that enhance communication and comprehension. These models translate medical documents, consent forms, and patient-provider interactions into multiple languages, ensuring clear and accurate information is delivered to patients, thus promoting more equitable and informed care. Real-time translation helps prevent misunderstandings and misdiagnoses that can occur due to language differences. LLMs also enhance equitable healthcare access and improve patient satisfaction by facilitating clear communication. These models support the delivery of culturally competent care, respecting patients' linguistic and cultural backgrounds. They also assist healthcare providers in learning essential phrases and medical terms in other languages, improving their ability to communicate effectively with diverse patient populations. The ability to offer translation services in real-time ensures that all patients, regardless of their language proficiency, can engage fully in their healthcare. Despite the benefits, it is important to ensure that translations are accurate and contextually appropriate. The ongoing development of LLMs promises to further enhance accessibility and inclusivity in healthcare [40, 51, 58].

6.3.7 Challenges and Future Directions

The deployment of LLMs in healthcare presents several challenges, particularly related to biases inherent in their training data. These biases can lead to unequal treatment recommendations and potentially exacerbate health disparities. Addressing these biases requires ongoing efforts to diversify training datasets and implement robust bias detection and mitigation strategies. Technical challenges also arise, such as ensuring seamless integration of LLMs with existing electronic health records and decision support systems. Ethical concerns, including maintaining patient privacy and ensuring transparency in AI-driven decisions, must be carefully managed to preserve public trust. The future development of LLMs will involve creating more refined regulatory frameworks to guide their use in healthcare. Collaborative research is essential to maximize the benefits of LLMs while mitigating potential risks. Additionally, continued advancements in LLM technology will likely lead to more sophisticated models that better address the complexities of healthcare. The successful integration of LLMs into healthcare systems will depend on addressing these challenges and leveraging collaborative efforts to advance the field [17, 19–22, 47].

6.4 INTEGRATION OF LLMS INTO ELECTRONIC HEALTH RECORD SYSTEMS

The integration of large language models into electronic health record systems holds considerable promise for enhancing various facets of healthcare delivery, including improved clinical decision support and more personalized patient interactions, as shown in Figure 6.3. However, documented examples of successful implementations are still relatively sparse. Challenges such as data interoperability, system compatibility, and the need for robust privacy protections have hindered widespread adoption. Addressing these issues is crucial for realizing the full benefits of LLM integration. As research and development continue, overcoming these barriers will be key to leveraging LLMs effectively within EHR systems. The progress in this area will likely shape the future of more efficient and personalized healthcare delivery.

6.4.1 Support for Clinical Documentation

One of the primary applications of LLMs in EHR systems is in supporting clinical documentation. LLMs can automate the transcription and organization of patient interactions, thus significantly reducing the administrative burden on healthcare providers. By generating accurate and comprehensive documentation from patient consultations, LLMs enable clinicians to allocate more time and focus to direct patient care rather than clerical tasks. This automation not only enhances efficiency but also reduces the likelihood of errors associated with manual data entry. Virtual health assistants powered by LLMs are increasingly recognized for their potential to streamline documentation processes and improve the overall quality of patient records [59, 60]. The successful application of LLMs in this domain highlights their capability to transform clinical workflows and enhance provider productivity.

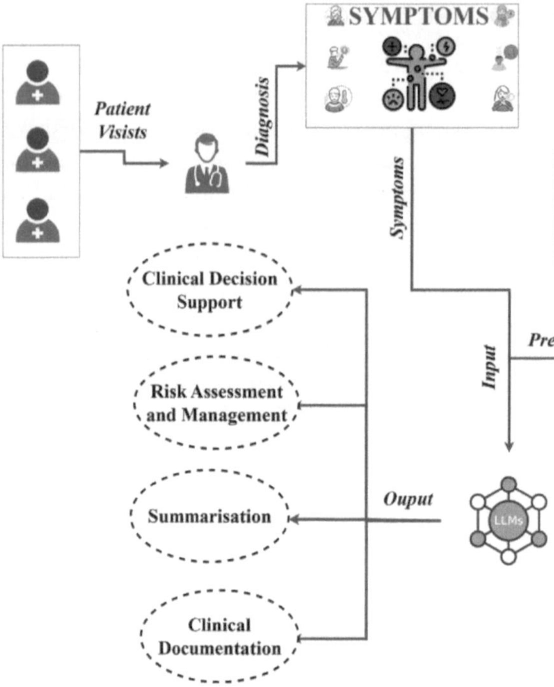

FIGURE 6.3 LLMs in healthcare.

6.4.2 Enhancing Clinical Decision Support

LLMs are revolutionizing clinical decision support systems by analyzing patient data and providing evidence-based recommendations. These models integrate and interpret information from electronic health records to offer insights that align with clinical guidelines. For example, LLMs can propose potential diagnoses and recommend treatment options based on a patient's medical history and current symptoms. This functionality improves the accuracy and speed of clinical decision-making, enhancing patient outcomes. Integrating LLMs into CDSSs enables a data-driven approach to patient care, allowing healthcare providers to make informed decisions more efficiently. LLMs can identify patterns and trends that may not be immediately visible to clinicians. Their inclusion in CDSSs supports a more systematic decision-making process, leading to better management of patient care. The overall impact is a more effective and responsive healthcare system, with the potential for significant improvements in patient outcomes [61, 62].

6.4.3 Risk Assessment and Management

Large language models have emerged as transformative tools in the field of healthcare, particularly in risk assessment and management. Leveraging historical patient data from electronic health records, LLMs can analyze complex patterns and relationships that might be missed by traditional methods. Through predictive analytics, these models can forecast the likelihood of disease development in individuals, enabling healthcare providers to identify high-risk patients early on. This foresight allows for the implementation of proactive care strategies, such as targeted screenings and preventive interventions, which can significantly reduce the incidence of severe health conditions. The predictive capability of LLMs not only enhances patient care by addressing potential health issues before they escalate but also optimizes the allocation of healthcare resources. By focusing on high-risk populations, health care systems can allocate their resources more efficiently, leading to better overall patient outcomes. Furthermore, the integration of LLMs in risk management practices supports a shift towards a more anticipatory approach to healthcare, ultimately contributing to more personalized and effective care delivery. As these models continue to evolve, their role in improving patient outcomes and resource management is expected to grow, solidifying their place in modern healthcare practices [59, 63].

6.4.4 Personalization of Patient Care

The potential of LLMs to personalize patient care is a noteworthy advantage of their integration into EHR systems. Analyzing a comprehensive range of patient records and individual preferences allows LLMs to assist in developing customized care plans that address specific patient needs. Personalized care plans enhance treatment efficacy and patient satisfaction by tailoring interventions to the unique characteristics and circumstances of each patient. The ability of LLMs to synthesize vast amounts of data enables a more nuanced and individualized approach to healthcare, promoting better alignment between patient needs and care strategies [1, 14].

6.4.5 Summary of Adoption Challenges

The adoption of LLMs in electronic health record systems presents several notable challenges. Data privacy and security are paramount concerns, as integrating LLMs raises risks related to patient data breaches and unauthorized access. This necessitates robust security measures and strict adherence to regulatory standards to protect sensitive information. Additionally, integrating LLMs with existing EHR systems can be complicated, with potential issues arising from compatibility with legacy systems and the need for extensive IT adjustments. Ensuring the accuracy and reliability of LLM-generated outputs is critical, as inaccuracies or biases could adversely affect patient care, highlighting the need for ongoing validation and refinement of these models. Financial considerations also pose a significant barrier, as the costs associated with acquiring, implementing, and maintaining LLM systems can be substantial. Smaller healthcare providers find these expenses challenging to manage. Ethical and regulatory concerns further complicate adoption, requiring careful navigation to ensure transparency, accountability, and patient consent in the use of LLMs. Aligning LLM applications with legal and ethical standards is essential to gain trust and acceptance among stakeholders. Additionally, challenges related to the effective training of healthcare staff to use these new technologies proficiently must be addressed. Overcoming these obstacles demands strategic planning and a commitment to continuous evaluation and improvement. Engaging stakeholders throughout the process can facilitate smoother integration and address concerns as they arise. Overall, addressing these challenges is crucial for realizing the full potential of LLMs in improving clinical workflows and patient care. Successful adoption will depend on a balanced approach that considers technical, financial, ethical, and regulatory factors. Tackling these issues effectively allows healthcare organizations to harness the benefits of LLMs while mitigating risks, requiring a concerted effort from all involved parties to ensure that LLMs can be integrated seamlessly into existing systems and used to their fullest potential.

6.5 LLMS IN PERSONALIZED CARE

Large language models offer transformative potential in personalized health care through their advanced capabilities in natural language processing. This section outlines the structured approach to integrating LLMs into personalized care, detailing each step (Figure 6.4) from data collection to implementation and systematically addressing data handling, model training, clinical integration, and continuous improvement, this approach ensures that LLMs enhance the precision and effectiveness of personalized healthcare. In the design, each step's objective is to optimize the utility of LLMs while addressing practical, ethical, and regulatory considerations essential for successful deployment.

6.5.1 Data Collection and Integration

Data collection begins with gathering comprehensive patient information, including medical history, genetic data, lifestyle factors, and treatment preferences. This diverse data pool is integrated from various sources such as electronic health records, wearable devices, and patient-reported outcomes to form a unified patient profile. Proper data integration enhances the accuracy of the patient profile, providing a holistic view necessary for personalized recommendations. Ensuring data privacy

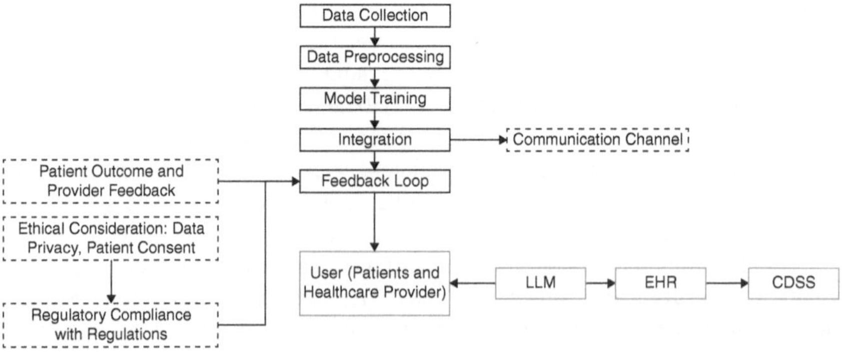

FIGURE 6.4 Design overview: LLMs in personalized care.

and security is crucial; compliance with regulations like HIPAA and the implementation of encryption and access controls safeguard sensitive patient information and maintain trust.

6.5.2 Data Preprocessing

Data preprocessing is a fundamental step in preparing data for effective use by LLMs. It begins with data cleaning, which addresses inconsistencies, fills in missing values, and standardizes formats to ensure high-quality input. This step is crucial for eliminating errors and ensuring that the data is reliable. Feature engineering follows, where relevant features such as biomarkers and symptoms are identified and extracted. These features are essential for enhancing the LLM's predictive capabilities and relevance. Normalization and scaling adjust different data types to a common scale, which facilitates uniform processing and improves the model's performance. Transforming data into a consistent format helps the LLM interpret and analyze it more effectively. Handling categorical data, dealing with outliers, and ensuring data privacy are also key considerations during preprocessing. The thorough preprocessing of data ensures that the LLM can provide accurate and meaningful predictions. Ultimately, well-prepared data is critical for the success of the LLM in delivering effective and personalized healthcare solutions.

6.5.3 Model Training and Fine-Tuning

Model training and fine-tuning are crucial for adapting LLMs to personalized care. Initially, the LLM undergoes pretraining on extensive medical datasets to establish a foundational understanding of medical terminology and scenarios. This pretraining phase builds the model's general knowledge base. Fine-tuning then customizes the LLM using specific patient data or defined cohorts, which enhances its relevance and accuracy for individual needs. This step involves adjusting the model to better align with the particular characteristics and requirements of different patient groups. Validation with separate, independent datasets is essential for evaluating the model's performance and ensuring its generalizability. Rigorous testing assesses how well the model delivers accurate, personalized recommendations across diverse patient populations. Continuous monitoring and iterative refinement further improve the model's precision and utility. Ensuring that the LLM adapts effectively to new information and patient-specific data is critical for maintaining high-quality care. Ultimately, a well trained and finely tuned LLM can significantly enhance the personalization of medical recommendations and treatments.

6.5.4 Implementation in Clinical Workflows

Successful integration of LLMs into clinical workflows demands effective coordination with existing systems, such as clinical decision support systems and EHRs. This integration ensures smooth interaction between healthcare providers and the AI system, thereby enhancing the decision-making process. Real-time deployment of LLMs through applications like chatbots or mobile health apps offers personalized advice and support during patient interactions. Such applications can assist in answering patient queries and providing tailored health recommendations. Additionally, tools designed for healthcare providers facilitate treatment planning and risk assessment, customizing recommendations to fit individual patient needs. Ensuring seamless integration helps in optimizing the use of LLMs, improving efficiency, and supporting high-quality care. Continuous feedback and adjustment of these tools are necessary to align with evolving clinical practices. Ultimately, effective implementation enhances both patient outcomes and provider efficiency.

6.5.5 Continuous Learning and Adaptation

Maintaining the effectiveness of large language models requires ongoing learning and adaptation. Establishing a feedback loop that integrates new patient data and outcomes is essential for refining the model's predictions and recommendations. Regular monitoring and evaluation ensure that the model's performance remains high and relevant. Periodic updates with the latest data and emerging research keep the LLM aligned with current healthcare developments. This continuous process enables the model to address evolving patient needs and clinical practices effectively. Incorporating real-world feedback further enhances the model's accuracy and utility. Staying responsive to new information and trends ensures that the LLM remains a valuable tool in personalized care. Ongoing learning and adaptation are crucial for maximizing the model's impact and effectiveness. Ultimately, these practices help sustain the model's relevance and improve its contributions to patient care.

6.5.6 Ethical and Regulatory Compliance

Ethical and regulatory concerns must be addressed for the responsible use of LLMs in healthcare. Implementing strategies to identify and mitigate biases ensures that the model provides fair and equitable care to all patients. Transparency and explainability mechanisms make the model's decision-making process understandable to both providers and patients, fostering trust. Compliance with healthcare regulations and ethical standards, including patient consent and data protection laws, ensures the model's legality and ethical use.

Education for both patients and healthcare providers is crucial for the successful integration of LLMs into healthcare. Providers need comprehensive training on effectively utilizing LLMs, understanding their strengths, limitations, and how they complement clinical practice. Patients should be informed about the role of LLMs in their care, including how their data is used and the benefits of personalized treatment. This education fosters trust and transparency, ensuring both parties are well informed and engaged. Enhancing understanding through education helps integrate LLMs smoothly into clinical workflows. Ultimately, informed patients and providers are better equipped to leverage AI for improved healthcare outcomes.

6.5.7 Outcome Measurement and Optimization

Measuring outcomes and optimizing large language models is crucial for ensuring their effectiveness in personalized care. To gauge the impact of LLMs, it is essential to track metrics such as treatment success rates, patient satisfaction, and adherence to recommendations. This data provides insights into how well the LLM contributes to personalized treatment plans and identifies areas for improvement. Continuous refinement of the LLM's algorithms, based on outcome data, enhances its performance and accuracy over time. Engaging in an iterative improvement process allows the model to adapt to changing healthcare needs and incorporate the latest medical knowledge. Regular assessment of the LLM's effectiveness in clinical settings helps maintain its relevance and utility. This process also involves updating training data and algorithms to reflect emerging trends and evidence in healthcare. Ensuring that LLMs are regularly optimized and evaluated keeps them valuable tools for personalized care. Ultimately, this approach supports high-quality, patient-centered outcomes by aligning LLM capabilities with evolving patient needs and treatment practices.

6.6 CHALLENGES OF LLM IN PERSONALIZED CARE

LLMs face significant challenges in accurately parsing the complex and varied clinical language used in healthcare settings. Medical terminology often includes specialized jargon, abbreviations, and context-specific nuances that are not easily understood by traditional natural language processing methods. These models may struggle with the dense and technical nature of clinical language, which can impede their ability to fully comprehend patient interactions and clinical notes. For example, medical records often contain shorthand notations and unique phrases specific to different specialties, which can lead to misinterpretation by LLMs. Furthermore, variations in language use across different healthcare providers and institutions can introduce inconsistencies that complicate text understanding. As a result, the ability of LLMs to support clinical decision-making and patient care may be significantly compromised if they cannot accurately interpret the nuances of medical language. This limitation can affect the precision of recommendations and the overall effectiveness of the model in real-world clinical applications. Addressing these challenges requires targeted efforts to enhance the model's language capabilities, including specialized training on medical datasets and the development of advanced NLP techniques. Improving the model's understanding of clinical language is essential for ensuring that LLMs can effectively contribute to personalized care and support healthcare professionals. Ongoing research and refinement are crucial to overcoming these linguistic barriers and maximizing the potential benefits of LLMs in healthcare.

6.6.1 Ethical Considerations

The deployment of LLMs in personalized care raises significant ethical concerns, particularly in relation to the accountability of AI-driven recommendations in clinical settings. Issues of bias in training data can result in skewed outcomes, which may disproportionately affect certain patient groups and exacerbate health disparities. Transparency in AI decision-making is crucial to ensure that patients and healthcare providers understand how recommendations are generated. Fairness in treatment recommendations is also essential to prevent discriminatory practices. Ethical guidelines must be developed and rigorously enforced to address these challenges. Continuous monitoring and auditing of AI systems can help identify and correct biases that may emerge over time. Additionally, the role of human oversight in AI-driven care must be clearly defined to maintain accountability. Informed consent should be prioritized, ensuring patients are aware of the involvement of AI in their care. Collaboration among ethicists, clinicians, and AI developers is necessary to create a robust ethical framework. Ultimately, responsible AI use in healthcare depends on balancing innovation with a commitment to patient welfare and equity.

6.6.2 Data Privacy and Security

Ensuring the privacy and security of patient data presents a critical challenge when integrating LLMs into personalized care. These models often handle sensitive medical information, necessitating strict adherence to data protection regulations such as HIPAA. Protecting patient data through encryption and controlled access is essential but can complicate the implementation of LLM-driven systems. Unauthorized access or data breaches could severely impact patient confidentiality and trust. Therefore, robust security measures, including advanced encryption and strict access controls, are necessary to safeguard patient information. Regular audits and updates to security protocols are vital to addressing potential vulnerabilities. Anonymization techniques should also be employed to minimize the risk of data exposure. Compliance with legal and ethical standards requires proactive management of these privacy concerns. Patient trust depends on the assurance that their data remains secure and is handled responsibly. Ultimately, the successful integration of LLMs in healthcare hinges on balancing innovation with stringent privacy and security safeguards.

6.6.3 Integration with Existing Systems

Integrating LLMs with existing electronic health record systems presents significant challenges due to potential compatibility issues. Discrepancies between new AI technologies and legacy systems can lead to workflow disruptions or require substantial customization efforts. Ensuring seamless operation within the established healthcare infrastructure is crucial to prevent interruptions in clinical processes and enhance overall efficiency. Effective integration demands careful collaboration between AI developers and healthcare IT teams to overcome technical obstacles like data format mismatches and system interoperability. Training healthcare staff on the new systems is also essential to ensure a smooth transition and minimize resistance. Continuous monitoring and iterative refinements can further optimize the integration process over time. Successfully navigating these challenges is key to unlocking the full potential of LLMs in personalized care. A well-executed integration will ultimately improve patient outcomes and streamline operations within the healthcare system.

6.6.4 Continuous Improvement and Adaptation

LLMs must undergo continuous improvement and adaptation to stay effective in the rapidly evolving healthcare landscape. As new medical knowledge and patient needs emerge, regular updates are essential to incorporate the latest research and best practices. Without ongoing refinement, the relevance and accuracy of these models can diminish, potentially compromising patient care. Implementing mechanisms for continuous learning is crucial to maintaining their effectiveness in personalized care applications. This process should include periodic retraining with updated data and integration of the latest clinical guidelines. Collaboration with healthcare professionals is necessary to ensure that the models align with current practices. Additionally, monitoring the performance of LLMs in real-world settings can identify areas for improvement. Adapting to new developments in medicine will keep the models relevant and useful. Ultimately, a commitment to continuous learning will enhance the impact of LLMs in delivering high-quality, personalized care.

6.7 RESEARCH DIRECTIONS

6.7.1 Understanding Ethical Implications

A critical area of research in applying large language models within healthcare revolves around the ethical considerations of their deployment, especially concerning personalized care. Key issues include the potential biases embedded in LLMs that could influence individualized treatment plans, impacting fairness and equity in patient care. Transparency of AI-driven recommendations is another major concern, as patients and providers must understand how decisions are made to trust and effectively use these systems. Accountability in clinical decision-making is also crucial, ensuring that the use of LLMs does not undermine responsibility for patient outcomes. Ongoing research aims to address these challenges by developing comprehensive ethical guidelines for integrating LLMs into personalized care frameworks. This includes creating standards for transparency and bias mitigation, as well as ensuring that LLMs operate within a framework that protects sensitive patient data. Additionally, efforts are focused on establishing protocols for responsible AI use, balancing innovation with ethical considerations. Researchers are also exploring the impact of LLMs on the doctor patient relationship and how to maintain human oversight. The goal is to ensure that the deployment of LLMs enhances, rather than compromises, the ethical standards of personalized healthcare. These issues are addressed by the research, which aims to foster trust and efficacy in the use of AI technologies in healthcare settings.

6.7.2 Enhancing Telehealth Services

The integration of large language models in telehealth is an emerging research frontier with significant potential for personalized healthcare. Ongoing studies are exploring how LLMs can improve telehealth services by enhancing communication between patients and providers, offering tailored diagnostic insights based on individual profiles, and optimizing management protocols with personalized health data. The aim is to integrate models like ChatGPT into telehealth platforms to boost the efficiency, personalization, and accessibility of healthcare delivery. Refining how LLMs are utilized in telehealth seeks to make interactions more meaningful and responsive to patient needs. This includes improving the accuracy and relevance of diagnostic support and ensuring that patient management is customized and effective. The goal is to create telehealth systems that are not only more efficient but also more attuned to the unique needs of each patient. The ongoing research is crucial for developing telehealth solutions that offer a higher level of personalized care.

6.7.3 Investigating User Modeling

User modeling in personalized healthcare represents a pivotal area of research where large language models are poised to offer substantial advancements. Meticulously analyzing patient interactions, preferences, and individual health data allows researchers to craft healthcare solutions tailored to each patient's unique needs. This approach leverages LLMs to enhance our comprehension of patient behavior and preferences, which is critical for developing targeted interventions. Through sophisticated analysis of diverse patient data, LLMs can identify subtle patterns and trends that may otherwise go unnoticed. This capability allows for the creation of highly personalized healthcare strategies that align with individual patient profiles. Additionally, LLMs can assist in predicting patient responses to various treatments based on historical data, leading to more effective and proactive healthcare management. The integration of LLMs into user modeling can also facilitate real-time adjustments to healthcare plans, improving their relevance and efficacy. As research progresses, the ability of LLMs to process and interpret vast amounts of data will continue to enhance their role in personalized healthcare. This evolution underscores the potential for LLMs to drive significant improvements in patient care through more nuanced and individualized approaches. Ultimately, this research direction highlights the transformative impact that LLMs could have on the future of personalized healthcare interventions.

6.7.4 Improving Documentation and Workflow

Investigating how large language models can transform healthcare documentation and workflow processes is essential, particularly within personalized care contexts. This involves evaluating LLMs' ability to automate routine administrative tasks, such as customizing medical documentation to individual patient needs, which can alleviate clerical burdens on healthcare professionals. Understanding how LLMs enhance operational efficiency while supporting personalized care is crucial. Research should also focus on how LLMs can streamline documentation processes without compromising accuracy or completeness. Examining integration strategies to ensure LLMs complement existing workflows and do not disrupt clinical practices is necessary. Additionally, studying the adaptability of LLMs to various medical specialties and documentation standards is important. Investigating the training requirements for LLMs to handle diverse documentation needs will be valuable. Ultimately, this research aims to leverage LLMs to improve both operational efficiency and the quality of patient care.

6.7.5 Fostering Collaboration between AI and Healthcare Professionals

Exploring the collaborative dynamics between large language models and healthcare professionals is crucial for advancing personalized care. Developing frameworks that facilitate effective human-AI collaboration is essential, ensuring that AI tools enhance rather than replace the decision-making capabilities of healthcare practitioners. This collaboration is particularly important in personalized care settings, where integrating AI's analytical capabilities with the nuanced understanding of human professionals can create individualized treatment plans. Research should focus on how LLMs can provide real-time, data-driven insights while preserving essential human elements such as empathy and clinical judgment. Creating intuitive interfaces and workflows that seamlessly integrate AI outputs with clinical expertise will be key. Additionally, balancing AI-driven recommendations with professional judgment is necessary to avoid over-reliance on technology. Training programs must also be developed to help healthcare professionals effectively interact with AI systems. Fostering a synergistic relationship between AI and human expertise will enhance the quality and personalization of patient care.

6.8 CONCLUSION AND FUTURE WORK

This chapter has explored the transformative potential of large language models within healthcare information systems, emphasizing their impact on advancing personalized care. Traditional HISs often suffer from decentralization, which limits effective communication and the ability to deliver customized care. LLMs present a significant opportunity to overcome these limitations by facilitating improved communication across healthcare systems and harnessing historical patient data to tailor treatments and recommendations more precisely. Despite these advantages, the implementation of LLMs faces several challenges, including technical integration with existing systems, the protection of patient data privacy, and the maintenance of model relevance over time.

Overcoming these challenges is essential to harness the full potential of LLMs in personalized healthcare. Future research should focus on refining integration strategies to ensure compatibility with legacy systems, developing robust ethical frameworks to safeguard patient data, and continuously updating models to maintain their effectiveness. By addressing these issues, researchers can enhance the effectiveness of personalized care and improve patient outcomes. Successfully navigating these hurdles will unlock the transformative power of LLMs, leading to more personalized and effective treatment plans and significantly enhancing the overall quality of patient care.

REFERENCES

1. Abdulqadir J. Nashwan and Ahmad A. Abujaber. Harnessing large language models in nursing care planning: Opportunities, challenges, and ethical considerations. *Cureus*, 15(6), 2023.
2. Abid Haleem, Mohd Javaid, and Ravi Pratap Singh. An era of ChatGPT as a significant futuristic support tool: A study on features, abilities, and challenges. *BenchCouncil Transactions on Benchmarks, Standards and Evaluations*, 2(4):100089, 2022.
3. Jiancheng Yang, Hongwei Bran Li, and Donglai Wei. The impact of ChatGPT and LLMs on medical imaging stakeholders: Perspectives and use cases. *Meta-Radiology*, 100007, 2023.

4. Partha Pratim Ray. Timely need for navigating the potential and downsides of LLMs in healthcare and biomedicine. *Briefings in Bioinformatics*, 25(3):bbae214, 2024.
5. Senay A. Gebreab, Khaled Salah, Raja Jayaraman, Muhammad Habib ur Rehman, and Samer Ellaham. LLM-based framework for administrative task automation in healthcare. In *2024 12th International Symposium on Digital Forensics and Security (ISDFS)*, pp. 1–7. IEEE, 2024.
6. Avishek Choudhury and Zaria Chaudhry. Large language models and user trust: Focus on healthcare. *arXiv preprint* arXiv:2403.14691, 2024.
7. Satvik Tripathi, Rithvik Sukumaran, and Tessa S. Cook. Efficient healthcare with large language models: Optimizing clinical workflow and enhancing patient care. *Journal of the American Medical Informatics Association*, 31(6):1436–1440, 2024.
8. Jan Oldenburg, Dave Chase, Kate T. Christensen, and Brad Tritle. *Engage!: Transforming Healthcare Through Digital Patient Engagement*. CRC Press, 2020.
9. Fekri Dureab, Taha Hussain, Rashad Sheikh, Najwa Al-Dheeb, Sameh Al-Awlaqi, and Albrecht Jahn. Forms of health system fragmentation during conflict: The case of Yemen. *Frontiers in Public Health*, 9:659980, 2021.
10. Monika Martens, Katrien Danhieux, Sara Van Belle, Edwin Wouters, Wim Van Damme, Roy Remmen, Sibyl Anthierens, and Josefien Van Olmen. Integration or fragmentation of health care? Examining policies and politics in a Belgian case study. *International Journal of Health Policy and Management*, 11(9):1668, 2022.
11. Petronille Bogaert, Marieke Verschuuren, Herman Van Oyen, and Hans Van Oers. Identifying common enablers and barriers in European health information systems. *Health Policy*, 125(12):1517–1526, 2021.
12. Hilal Atasoy, Emre M. Demirezen, and Pei-Yu Chen. Impacts of patient characteristics and care fragmentation on the value of HIEs. *Production and Operations Management*, 30(2):563–583, 2021.
13. Mark L. Braunstein. *Health Informatics on FHIR: How HL7's New API is Transforming Healthcare*. Springer, 2018.
14. Daryl E. Pritchard, Franziska Moeckel, Mary Susan Villa, Laura T. Housman, Catherine A. McCarty, and Howard L. McLeod. Strategies for integrating personalized medicine into healthcare practice. *Personalized Medicine*, 14(2):141–152, 2017.
15. Nicos Maglaveras, Vassilis Kilintzis, Vassilis Koutkias, and Ioanna Chouvarda. Integrated care and connected health approaches leveraging personalised health through big data analytics. In *pHealth 2016*, pp. 117–122. IOS Press, 2016.
16. Fabian Prasser, Oliver Kohlbacher, Ulrich Mansmann, Bernhard Bauer, and Klaus A. Kuhn. Data integration for future medicine (difuture). *Methods of Information in Medicine*, 57(S 01):e57–e65, 2018.
17. Amy Sitapati, Hyeoneui Kim, Barbara Berkovich, Rebecca Marmor, Siddharth Singh, Robert El-Kareh, Brian Clay, and Lucila Ohno-Machado. Integrated precision medicine: The role of electronic health records in delivering personalized treatment. *Wiley Interdisciplinary Reviews: Systems Biology and Medicine*, 9(3):e1378, 2017.
18. Lucia Sacchi, Giordano Lanzola, Natalia Viani, and Silvana Quaglini. Personalization and patient involvement in decision support systems: Current trends. *Yearbook of Medical Informatics*, 24(01):106–118, 2015.
19. Alan H. Morris, Christopher Horvat, Brian Stagg, David W. Grainger, Michael Lanspa, James Orme Jr., Terry P. Clemmer, Lindell K. Weaver, Frank O. Thomas, Colin K. Grissom, et al. Computer clinical decision support that automates personalized clinical care: A challenging but needed healthcare delivery strategy. *Journal of the American Medical Informatics Association*, 30(1):178–194, 2023.
20. Arnaud Belard, Timothy Buchman, Jonathan Forsberg, Benjamin K. Potter, Christopher J. Dente, Allan Kirk, and Eric Elster. Precision diagnosis: A view of the clinical decision support systems (CDSS) landscape through the lens of critical care. *Journal of Clinical Monitoring and Computing*, 31:261–271, 2017.

21. Don Detmer, Meryl Bloomrosen, Brian Raymond, and Paul Tang. Integrated personal health records: Transformative tools for consumer-centric care. *BMC Medical Informatics and Decision Making*, 8:1–14, 2008.
22. Emil Chiauzzi, Carlos Rodarte, and Pronabesh DasMahapatra. Patient-centered activity monitoring in the self-management of chronic health conditions. *BMC Medicine*, 13:1–6, 2015.
23. Chioma Anthonia Okolo, Oloruntoba Babawarun, Jeremiah Olawumi Arowoogun, Adekunle Oyeyemi Adeniyi, Rawlings Chidi. The role of mobile health applications in improving patient engagement and health outcomes: A critical review. *International Journal of Science and Research Archive*, 11(1):2566–2574, 2024.
24. Jorge Cancela, Iliàs Charlafti, Seya Colloud, and Catherine Wu. Digital health in the era of personalized healthcare: Opportunities and challenges for bringing research and patient care to a new level. *Digital Health*, 7–31, 2021.
25. José Luis Fernández-Alemán, Inmaculada Carrión Señor, Pedro Ángel Oliver Lozoya, and Ambrosio Toval. Security and privacy in electronic health records: A systematic literature review. *Journal of Biomedical Informatics*, 46(3):541–562, 2013.
26. Antonio López Martínez, Manuel Gil Pérez, and Antonio Ruiz-Martínez. A comprehensive review of the state-of-the-art on security and privacy issues in healthcare. *ACM Computing Surveys*, 55(12):1–38, 2023.
27. Indu Bala, Irfan Pindoo, Maad M. Mijwil, Mostafa Abotaleb, and Wang Yundong. Ensuring security and privacy in healthcare systems: A review exploring challenges, solutions, future trends, and the practical applications of artificial intelligence. *Jordan Medical Journal*, 58(2), 2024.
28. Amir Torab-Miandoab, Taha Samad-Soltani, Ahmadreza Jodati, and Peyman Rezaei Hachesu. Interoperability of heterogeneous health information systems: A systematic literature review. *BMC Medical Informatics and Decision Making*, 23(1):18, 2023.
29. Vasundra Touré, Philip Krauss, Kristin Gnodtke, Jascha Buchhorn, Deepak Unni, Petar Horki, Jean Louis Raisaro, Katie Kalt, Daniel Teixeira, Katrin Crameri, et al. Fairification of health-related data using semantic web technologies in the Swiss personalized health network. *Scientific Data*, 10(1):127, 2023.
30. Penelope Schofield, Tim Shaw, and Michaela Pascoe. Toward comprehensive patient centric care by integrating digital health technology with direct clinical contact in Australia. *Journal of Medical Internet Research*, 21(6):e12382, 2019.
31. Gokce B. Laleci Erturkmen, Mustafa Yuksel, Bunyamin Sarigul, Theodoros N. Arvanitis, Pontus Lindman, Rong Chen, Lei Zhao, Eric Sadou, Jacques Bouaud, Lamine Traore, et al. A collaborative platform for management of chronic diseases via guideline-driven individualized care plans. *Computational and Structural Biotechnology Journal*, 17:869–885, 2019.
32. Lea Davidson, Jason Scott, and Natalie Forster. Patient experiences of integrated care within the United Kingdom: A systematic review. *International Journal of Care Coordi Nation*, 24(2):39–56, 2021.
33. Tsipi Heart, Ofir Ben-Assuli, and Itamar Shabtai. A review of PHR, EMR and EHR integration: A more personalized healthcare and public health policy. *Health Policy and Technology*, 6(1):20–25, 2017.
34. Cong Peng, Prashant Goswami, and Guohua Bai. A literature review of current technologies on health data integration for patient-centered health management. *Health in Formatics Journal*, 26(3):1926–1951, 2020.
35. Mana Azarm, Chantal Backman, Craig Kuziemsky, and Liam Peyton. Breaking the healthcare interoperability barrier by empowering and engaging actors in the healthcare system. *Procedia Computer Science*, 113:326–333, 2017.
36. Rajiv Kapur. *Digital Platforms and Transformation of Healthcare Organizations: Integrating Digital Platforms with Advanced IT Systems and Work Transformation*. CRC Press, 2023.

37. Ethan Goh, Bryan Bunning, Elaine Khoong, Robert Gallo, Arnold Milstein, Damon Cen tola, and Jonathan H. Chen. ChatGPT influence on medical decision-making, bias, and equity: A randomized study of clinicians evaluating clinical vignettes. *medRxiv*, 2023.
38. Shahriar Akter, Mujahid Mohiuddin Babu, Umme Hani, Saida Sultana, Ruwan Bandara, and David Grant. Unleashing the power of artificial intelligence for climate action in industrial markets. *Industrial Marketing Management*, 117:92–113, 2024.
39. Rui Yang, Ting Fang Tan, Wei Lu, Arun James Thirunavukarasu, Daniel Shu Wei Ting, and Nan Liu. Large language models in health care: Development, applications, and challenges. *Health Care Science*, 2(4):255–263, 2023.
40. Brenna Li, Amy Wang, Patricia Strachan, Julie Anne Séguin, Sami Lachgar, Karyn C. Schroeder, Mathias S. Fleck, et al. Conversational AI in health: Design considerations from a Wizard-of-Oz dermatology case study with users, clinicians and a medical LLM. In *Extended Abstracts of the CHI Conference on Human Factors in Computing Systems*, pp. 1–10. ACM, 2024.
41. M. Sreenivasan, Sayan Dhar, and Anu Chacko. PCPS: Personalized care through patient similarity. In *2022 IEEE Region 10 Symposium (TENSYMP)*, pp. 1–6. IEEE, 2022.
42. J.E. O'Connell, E. Gilmartin, D. Roche, and S.N. Rogers. Conversational artificial intelligence: The interface with the patient concerns inventory. *British Journal of Oral and Maxillofacial Surgery*, 62(7), 2024.
43. Paul Hager, Friederike Jungmann, Robbie Holland, Kunal Bhagat, Inga Hubrecht, Manuel Knauer, Jakob Vielhauer, Marcus Makowski, Rickmer Braren, Georgios Kaissis, et al. Evaluation and mitigation of the limitations of large language models in clinical decision making. *Nature Medicine*, 1–10, 2024.
44. Jong-Lyul Ghim and Sangzin Ahn. Transforming clinical trials: The emerging roles of large language models. *Translational and Clinical Pharmacology*, 31(3):131, 2023.
45. Mohammad Abu-Jeyyab, Sallam Alrosan, and Ibraheem Alkhawaldeh. Harnessing large language models in medical research and scientific writing: A closer look to the future: LLMs in medical research and scientific writing. *High Yield Medical Reviews*, 1(2), 2023.
46. Conrad W. Safranek, Anne Elizabeth Sidamon-Eristoff, Aidan Gilson, and David Chartash. The role of large language models in medical education: Applications and implications. *JMIR Medical Education*, 9, 2023.
47. Vaibhav Gulati, Shambo Guha Roy, Ahmed Moawad, Daniela Garcia, Aparna Babu, Jeffrey D. Poot, and Oleg M. Teytelboym. Transcending language barriers: Can ChatGPT be the key to enhancing multilingual accessibility in healthcare? *Journal of the American College of Radiology*, 2024.
48. Jiyeon Han, Jimin Park, Jinyoung Huh, Uran Oh, Jaeyoung Do, and Daehee Kim. AscleAI: A LLM-based clinical note management system for enhancing clinician productivity. In *Extended Abstracts of the CHI Conference on Human Factors in Computing Systems*, pp. 1–7. 2024.
49. Emma Urquhart, John Ryan, Sean Hartigan, Ciprian Nita, Ciara Hanley, Peter Moran, John Bates, Rachel Jooste, Conor Judge, John G. Laffey, et al. A pilot feasibility study comparing large language models in extracting key information from ICU patient text records from an Irish population. *Intensive Care Medicine Experimental*, 12(1):71, 2024.
50. Grady McPeak, Anja Sautmann, Ohia George, Adham Hallal, Eduardo Arancón Simal, Aaron L. Schwartz, Jason Abaluck, Nirmal Ravi, and Robert Pless. An LLM's medical testing recommendations in a Nigerian clinic: Potential and limits of prompt engineering for clinical decision support. In *2024 IEEE 12th International Conference on Healthcare Informatics (ICHI)*, pp. 586–591. IEEE, 2024.
51. Gabriele De Vito. Assessing healthcare software built using IoT and LLM technologies. In *Proceedings of the 28th International Conference on Evaluation and Assessment in Software Engineering*, pp. 476–481. 2024.

52. Kerstin Denecke, Richard May, LLMHealthGroup, and Octavio Rivera Romero. Potential of large language models in health care: Delphi study. *Journal of Medical Internet Research*, 26:e52399, 2024.
53. Luis Cardenas, Katherine Parajes, Ming Zhu, and Shengjie Zhai. AutoHealth: Advanced LLM-empowered wearable personalized medical Butler for Parkinson's disease management. In *2024 IEEE 14th Annual Computing and Communication Workshop and Conference (CCWC)*, pp. 0375–0379. IEEE, 2024.
54. Umesh Gupta, Ayushman Pranav, Anvi Kohli, Sukanta Ghosh, and Divya Singh. The contribution of artificial intelligence to drug discovery: Current progress and prospects for the future. *Microbial Data Intelligence and Computational Techniques for Sustainable Computing*, 1–23, 2022.
55. D. Gupta, U. Gupta, and H.J. Sarma. Functional iterative approach for Universum-based primal twin bounded support vector machine to EEG classification (FUPTBSVM). *Multimedia Tools and Applications*, 83(8):22119–22151, 2024.
56. U. Gupta and V. Jain. Social neuroscience: Inferring mental states in social media. In *Emotional AI and Human-AI Interactions in Social Networking*, pp. 15–39. Elsevier, 2024.
57. M. Sharma, S. Deswal, U. Gupta, M. Tabassum, and I. Lawal, eds. *Soft Computing Techniques in Connected Healthcare Systems*. CRC Press, 2023.
58. K. Malik, H. Sadawarti, M. Sharma, U. Gupta, and P. Tiwari, eds. *Computational Techniques in Neuroscience*. CRC Press, 2023.
59. D. Singh, D. Singh, Manju, and U. Gupta. Smart healthcare: A breakthrough in the growth of technologies. In *Artificial Intelligence-based Healthcare Systems*, pp. 73–85. Cham: Springer Nature Switzerland, 2023.
60. M. Gupta, D. Srivastava, D. Pantola, and U. Gupta. Brain tumor detection using improved Otsu's thresholding method and supervised learning techniques at early stage. In *Proceedings of Emerging Trends and Technologies on Intelligent Systems: ETTIS 2022*, pp. 271–281. Singapore: Springer Nature Singapore, 2022.
61. U. Gupta, D. Gupta, and U. Agarwal. Analysis of randomization-based approaches for autism spectrum disorder. In *Pattern Recognition and Data Analysis with Applications*, pp. 701–713. Singapore: Springer Nature Singapore, 2022.
62. D. Gupta, A. Choudhury, U. Gupta, P. Singh, and M. Prasad. Computational approach to clinical diagnosis of diabetes disease: A comparative study. *Multimedia Tools and Applications*, 1–26, 2021.
63. D. Gupta and U. Gupta. On robust asymmetric Lagrangian ν-twin support vector regression using pinball loss function. *Applied Soft Computing*, 102:107099, 2021.

7 Predictive Analytics for Early Cancer Detection Using Machine Learning and Generative AI

Ritu Gautam, Prableen Kaur, and Manik Sharma

7.1 INTRODUCTION

A chronic disorder is a long-lasting illness that has a major impact on a person's physical and mental health [1]. The primary causes of human impairment and casualties are the ones mentioned earlier [1]. There are several chronic diseases that affect people. Stroke, cancer, diabetes, arthritis, Alzheimer's, epilepsy, Parkinson's, HIV, schizophrenia, glaucoma, obesity, and hypertension are a few of the major chronic diseases [2, 3]. Of these, cancer is a common chronic human disease with high fatality rates. Additionally, there are a sizable number of cancer victims worldwide. Therefore, it is important to get a diagnosis for this lethal condition as quickly as feasible [4, 5].

Cancer is a condition when a few of the body's cells grow out of control and spread to other bodily regions. In the millions of cells that make up the human body, cancer can develop practically anywhere [6]. Human cells often divide (via a process known as cell growth and multiplication) to create new cells as the body requires them. New cells replace old ones when they die as a result of aging or damage. When cells in the body proliferate abnormally and uncontrollably, a chronic condition known as cancer results. Blood is used by cancerous cells to travel throughout the body and to rip apart healthy tissues [7, 8]. The process is shown in Figure 7.1. Fever, exhaustion, heavy perspiration, anemia, unexplained weight loss, recurrent headaches, severe coughing, and hoarseness are some of the typical cancer symptoms [9, 10]. There are more than 200 different varieties of cancer, and we can divide them into five groups based on where in the body they first manifest, such as breast cancer or lung cancer [11]. The classifications of this harmful illness are shown in Figure 7.2.

7.1.1 Types of Cancer

A genetic disorder, cancer takes place when genes that control cell activity change, resulting in aberrant cells that divide and grow uncontrollably, ultimately interfering with how your body functions [12]. According to medical specialists, inherited

DOI: 10.1201/9781003539483-7

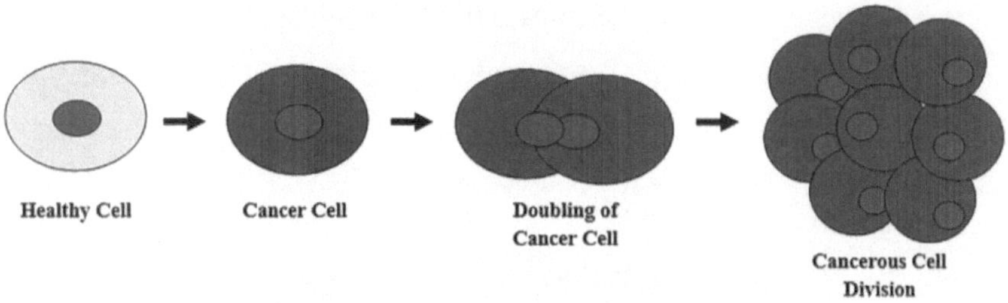

FIGURE 7.1 Development of cancerous cells in the human body.

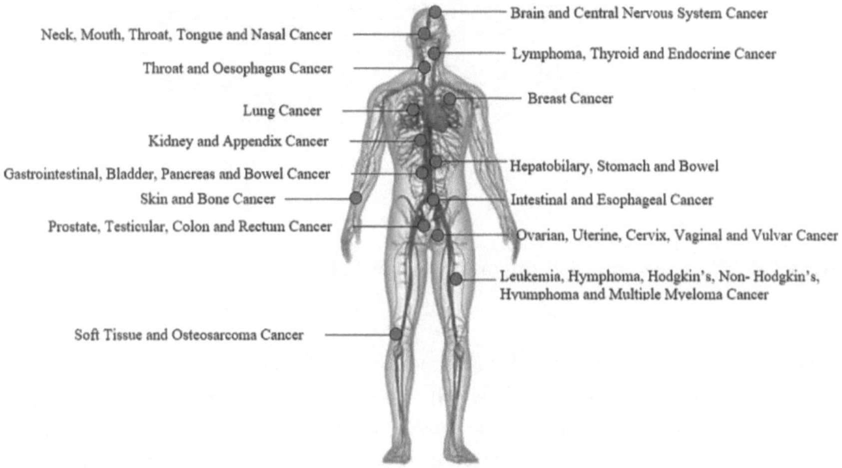

FIGURE 7.2 Types of cancer [20].

genetic abnormalities that are uncontrollable account for 5% to 12% of all cancers [13]. Cancer is more usually caused by an acquired genetic mutation. You can acquire genetic mutations throughout your life. Numerous risk factors that raise your chances of acquiring cancer have been found by medical researchers. Cancer is a challenging condition. Years can pass when you have cancer without showing any signs of it. Other times, cancer may show obvious symptoms that deteriorate rapidly. Many cancer symptoms are similar to those of other, less dangerous conditions. Certain symptoms do not necessarily indicate malignancy. Generally, any alteration in your body that lasts longer than two weeks should be discussed with a healthcare professional [14]. The American Cancer Society estimates that 1 in 2 males and persons assigned male at birth (AMAB) and 1 in 3 women and people assigned female at birth (AFAB) will acquire cancer [15]. A number of clinical terms are employed for certain cancer types in general, such as lymphomas, sarcomas, leukemia, and adenomas. Lymphomas are found in immune system tissues, sarcomas are found in bones, muscles, and connective tissues, leukemia starts in bone marrow, and adenomas cover both interior and external body parts (located in the thyroid and pituitary glands) [16, 17]. Men most frequently develop lung, prostate, colon, rectum, stomach,

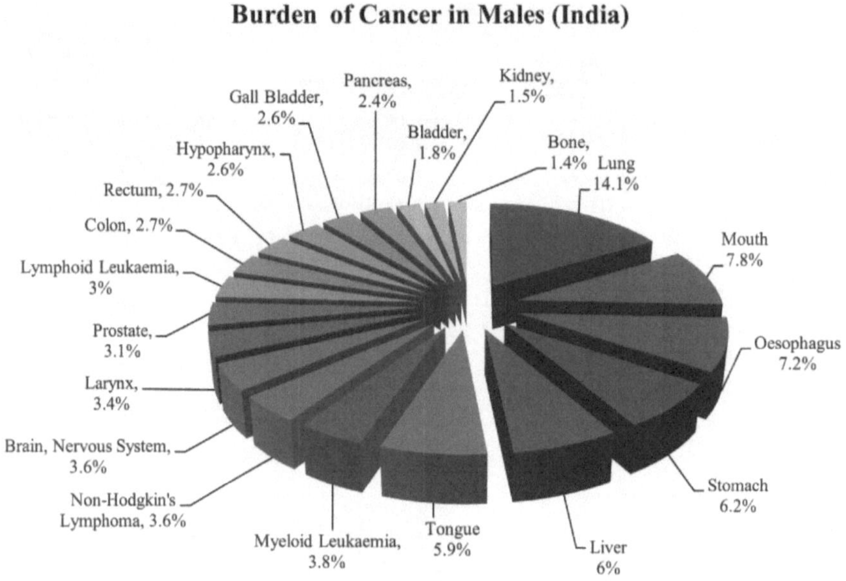

FIGURE 7.3 Prevalence of cancer in males in India [24].

and liver cancers. However, breast, colon, rectum, lung, cervix, and stomach cancer typically affect women. The World Health Organization (WHO) predicts that cancer incidence will increase by 70% by the end of 2035 [18]. Using a variety of imaging procedures, including X-rays, computed tomography (CT) scans, MRIs, PET scans, ultrasounds, and endoscopies, doctors can identify anomalies within the body and the organs that are impacted by cancer. SamCN, ClumpThick, U_cShape, U_cSize, M_Adhesion, SE_cSize, B_Nuclei, B_Chromatin, N_Nucleoli, Mitosis, and Class are some of the crucial parameters utilized in cancer detection [19].

The fight against cancer presents obstacles for both researchers and medical professionals [21]. The American Cancer Society estimates that in 2019 there will be 96,480 deaths from skin cancer, 142,670 deaths from lung cancer, 42,260 deaths from breast cancer, 31,620 deaths from prostate cancer, and 17,760 deaths from brain cancer [22]. The best chance of saving many lives is through early identification of cancer. The treatment and survival of cancer patients can be enhanced by early detection. For these kinds of cancer diagnoses, visual inspection and manual procedures are frequently employed. This manual assessment of medical images requires a significant amount of time and is quite error prone. Computer-aided diagnostic (CAD) systems were introduced to help clinicians interpret medical images more effectively in the early 1980s [23] because of this.

7.1.2 Statistics of Cancer

In 91 out of 172 nations worldwide, cancer is either the top or second leading cause of mortality before the age of 70. Globally, 9.6 million people died from cancer in

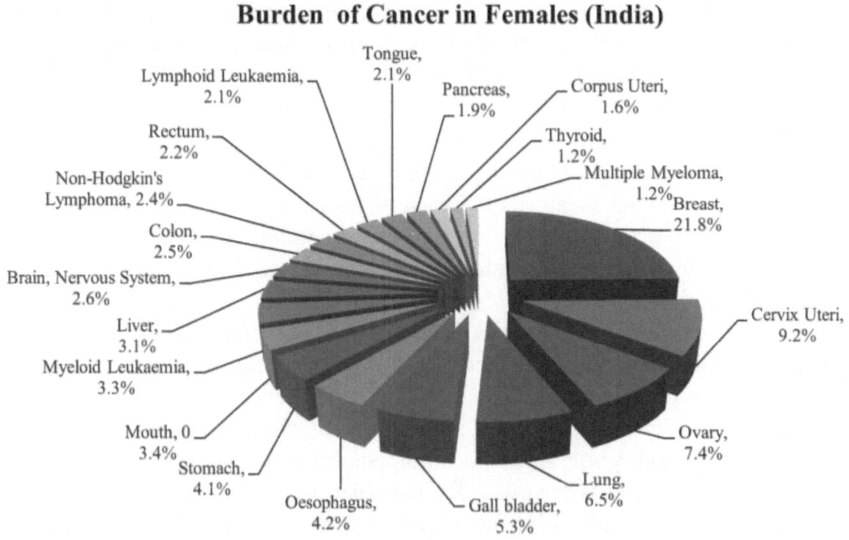

FIGURE 7.4 Prevalence of cancer in females in India [24].

2018, according to GLOBOCAN [24]. The predicted increases in cancer incidence and death are 29.5 million and 16.3 million, respectively, by 2040 [25]. Rapid urbanization, population aging, sedentary and unhealthy lifestyles, and indoor and outdoor air pollution are among the new and difficult problems causing the rising cancer burden worldwide, which primarily affects middle-to-low socio-economic countries like India.

In past years, men from the country's southern, northern, and eastern areas had the greatest crude incidence rates of lung cancer, while the western, central, and northeastern regions had the highest rates of oral and esophageal cancers, followed by lung cancer. Esophageal cancer incidence ranged from sixth to tenth in different regions. No matter the area, ovarian cancer came in third among female cancers in terms of incidence, followed by breast cancer and cervical cancer, with the exception of India's north and northeast. Esophageal cancer's incidence ranged from fifth to eleventh, whereas mouth cancer's incidence ranged from fourth to eighth.

7.2 COMPUTATIONAL TECHNIQUES

The primary reason we create computer programs is to automate certain tasks. Computers are used in approaches that use step-by-step, repeating, and iterative processes to tackle issues that would otherwise be laborious or impossible to solve by manual computations. The variety of engineering problems that can be reliably solved has considerably expanded with the emergence of quick, cheap, and efficient computers. The term "computational techniques" refers to a multidisciplinary field that includes advanced computational methods from the fields of computer science, statistical computation, and electronics engineering [26]. The fundamental tenet of sustainable computing is the application of algorithms, models, regulations, and protocols to enhance resource management, ecological balance, and biological sustenance, as well as other services in societal contexts [27].

It has been discovered that accurate and prompt diagnosis of human illnesses can significantly prolong human life [28]. Several deterministic and stochastic (computers influenced by nature) methodologies have used diagnostic techniques for this in recent years. Without using randomness, a deterministic model enables one to calculate the future occurrence precisely. When something is deterministic, one has all the information required to confidently anticipate (determine) the outcome. These techniques typically apply more quickly and easily, and thus are well suited for computer applications. Some of the traditional deterministic methods are naive Bayes, random forest, decision tree, and support vector machine. However, these are not the most thorough or precise reservoir models. On other hand, a stochastic model has the ability to deal with applied input uncertainty. Stochastic models include some intrinsic unpredictability; the identical initial conditions and parameter values will result in a variety of outputs. Heuristic and meta-heuristic techniques are two general categories of stochastic computing techniques. It is practicable to use heuristic methods to provide excellent results with less computing time [29, 30]. To solve enormous, complicated problems in the actual world, meta-heuristic methods can be used [31]. Additionally, there are two subcategories of meta-heuristic techniques: those that are inspired by nature and those that are not. There are over 100 meta-heuristic methods that draw inspiration from nature. Depending on their source of inspiration, these can be further divided into meta-heuristic techniques inspired by insects, people, animals, and other natural phenomena. The leading ones include GA, FA, ABC, ACO, GWO, ALO, and SA [32, 33]. The two main population-based meta-heuristic methodologies are evolutionary and swarm intelligence. Swarm intelligence is a cutting-edge optimization method that draws inspiration from the biological behavior of fish, birds, and other animals. The swarming, flocking, and herding processes in vertebrates are frequently the source of inspiration. Individual agents that communicate with one another and their surroundings collectively form swarms [34]. They adhere to the straightforward rule of not having a centralized control structure, which causes sophisticated global behavior to arise. By interacting with nearby neighbors, it primarily applies the self-organizing behavior of mechanical agents. ACO and PSO are two popular swarm intelligence algorithms. Swarm intelligence is being used to handle discrete and continuous optimization problems in addition to more traditional optimization problems using optimization-based data mining [35].

Deep learning models that can produce excellent writing, graphics, and other content from the training data are referred to as generative AI (GAI) [36]. It is a kind of artificial intelligence system that can generate text, images, audio, and synthetic data, among other kinds of content. The ease of use of new user interfaces that enable the creation of excellent text, pictures, and movies in a matter of seconds has been the driving force behind the recent excitement surrounding generative AI.

To represent and analyze content, GAI models mix several AI techniques. To produce text, for instance, different natural language processing methods convert raw characters (such as letters, punctuation, and words) into sentences, entities, and actions. These are then represented as vectors using a variety of encoding techniques [37]. In a similar way, vectors are used to express different visual aspects from photographs. A word of caution: the training data may contain bigotry, prejudice, deceit, and exaggeration that these techniques can also encode. The potential of GAI to completely transform the way knowledge work is done in industries and business operations throughout the economy has both shocked and delighted people worldwide. It has the potential to change jobs and improve performance in a variety of industries, including software development, customer operations, and sales and marketing. It might create trillions of dollars' worth of value in a variety of industries, including finance and the life sciences. [38–40]

For the purpose of developing GAI models and creating creative solutions in a variety of fields, GAI architecture is essential. This architecture offers the fundamental framework for creating complex tools and improving development procedures in GAI in software development. This architecture is utilized by GAI solutions with private LLMs to guarantee customized and safe applications [41]. The design of contact center GAI facilitates the development of effective, automated customer care systems. This design also helps GAI search, which yields more precise and contextually appropriate search results. Through the integration of these components, GAI architecture promotes efficiency and progress across several industries, demonstrating its pivotal significance in contemporary technological breakthroughs. The general framework and elements involved in creating and implementing GAI models are referred to as GAI architecture. A basic GAI architecture consists of four essential parts. The first is the data processing layer, which gathers, prepares, and processes data for the GAI model. However, changes may occur depending on particular use cases. It involves gathering data from diverse sources, cleaning and standardizing the data, and extracting features. The second element is generative: create new material or data by modelling it with machine learning models. It entails selecting the best model for the use case, training the models with pertinent data, and optimizing their performance through fine-tuning. The accuracy and efficiency of the generative model are continuously improved by the next component, the feedback and improvement layer [42]. It entails gathering user input, examining data that has been created, and applying learning to advance the model. The generative model is finally integrated and deployed into the finished system or product via the deployment and integration layer. It involves monitoring the model's performance, integrating it with application systems, and putting up a production infrastructure. Figure 7.5 presents the architecture of GAI [43, 44].

7.3 RELATED WORK

Yang et al. [44] suggested that the low accuracy of deep learning-based classification of breast tissues from histology images is due to a lack of training data as well as a lack of understanding of structural and textual data that can transcend multiple layers. Hematoxylin-eosin-stained breast microscope pictures are divided into four groups using the ensemble of the multiscale convolutional neural network (EMCN) approach described in this paper: benign lesion, normal tissue, invasive, and in-situ malignancy. Each image is translated to numerous scales before to training the pre-trained models, such as ResNet-152, DenseNet-161, and ResNet-101. During each scale, the amassed training bits are then put to work and improved. The EMS-net strategy outperforms the other three examined algorithms in terms of accuracy. Rajaguru et al. [45] used KNN and decision tree (DT) machine learning algorithms

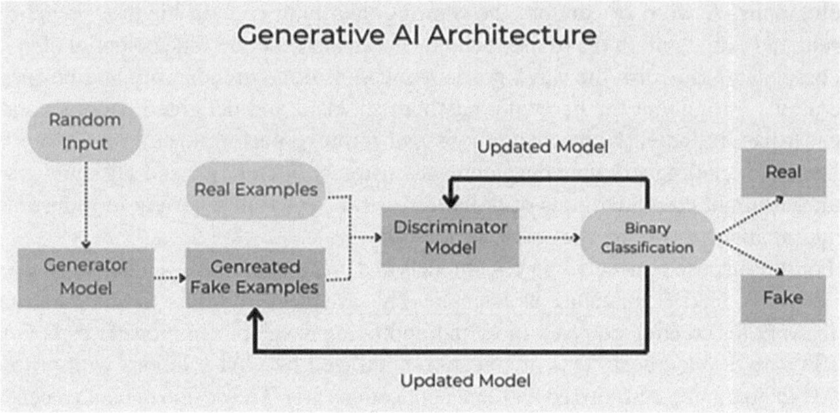

FIGURE 7.5 Architecture of generative AI.

to categorize the WDBC attributes to address the breast cancer prediction challenge. KNN performed better than the DT when the feature classification was done using the conventional principal component analysis (PCA) feature selection approach. Based on the shape, location, and size, Blanes-Vidal et al. [46] developed an algorithm to objectively measure the similarity between anticipated polyps and those categorized by OC, CCE, and HP. In addition, they suggested using a CNN for the autonomous localization and identification of colorectal polyps in WCE. The findings achieved by using WCE images from datasets were unexpectedly strong in terms of sensitivity (97.1%), accuracy (96.4%), and specificity (93.3%).

In the progression of colorectal cancer with the risk of malignancy, Nadimi et al. [47] introduced a CNN for autonomous colorectal tissue detection in pictures taken during WCE. With the help of Kvasir datasets and WCE pictures from separate datasets, authors were able to achieve sensitivity, accuracy, and specificity values of 98.1%, 98.0%, and 96.3%, respectively. Yu-Min Chiang et al. [48] designed a hybrid framework for detecting the data of cancer patients by fusing ACO with MLP and SVM. Prostate and lung cancer were diagnosed using the proposed framework. A classification rate of 97% was achieved using their hybridization. Kumar et al. [49] presented an extended ABC optimization method to identify early indications of breast cancer. Using data from the Mammography Image Analysis Society (MIAS) database, the authors applied bilateral subtraction to left and right mammographic breast images. With the proposed technique, a satisfactory prediction accuracy of 96.4% was attained. The enhanced firefly algorithm (EFA) and the adaptive-neuro-neutrosophic-inference-system (ANNIS) are two hybrid methodologies that has been presented by the authors to diagnose circulating tumor cells (CTCs) for the investigation of breast cancer. EFA is used to identify perceptual traits that can help in spotting early signs of breast cancer. In a shorter execution time of 0.72 s, the maximum prediction accuracy rate (92%) was attained (Umamaheswari et al.).

Moosa et al. [50] developed a modified ABC (mABC) cancer classifier to identify the ideal genes required for the early detection of cancer. Ten different datasets were used in the experiment. In comparison to GA, ACO, and ABC, the authors discovered that mABC was a more promising cancer diagnostic classifier. Banu et al. [51] focused on the combination of clustering, FA, and fuzzy approaches for identifying tumors and cancer in humans. The proposed method aids in the discovery of highly expressed and suppressed genes using five different datasets. PSO, FA, and fuzzy PSO were all found to be inferior to the fuzzy-firefly proposed method. Alickovic et al. [52] proposed a diagnostic method for identifying the risk of breast cancer in females. The dataset was classified using a variety of data mining methods, including logistic regression, decision trees, random forests, Bayesian networks, multilayer perceptron, radial basis function networks (RBFNs), SVM, and rotation forest. Rotation forest with GA produced the highest accuracy (99.48%) rate. Filho et al. [53] hybridized GA and SVM to predict lung cancer among patients. The proposed method's accuracy, sensitivity, and specificity predictions had predictive rates of 93.19%, 92.7%, and 93.3%, respectively.

Mansoori et al. [54] designed a technique using GA and SVM for diagnosis of ovarian cancer in patients. For categorization of data, SVM was used, whereas GA was used to minimize the features to achieve a better predictive rate of accuracy of 96.3%. For the diagnosis of lung cancer, Parag Deoskar et al. [55] developed a support-based ACO. The authors conducted research using UCI lung cancer databases. They began by identifying the support for each ant, calculated based on treatment symptoms. The support was calculated considering the symptoms of the treatment. Using three different cases of support, the authors achieved accuracies of 77%–81%, 89%–91%, and 20%–72%. Varsha Patankar et al. [56] designed an innovative ACO-based edge detection for the diagnosis of breast cancer. The authors found that an ACO-based edge detection technique can accurately identify an object and its associated boundaries. Vimaladevi et al. [57] compared a GA–back propagation neural network (BPNN) and hybrid PSO-BPNN for the diagnosis of three different cancers: lymphoma, leukemia, and SRBCT. The study found that for all three forms of cancer, accuracy utilizing the hybrid strategy of NN, GA, and PSO was greater than 80%, whereas accuracy using the GA-BPNN method was less than 80%. Furthermore, the hybrid approach's computation time was faster than that of GA-BPNN.

Aswini Kumar Mohanty et al. [58] designed a discrete PSO technique for the detection of breast cancer. Using DPSO, an accuracy of 97% was achieved. For the early diagnosis of breast cancer, Vijaylakshmi et al. [59] utilized a variety of techniques, including KNN, decision trees, SVM, and a hybrid approach combining PSO and GA. KNN, decision trees, and SVM all achieved predicted rates of accuracy of 86%, 89%, and 88%, respectively. Better diagnosis outcomes were made possible with the use of GA and PSO. PSO and GA achieved an accuracy rate of 95%. Mahsa Nazarian et al. [60] used an ABC nature-inspired technique for the diagnosis of cancer in patients. The rate of accuracy achieved using ABC was better than SVM, C 4.5, naive Bayes and a neural network. Table 7.1 depicts the rate of accuracies achieved by different classification techniques (traditional classifiers, metaheuristic techniques, and deep learning techniques) and by different authors in diagnosing breast cancer.

From Table 7.1, it can be seen that authors were successful in achieving a high predicted rate of accuracy by adopting a hybrid strategy. Convolutional neural networks

TABLE 7.1
MLT in Breast Cancer Diagnosis

Author	Published Year	Technique	Results
Abdur Rasool et al. [61]	2022	SVM	99.3%
Onyinyechi Jessica Egwom et al. [62]	2022	LDA and SVM	99.2%
Chandrashish Roy et al. [63]	2022	Extreme gradient boosting algorithms	98.24%
Jasti et al. [64]	2022	Least square SVM and AlexNet	90%
Nicolle Vigil et al. [65]	2022	Convolutional deep autoencoder	78.5%
Omid Fallahzadeh et al. [66]	2018	ACO	87.7%
Umamaheswari et al. [67]	2018	Enhanced FA, ANNIS	92%
Naresh Khuriwal et al. [68]	2018	PCA and CNN	**99.67%**
Senapati et al. [69]	2017	Firefly local linear wavelet neural network	98.14%
Kumar et al. [49]	2017	FA	98%
S. Shahbeig et al. [70]	2017	PSO and fuzzy logic	91.88%
E. Alickovic et al. [52]	2017	GA and rotation forest	99.48%
Zamani et al. [71]	2016	FA	98.54%
Mazen et al. [72]	2016	FA-GA	97.16%
Gehad Ismail Sayed et al. [73]	2016	FA	90%
Hala M. Alshamlan et al. [74]	2016	ABC	76.8%
S. Aalaei et al. [75]	2016	GA and ANN	96.6%
H. Turabieh [76]	2016	GA and ANFIS	88%
S. Anto et al. [77]	2015	ACO and fuzzy logic	95.72%
Sadeghipour et al. [78]	2015	FA	99.14%
Cinar et al. [79]	2015	FAGR	96%
Shah et al. [80]	2015	GGABC+NN	99.98%
Pourmandi et al. [81]	2015	Gbest-guided, ABC+fuzzy-Cmeans, neural network	99.16%
Varsha Patankar et al. [56]	2014	ACO	Not mentioned
Aboul Ella Hassanien et al. [82]	2014	ACO, MLPNN	98%
Gerald Schaefer [83]	2014	ACO	79.52%
Karnan [84]	2014	FA, fuzzy, MRF	99.13%
Bartosz Krawczyk et al. [85]	2013	FA	96.33%
Mahsa Nazarian et al. [86]	2013	ABC	96.5%
Ajay Sharma and Pramod Kumar Mishra [87]	2012	ANN, LR and SVM	99.41%
T. Kavitha et al. [88]	2012	OMLTS	98.50%
Kumar et al. [49]	2012	EABCO	96.40%
Aswini Kumar Mohanty et al. [58]	2011	Discrete PSO	97%

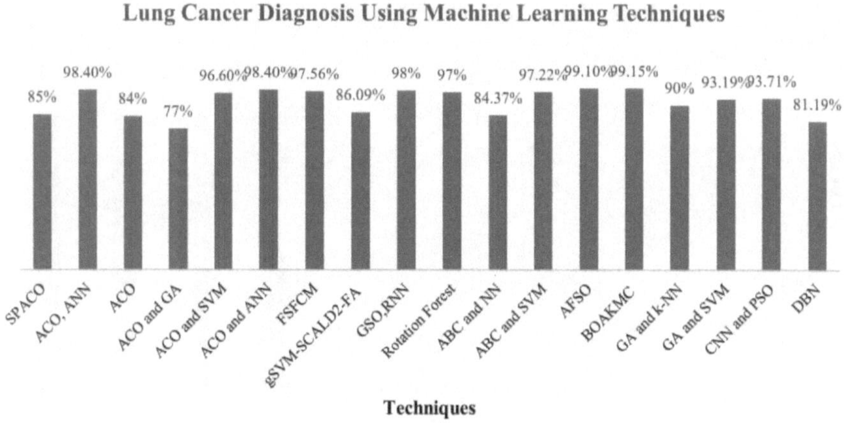

FIGURE 7.6 Lung cancer diagnosis using MLT.

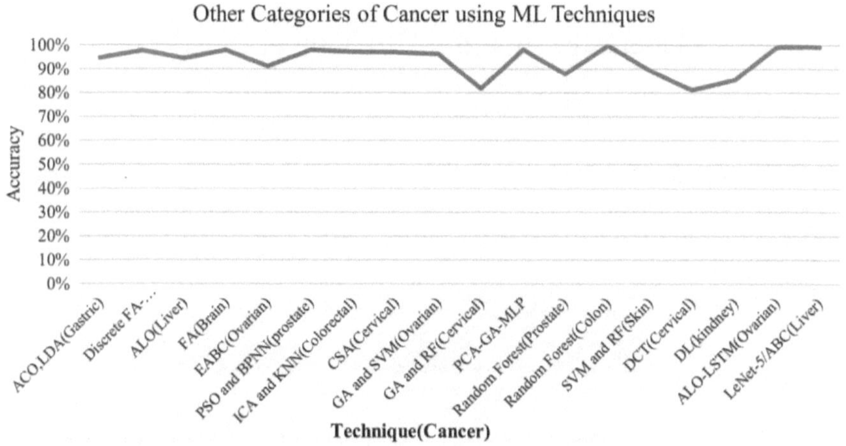

FIGURE 7.7 Different categories of cancer diagnosis using MLT.

and principal component analysis were combined to diagnose breast cancer at the highest rate of accuracy possible. Additionally, when compared to other machine learning techniques for cancer diagnosis, the findings of the firefly algorithm and SVM were also found to be superior. Furthermore, most authors attained strong predicted rates of accuracy of more than 90%.

The best lung cancer diagnostic accuracy is represented graphically in Figure 7.8. Figure 7.8 shows that artificial fish swarm optimization (AFSO) and butterfly optimization algorithm-based K-means clustering (BOAKMC) have the greatest predictive rates of accuracy of 99.15% and 99.10% for diagnosis of lung cancer.

It is shown in Figure 7.9 that the range of accuracies lies between 81.71% and 99.38% in diagnosis of 12 other types of cancer (colon cancer, prostate cancer, liver

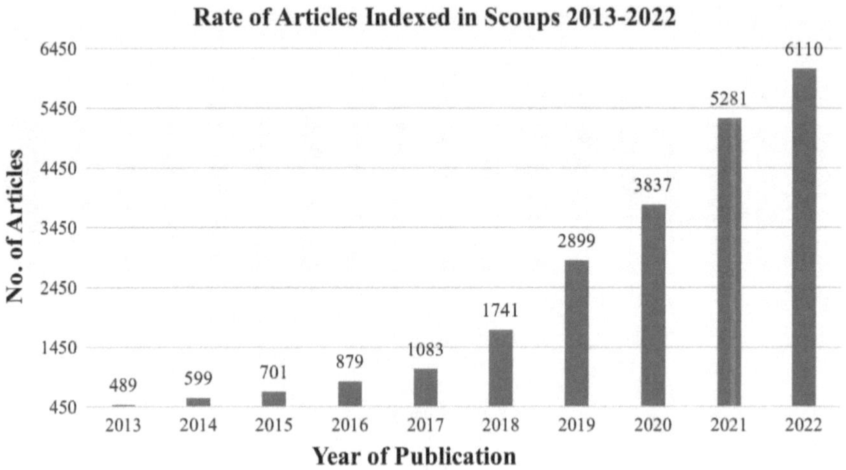

FIGURE 7.8 Publishing trends in cancer-related articles on MLT.

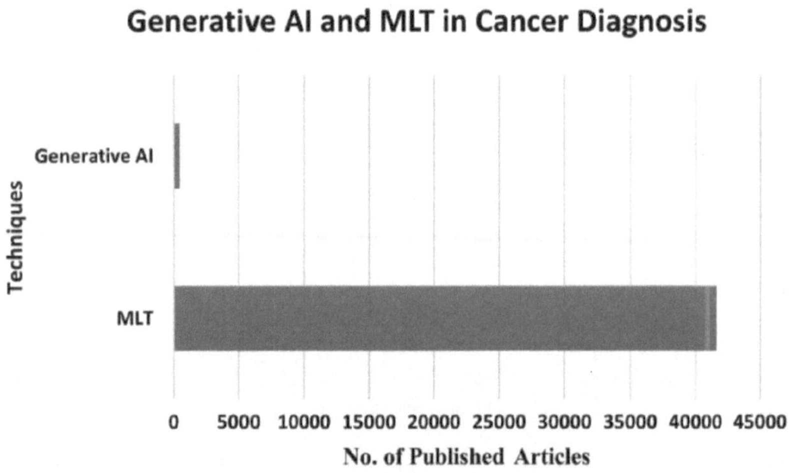

FIGURE 7.9 Publishing trends in cancer-related articles on MLT with GAI.

cancer, ovarian cancer, colorectal cancer, leukemia, skin cancer, kidney cancer, gastric cancer, brain tumor, and cervical cancer). Liver and colon cancer showed the highest performance of the cancers. The random forest classifier achieved excellent results in the diagnosis of colon cancer. Also, the hybridization of deep learning techniques with meta-heuristic techniques achieved superior results in the diagnosis of liver and ovarian cancer. Table 7.2 presents the diagnosis of cancer (without category) using machine learning techniques.

From Table 7.2, it can be seen that deep learning techniques outperform others in the diagnosis of cancer. The results of nature-inspired techniques are also found to be superior for cancer diagnosis.

TABLE 7.2
Cancer (without Categorization) Diagnosis Using MLT

Author	Published Year	Technique	Results
Rehman et al. [89]	2022	Deep learning	**98.9%**
Banu et al. [51]	2017	Fuzzy firefly	Not mentioned
Pramita et al. [90]	2016	FA	Not mentioned
Moosa et al. [50]	2015	mABC	98.65%
Hala Alshamlan et al. [74]	2015	ABC	76.8%
Habib Shah et al. [80]	2015	ABC	76.8%
Ritu Shukla et al. [91]	2014	Association rule, ACO	Not mentioned
Sunny et al. [92]	2014	FA, adaptive fuzzy neural network	Not mentioned
Yu-Min Chiang et al. [48]	2008	ACO	97%

7.3.1 Comparison of Studies with and without GAI

Shin et al. [93] addressed the imbalance issue in brain MRI data sets by using a GAN model and manufactured tumor MRI pictures, which led to enhanced performance on tumor segmentation findings. Wang et al. [94] investigated state-of-the-art Wasserstein GANs to solve a lung nodule image data imbalance issue. Liu et al. [95] proposed a GAN to create synthetic unlawful transaction data and combined these synthetic records into an enhanced training set in order to increase the efficacy of credit card fraud detection,

7.4 PUBLICATION TREND ANALYSIS

To evaluate publishing trends in cancer diagnosis using various machine learning approaches, several queries were developed and exploited over the Scopus indexing databases.

Compared to MLT with GAI, the number of publications about cancer diagnosis using MLT is significantly higher.

7.5 NEED FOR CANCER DIAGNOSIS SYSTEMS

The combination of generative AI with machine learning in cancer diagnostics offers transformative potential. It enhances data-driven decision-making, improves the accuracy and personalization of diagnostics, supports advanced research, and expands access to high-quality healthcare [111]. This synergy can significantly advance the fight against cancer, leading to better outcomes for patients worldwide [112]. The need for cancer diagnostic systems using machine learning (ML) is increasingly vital due to several critical factors.

The integration of generative artificial intelligence with machine learning in cancer diagnostic systems offers numerous advantages, addressing critical needs

TABLE 7.3
Comparison of Results with and without GAI

Author	Disease	Year	Generative Intelligence Methods	Generative Intelligence Used to Enhance Performance of MLT and DLT	Results without Generative AI	Results with Generative AI
Srivishnu M V et al. [96]	Cancer	2024	Generative adversarial network	XG Boost	95%	99.04%
Mehran Karimzadeh et al. [97]	Cancer	2024	Deep generative AI model	SVM	60%	92% sensitivity and 90% specificity
Mudassir Saeed et al. [98]	Skin cancer	2023	Generative adversarial networks+SVM	VGG16 VGG19	92% 93%	96%
Adrian B Levine et al. [99]	Cancer	2020	Generative adversarial network			No results
Yawen Xiao et al. [100]	Cancer	2021	Wasserstein generative adversarial network	GAN SMOTE Random oversampling	96.67% 96.67% 95.00	98.33%
Marco La Salvia et al. [101]	Skin cancer	2022	Deep convolutional generative adversarial network	ResNet18	-	-
Muhammad Sakib Khan Inan et al. [102]	Breast tumors	2023	Tabular variational autoencoder (TVAE) and the conditional generative adversarial network (CTGAN)	-	-	96.66%
Yufei Liu et al. [103]	Cancer	2018	DNN with Wasserstein GAN	NB with WGAN RF with WGAN RF NB	61% 29% 54% 32%	70%
Wessam M. Salama et al. [104]	Lung cancer	2022	Deep generative model	-	-	98.91%

(*Continued*)

TABLE 7.1 ***(Continued)***
Comparison of Results with and without GAI

Author	Disease	Year	Generative Intelligence Methods	Generative Intelligence Used to Enhance Performance of MLT and DLT	Results without Generative AI	Results with Generative AI
Marco Cascella et al. [105]	Enhancing the telemedicine approach to cancer pain management.	2023	Conditional GAN	GBM LASSO ANN	86% 62% 89%	87% 70% 92% Accuracy increased of all data set
Kaimin Wei et al. [106]	Cancer	2022	Deep generative AI model	GAN DC-GAN (updated)	-	79% 92.6%
Moulaei et al. [107]	Breast cancer	2021	Generative adversarial network with Siamese convolutional neural network	-	-	98.87%
Rajeev Kumar Gupta et al., 2022 [108]	Brain tumor	2022	Cyclic generative adversarial network	-	-	99%
Fan Zhang et al. [109]	Breast cancer	2022	PregGAN based on conditional generative adversarial network (CGAN)	-	-	90%
Ananjan Maiti et al. [110]	Skin cancer	2021	Generative adversarial network	RF with GAN		97.08%

in cancer detection, treatment planning, and research. Generative AI models, such as generative adversarial networks (GANs), can create synthetic data that mimics real patient data. This is particularly useful when dealing with rare cancers where actual data may be limited. These synthetic datasets can be used to train ML models, improving their accuracy and generalization capabilities. Generative AI can create variations of existing medical images (e.g., CT scans, MRIs) to train diagnostic models more effectively, helping to recognize cancer in diverse scenarios and

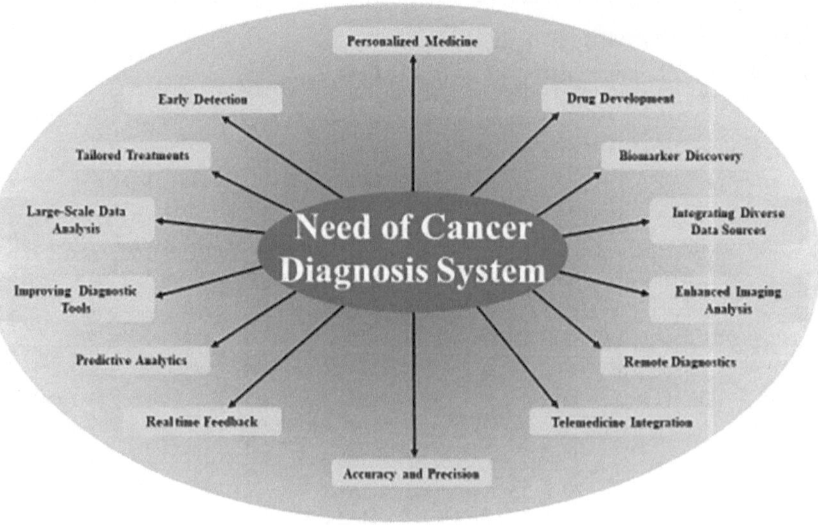

FIGURE 7.10 Need for cancer diagnostic systems.

improving model robustness. Generative AI can enhance the resolution of medical images, making it easier to detect subtle signs of cancer that may be missed in lower-quality scans [113, 114]. This can lead to more accurate diagnoses, especially in early stages. Generative models can be trained to understand what healthy tissue looks like and then identify deviations that might indicate cancerous growths. This can enhance the accuracy of detection by focusing on areas of concern that differ from the norm. Generative AI can simulate how different treatment options (e.g., chemotherapy, radiation) might affect a patient based on their unique biological data. This can assist oncologists in planning personalized treatment strategies with higher success probabilities. Generative models can predict how a patient's cancer might respond to specific drugs by generating molecular simulations, helping to tailor treatment plans more effectively. Generative models can provide insights into how a diagnosis was reached by generating visual or textual explanations, making the decision-making process more transparent and trustworthy for clinicians and patients alike. Generative AI can offer interactive diagnostic tools where clinicians can explore different hypothetical scenarios (e.g., "What if this tumor grows by 10%?") and visualize the potential outcomes, aiding in more informed decision-making [114]. By generating hypothetical patient profiles, generative AI can help in stratifying patients into different risk categories, leading to more precise monitoring and intervention strategies. Generative AI can synthesize multi-omics data (genomics, proteomics, metabolomics) to create comprehensive patient profiles that enhance the precision of cancer diagnostics. This holistic view is crucial for understanding cancer at a molecular level. Generative models can simulate interactions between genes, proteins, and other molecules to predict how these interactions might lead to cancer, aiding in the discovery of new biomarkers and therapeutic targets. Generative AI can offer real-time assistance to clinicians by generating potential diagnostic outcomes and treatment suggestions based on the latest patient data, facilitating quicker and more accurate decisions. Generative AI can enhance remote diagnostics by generating detailed patient reports and treatment simulations that can be shared with clinicians across the globe, facilitating better care even from a distance. Generative AI can create realistic yet anonymous patient data, allowing researchers and developers to work with high-quality data without compromising patient privacy. By generating diverse datasets that represent different populations, generative AI can help mitigate biases in diagnostic models, leading to more equitable healthcare outcomes. In summary, the combination of generative AI with machine learning in cancer diagnostics offers transformative potential. It enhances data-driven decision-making, improves the accuracy and personalization of diagnostics, supports advanced research, and expands access to high-quality healthcare. This synergy can significantly advance the fight against cancer, leading to better outcomes for patients worldwide [115–123].

7.5.1 Design of Smart and Intelligent Cancer Diagnostic Systems

A comprehensive analysis has led to the proposal of a diagnostic model for cancer illnesses. The suggested model has several crucial elements, including data sources, pre-processing, model development, testing and validation, model deployment [118, 124]. The remainder of this section presents the model's operation. Initially, the patients' data must be gathered. Among the crucial data sources are medical equipment, electronic medical records (EMRs), diagnostic and research facilities, healthcare applications, and social media. Despite this, real-time data collection from patients will also be facilitated by the Internet of Things (IoT), enabling routine monitoring of individuals with cancer. Pre-processing will be done on the gathered data to eliminate any ambiguity. Appropriate feature selection methods will be used to raise the diagnosis prediction rate. In order to diagnose cancer, clustering approaches aid in the examination of various biological, social, psychological, and emotional aspects [118, 125]. Furthermore, the suggested model's predictive module performs the illness prediction. Random forests, SVMs, and CNNs are used for feature selection, binary classification, segmentation, and image classification, as well as for feature interpretation and convolutional neural network. On the other hand, generative adversarial networks and variational autoencoders (VAEs) are utilized for anomaly detection and creating synthetic medical images to enhance datasets. When creating generative AI models, training and validation are essential phases. In order for the generative model to produce new, comparable data, training must let it recognize the underlying patterns and structures of the training set [126, 127]. The generator and discriminator in a GAN are trained in tandem, with the generator attempting to produce realistic data and the discriminator attempting to discern between authentic and fraudulent data. Validation is done using a different dataset that wasn't utilized for training [119, 128]. The distribution of this dataset ought to resemble that of the training dataset. The metrics used for the generating task are used to assess the model's performance. Hyperparameters and model retraining may be done in response to validation findings in order to enhance performance. Finally, both the patient and medical providers will receive a graphic representation of the

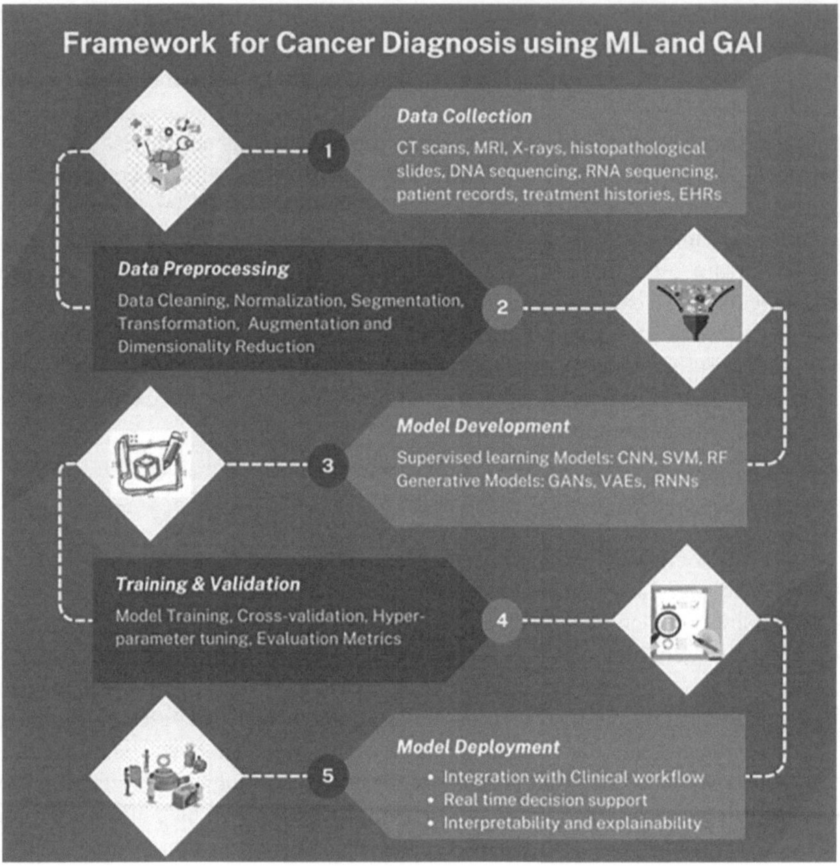

FIGURE 7.11 Design of smart and intelligent cancer diagnostic systems.

patient's final health state. By integrating the AI model into a picture archiving and communication system (PACS) or hospital information system (HIS), clinicians can interact with AI tools through intuitive interfaces, implementing models for real-time cancer diagnosis and detection on edge or cloud devices [120, 129].

7.6 RESULTS AND DISCUSSION

Cancer identification is crucial to patient outcomes. Traditional diagnostics use imaging, histology, and biomarkers. These approaches take time, need expert interpretation, and aren't always precise. ML algorithms, especially deep learning models, have excelled at analyzing X-rays, MRIs, and CT scans. Convolutional neural networks can recognize tumors in images, discriminate benign from malignant growths, and diagnose cancer early. From massive labelled image datasets, these models improve their accuracy. DeepMind's AI systems can outperform doctors in mammography breast cancer detection, showing ML's therapeutic promise.

Algorithms can predict outcomes and customize treatment approaches using gene expression data. This method is essential to personalized medicine, which tailors therapies to each patient's genetics. Historical data can be utilized to predict patient outcomes with ML models. ML can predict cancer recurrence, survival, and therapy responses by analyzing patient demographics, treatment history, and genetic data. This predictive power is essential for long-term therapy planning and patient management.

Generative AI like generative adversarial networks may create synthetic data that looks like actual data. This is useful in medical imaging, since large datasets are hard to get. GANs can create realistic medical images for ML model training, especially when labelled data is scarce. Generative AI enhances datasets to make ML models more robust and generalizable across populations and environments. Generative AI can model and simulate how cancer evolves over time, providing vital insights into disease dynamics. These models can produce synthetic patient trajectories to help clinicians make informed decisions about future scenarios. This is valuable for studying uncommon tumors or predicting new therapy responses when real-world data is limited. Generative AI improves medical image clarity and resolution to improve diagnosis. GAN-driven super-resolution imaging improves low-resolution pictures for malignant lesion analysis and detection. These models also reduce image noise and artefacts, improving diagnosis.

7.7 CONCLUSION

Machine learning and generative AI are transforming cancer diagnosis, offering new avenues for early detection, personalized treatment, and improved patient outcomes. While challenges remain, ongoing research and development hold the promise of more accurate, accessible, and equitable cancer care in the future. This framework provides a structured approach to leveraging machine learning and generative AI techniques in cancer diagnosis. By systematically integrating these advanced technologies, it is possible to develop more accurate, efficient, and accessible diagnostic tools that can significantly impact patient outcomes. For ML and generative AI to be fully effective, they need to be seamlessly integrated into clinical workflows. This includes developing user-friendly interfaces and ensuring compatibility with existing medical systems. The future may see the rise of collaborative AI systems where ML and generative AI models work alongside healthcare professionals, augmenting their decision-making processes rather than replacing them. This synergy can lead to more accurate, timely, and personalized cancer care. As new data becomes available, AI models must be capable of continual learning, adapting to new information, and improving over time. This will require developing robust frameworks for model updating and validation.

REFERENCES

1. Schlenk, E. A., Erlen, J. A., Dunbar-Jacob, J., McDowell, J., Engberg, S., Sereika, S. M., . . . Bernier, M. J. (1997). Health-related quality of life in chronic disorders: A comparison across studies using the MOS SF-36. *Quality of Life Research*, 7, 57–65.

2. Gautam, R., Kaur, P., & Sharma, M. (2019). A comprehensive review on nature inspired computing algorithms for the diagnosis of chronic disorders in human beings. *Progress in Artificial Intelligence*, 8(4), 401–424.
3. Arbelle, J. E., Chodick, G., Goldstein, A., & Porath, A. (2014). Multiple chronic disorders-health care system's modern challenge in the Maccabi health care system. *Israel Journal of Health Policy Research*, 3, 1–8.
4. Daré, L. O., Bruand, P. E., Gérard, D., Marin, B., Lameyre, V., Boumédiène, F., & Preux, P. M. (2019). Co-morbidities of mental disorders and chronic physical diseases in developing and emerging countries: A meta-analysis. *BMC Public Health*, 19, 1–12.
5. Stefanaki, C., Pervanidou, P., Boschiero, D., & Chrousos, G. P. (2018). Chronic stress and body composition disorders: Implications for health and disease. *Hormones*, 17, 33–43.
6. Zugazagoitia, J., Guedes, C., Ponce, S., Ferrer, I., Molina-Pinelo, S., & Paz-Ares, L. (2016). Current challenges in cancer treatment. *Clinical Therapeutics*, 38(7), 1551–1566.
7. Hassanpour, S. H., & Dehghani, M. (2017). Review of cancer from perspective of molecular. *Journal of Cancer Research and Practice*, 4(4), 127–129.
8. Dunn, G. P., Old, L. J., & Schreiber, R. D. (2004). The immunobiology of cancer immunosurveillance and immunoediting. *Immunity*, 21(2), 137–148.
9. Coughlin, S. S., & Ekwueme, D. U. (2009). Breast cancer as a global health concern. *Cancer Epidemiology*, 33(5), 315–318.
10. Guan, X. (2015). Cancer metastases: Challenges and opportunities. *Acta Pharmaceutica Sinica B*, 5(5), 402–418.
11. Fass, L. (2008). Imaging and cancer: A review. *Molecular Oncology*, 2(2), 115–152.
12. Carroll, K. K. (1998). Obesity as a risk factor for certain types of cancer. *Lipids*, 33(11), 1055–1059.
13. https://www.cancer.gov/about-cancer/causes-prevention/genetics [accessed on 12 April 2024].
14. Preethi, K. A., Lakshmanan, G., & Sekar, D. (2021). Antagomir technology in the treatment of different types of cancer. *Epigenomics*, 13(7), 481–484.
15. Jodry, D., Obedin-Maliver, J., Flowers, L., Jay, N., Floyd, S., Teoh, D., . . . Khan, M. J. (2023). Understanding sexual and gender minority populations and organ-based screening recommendations for human papillomavirus–related cancers. *Journal of Lower Genital Tract Disease*, 27(4), 307–321.
16. Alzahrani, S. M., Al Doghaither, H. A., & Al-Ghafari, A. B. (2021). General insight into cancer: An overview of colorectal cancer. *Molecular and Clinical Oncology*, 15(6), 271.
17. Kaur, B., Kumar, S., & Kaushik, B. K. (2022). Recent advancements in optical biosensors for cancer detection. *Biosensors and Bioelectronics*, 197, 113805.
18. https://www.who.int/news/item/01-02-2024-global-cancer-burden-growing—amidst-mounting-need-for-services [accessed on 16 April 2024].
19. Auyang, Y. S. (2006). Cancer causes and cancer research on many levels of complexity. *Creating Technology*, 1–15.
20. Preethi, K. A., Lakshmanan, G., & Sekar, D. (2021). Antagomir technology in the treatment of different types of cancer. *Epigenomics*, 13(7), 481–484.
21. Wang, Y., & Feng, W. (2022, Oct 6). Cancer-related psychosocial challenges. *General Psychiatry*, 35(5), e100871. doi:10.1136/gpsych-2022-100871. PMID: 36311374; PMCID: PMC9540834.
22. Munir, K., Elahi, H., Ayub, A., Frezza, F., & Rizzi, A. (2019, Aug 23). Cancer diagnosis using deep learning: A bibliographic review. *Cancers (Basel)*, 11(9), 1235. doi:10.3390/cancers11091235. PMID: 31450799; PMCID: PMC6770116.
23. Youneszade, N., Marjani, M., & Pei, C. P. (2023). Deep learning in cervical cancer diagnosis: Architecture, opportunities, and open research challenges. *IEEE Access*, 11, 6133–6149.

24. Sung, H., Ferlay, J., Siegel, R. L., Laversanne, M., Soerjomataram, I., Jemal, A., & Bray, F. (2021). Global cancer statistics 2020: GLOBOCAN estimates of incidence and mortality worldwide for 36 cancers in 185 countries. *CA: A Cancer Journal for Clinicians*, 71(3), 209–249.
25. Kulothungan, V., Sathishkumar, K., Leburu, S., et al. (2022). Burden of cancers in India—estimates of cancer crude incidence, YLLs, YLDs and DALYs for 2021 and 2025 based on National Cancer Registry Program. *BMC Cancer*, 22, 527.
26. Shreyas, J., Jumnal, A., Kumar, S. D., & Venugopal, K. R. (2020). Application of computational intelligence techniques for internet of things: An extensive survey. *International Journal of Computational Intelligence Studies*, 9(3), 234–288.
27. Rajkumar, S., Sujay, D. J., Sangeetha, R., Sudhakar, G., Muralikrishna, K., & Kumaraswamy, D. (2024). An overview of computer science and engineering and its latest technologies. *International Research Journal on Advanced Engineering Hub (IRJAEH)*, 2(04), 683–698.
28. Kaur, S., Singla, J., Nkenyereye, L., Jha, S., Prashar, D., Joshi, G. P., . . . Islam, S. R. (2020). Medical diagnostic systems using artificial intelligence (AI) algorithms: Principles and perspectives. *IEEE Access*, 8, 228049–228069.
29. SS, V. C., & HS, A. (2022). Nature inspired meta heuristic algorithms for optimization problems. *Computing*, 104(2), 251–269.
30. Abd Elaziz, M., Dahou, A., Abualigah, L., Yu, L., Alshinwan, M., Khasawneh, A. M., & Lu, S. (2021). Advanced metaheuristic optimization techniques in applications of deep neural networks: A review. *Neural Computing and Applications*, 1–21.
31. Lu, P., Ye, L., Zhao, Y., Dai, B., Pei, M., & Tang, Y. (2021). Review of meta-heuristic algorithms for wind power prediction: Methodologies, applications and challenges. *Applied Energy*, 301, 117446.
32. Karimi-Mamaghan, M., Mohammadi, M., Meyer, P., Karimi-Mamaghan, A. M., & Talbi, E. G. (2022). Machine learning at the service of meta-heuristics for solving combinatorial optimization problems: A state-of-the-art. *European Journal of Operational Research*, 296(2), 393–422.
33. Ezugwu, A. E., Shukla, A. K., Nath, R., Akinyelu, A. A., Agushaka, J. O., Chiroma, H., & Muhuri, P. K. (2021). Metaheuristics: A comprehensive overview and classification along with bibliometric analysis. *Artificial Intelligence Review*, 54, 4237–4316.
34. Long, N. K., Sammut, K., Sgarioto, D., Garratt, M., & Abbass, H. A. (2020). A comprehensive review of shepherding as a bio-inspired swarm-robotics guidance approach. *IEEE Transactions on Emerging Topics in Computational Intelligence*, 4(4), 523–537.
35. Feng, Y. (2023). *Collective behaviors of swarms and flocks* (Doctoral dissertation, Stanford University).
36. Bandi, A., Adapa, P. V. S. R., & Kuchi, Y. E. V. P. K. (2023). The power of generative AI: A review of requirements, models, input–output formats, evaluation metrics, and challenges. *Future Internet*, 15(8), 260.
37. Epstein, Z., Hertzmann, A., Investigators of Human Creativity, Akten, M., Farid, H., Fjeld, J., . . . Smith, A. (2023). Art and the science of generative AI. *Science*, 380(6650), 1110–1111.
38. Jo, A. (2023). The promise and peril of generative AI. *Nature*, 614(1), 214–216. Brynjolfsson, E., Li, D., & Raymond, L. R. (2023). *Generative AI at work* (No. w31161). National Bureau of Economic Research.
39. Lim, W. M., Gunasekara, A., Pallant, J. L., Pallant, J. I., & Pechenkina, E. (2023). Generative AI and the future of education: Ragnarök or reformation? A paradoxical perspective from management educators. *The International Journal of Management Education*, 21(2), 100790.
40. Liang, C., Du, H., Sun, Y., Niyato, D., Kang, J., Zhao, D., & Imran, M. A. (2024). Generative AI-driven semantic communication networks: Architecture, technologies and applications. *IEEE Transactions on Cognitive Communications and Networking*. https://doi.org/10.1109/TCCN.2024.3435524

41. Bandi, A., Adapa, P. V. S. R., & Kuchi, Y. E. V. P. K. (2023). The power of generative AI: A review of requirements, models, input–output formats, evaluation metrics, and challenges. *Future Internet*, 15(8), 260.
42. Sengar, S. S., Hasan, A. B., Kumar, S., & Carroll, F. (2024). Generative artificial intelligence: A systematic review and applications. *arXiv preprint* arXiv:2405.11029.
43. Foster, D. (2022). *Generative deep learning*. O'Reilly Media, Inc.
44. Yang, Z., Ran, L., Zhang, S., Xia, Y., & Zhang, Y. (2019). EMS-net: Ensemble of Multiscale convolutional neural networks for classification of breast cancer histology images. *Neurocomputing*, 366, 46–53.
45. Rajaguru, H. (2019). Analysis of decision tree and k-nearest neighbor algorithm in the classification of breast cancer. *Asian Pacific Journal of Cancer Prevention (APJCP)*, 20, 3777.
46. Blanes-Vidal, V., Baatrup, G., & Nadimi, E. S. (2019). Addressing priority challenges in the detection and assessment of colorectal polyps from capsule endoscopy and colonoscopy in colorectal cancer screening using machine learning. *Acta Oncologica*, 58, S29–S36.
47. Nadimi, E. S., Buijs, M. M., Herp, J., Kroijer, R., Kobaek-Larsen, M., Nielsen, E., Pedersen, C. D., Blanes-Vidal, V., & Baatrup, G. (2020). Application of deep learning for autonomous detection and localization of colorectal polyps in wireless colon capsule endoscopy. *Computers & Electrical Engineering*, 81, 106531.
48. Chiang, Y. M., Chiang, H. M., & Lin, S. Y. (2008). The application of ant colony optimization for gene selection in microarray-based cancer classification. *Proceedings of the Seventh International Conference on Machine Learning and Cybernetics*, Kunming, pp. 4001–4006.
49. Saravana Kumar, K., & Arthanariee, A. M. (2017). *Breast Cancer Risk Evaluation by Firefly Optimization*.
50. Moosa, J. M., Shakur, R., Kaykobad, M., Rahman, M. S. (2015). Gene selection for cancer classification with the help of bees. *BMC Medical Genomics*, 9(2), 136–204.
51. Banu, P. K. N., Azar, A. T., & Inbarani, H. H. (2017). Fuzzy firefly clustering for a tumour and cancer analysis. *International Journal of Modelling, Identification, and Control*, 27(2), 92–103.
52. Alickovic, E., & Subasi, A. (2017). Breast cancer diagnosis using GA feature selection and Rotation Forest. *Neural Computing & Applications*, 28(4), 753–763. doi:10.1007/s00521-015-2103-9.
53. De Carvalho Filho, A. O., Silva, A. C., De Paiva, A. C., Nunes, R. A., & Gattass, M. (2017). Computer-aided diagnosis system for lung nodules based on computed tomography using shape analysis, a genetic algorithm, and SVM. *Medical & Biological Engineering & Computing*, 55(8), 1129–1146. doi:10.1007/s11517-016-1577-7. PMID:27699621.
54. Mansoori, T. K., Suman, A., & Mishra, S. K. (2014). Feature selection by genetic algorithm and SVM classification for cancer detection. *International Journal of Advanced Research in Computer Science and Software Engineering*, 4(9), 357–365.
55. Deoskar, P., Singh, D. D., & Singh, D. A. (2013). An efficient support based ant colony optimization technique for lung cancer data. *International Journal of Advanced Research in Computer and Communication Engineering*, 2(9).
56. Patankar, V., Nawgaje, D., & Kanphade, R. (2014). An implementation of ant colony optimization technique for cancer diagnosis. *International Journal of Current Engineering and Technology*, 4, 568–570.
57. Vimaladevi, M., & Kalaavathi, B. (2014). Cancer classification using hybrid fast particle swarm optimization with back propagation neural network. *International Journal of Advanced Research in Computer and Communication Engineering*, 3, 8410–8414. doi:10.17148/IJARCCE.2014.31112.

58. Mohanty, A. K., Sahoo, S., Pradhan, A., & Lenka, S. K. (2011). Breast cancer assessment and diagnosis using particle swarm optimization. *International Journal of Computer Science and Technology*, 2, 37–41.
59. Vijaylakshmi, S., & Priyadarshini, J. (2016). An analysis of particle swarm optimization technique for breast cancer dataset. *International Journal of Computer Technology and Applications*, 9, 279–306.
60. Nazarian, M., Dezfouli, M. A., & Haronabadi, A. (2013). Classification of breast cancer samples through using the artificial bee colony algorithm. *International Journal of Computer Applications Technology and Research*, 2(5), 522–525. doi:10.7753/IJCATR0205.1004.
61. Rasool, A., Bunterngchit, C., Tiejian, L., Islam, M. R., Qu, Q., & Jiang, Q. (2022). Improved machine learning-based predictive models for breast cancer diagnosis. *International Journal of Environmental Research and Public Health*, 19(6), 3211.
62. Egwom, O. J., Hassan, M., Tanimu, J. J., Hamada, M., & Ogar, O. M. (2022). An LDA–SVM machine learning model for breast cancer classification. *BioMedInformatics*, 2(3), 345–358.
63. Roy, C., Mazumder, I., Debdas, S., Samanta, S., & Roy, S. S. (2022, Feb). Framework for breast cancer diagnosis using machine learning and IoT. In *2022 First international conference on electrical, electronics, information and communication technologies (ICEEICT)*, pp. 1–4. IEEE.
64. Jasti, V. D. P., Zamani, A. S., Arumugam, K., Naved, M., Pallathadka, H., Sammy, F., Raghuvanshi, A. Kaliyaperumal, K., & Thippa Reddy, G. (2022). Computational technique based on machine learning and image processing for medical image analysis of breast cancer diagnosis. *Security and Communication Networks*, 2022, 1–7. https://doi.org/10.1155/2022/1918379
65. Vigil, N., Barry, M., Amini, A., Akhloufi, M., Maldague, X. P., Ma, L., . . . Yousefi, B. (2022). Dual-intended deep learning model for breast cancer diagnosis in ultrasound imaging. *Cancers*, 14(11), 2663.
66. Fallahzadeh, O., Dehghani-Bidgoli, Z., & Assarian, M. (2018). Raman spectral feature selection using ant colony optimization for breast cancer diagnosis. *Lasers in Medical Science*, 1–8.
67. Umamaheswari, T. S., & Sumathi, P. (2018). Enhanced firefly algorithm (EFA) based gene selection and adaptive neuro neutrosophic inference system (ANNIS) prediction model for detection of circulating tumour cells (CTCs) in breast cancer analysis. *Cluster Computing*, 1–13.
68. Khuriwal, N., & Mishra, N. (2018, Oct). Breast cancer diagnosis using deep learning algorithm. In *2018 International conference on advances in computing, communication control and networking (ICACCCN)*, pp. 98–103. IEEE.
69. Senapati, M. R., & Dash, P. K. (2013). Local linear wavelet neural network based breast tumour classification using firefly algorithm. *Neural Computing and Applications*, 22(7), 1591–1598.
70. Shahbeig, S., Helfroush, M. S., & Rahideh, A. (2017). A fuzzy multi-objective hybrid TLBO–PSO approach to select the associated genes with breast cancer. *Signal Processing*, 131, 58–65. doi:10.1016/j.sigpro.2016.07.035.
71. Zamani, H., Hossein, M., & Shahrak, N. (2016). Swarm intelligence approach for breast cancer diagnosis. *International Journal of Computer Applications*, 151(1), 40–44.
72. Mazen, F., AbulSeoud, R. A., & Gody, A. M. (2016). Genetic algorithm and firefly algorithm in a hybrid approach for breast cancer diagnosis. *International Journal of Computer Trends and Technology*, 32(2), 62–68.
73. Sayed, G. I., Soliman, M., & Hassanien, A. E. (2016). Bio-inspired Swarm Techniques for thermogram breast cancer detection. In *Medical imaging in clinical applications, algorithmic and computer-based approaches*, pp. 487–506. Springer International Publishing.

74. Alshamlan, H., Badr, G., & Alohali, A. (2015). mRMR-ABC: A hybrid gene selection algorithm for cancer classification using microarray gene expression profiling. *BioMed Research International*, 2015, 1–15. doi:10.1155/2015/604910. PMID:25961028.
75. Aalaei, S., Shahraki, H., Rowhanimanesh, A., & Eslami, S. (2016). Feature selection using genetic algorithm for breast cancer diagnosis: Experiment on three different datasets. *Iranian Journal of Basic Medical Sciences*, 19, 476–482. PMID:27403253.
76. Turabieh, H. (2016). GA-based feature selection with ANFIS approach to breast cancer recurrence. *International Journal of Computer Science Issues*, 13(1), 36–41. doi:10.20943/IJCSI-201602-3641.
77. Anto, S., & Chandramathi, S. (2015). An expert system for breast cancer diagnosis using fuzzy classifier with ant colony optimization. *Australian Journal of Basic and Applied Sciences*, 9(13), 172–177.
78. Sadeghipour, E., Sahragard, N., Sayebani, M. R., & Mehdizadeh, R. (2015). Breast cancer detection based on a hybrid approach of firefly algorithm and intelligent systems. *Indian Journal of Fundamental and Applied Life Sciences*, 5, 468–472.
79. Cinar, M., Engin, M., Engin, E. Z., & Ziya, Y. (2009). Early prostate cancer diagnosis by using artificial neural networks and support vector machine. *Experts System with Applications*, 36(3), 6357–6361.
80. Shah, H., Chiromab, H., Herawan, T., & Ghazalic, R. (2015). An efficient bio-inspired bees colony for breast cancer prediction. In *Lecture notes in electrical engineering*, pp. 1–9. Springer.
81. Pourmandi, M., & Addeh, J. (2015). Breast cancer diagnosis using fuzzy feature and optimized neural network via the Gbest-guided artificial bee colony algorithm. *Computational Research Progress in Applied Science & Engineering*, 1(4), 152–159.
82. Hassanien, A. E., Moftah, H. M., Azar, A. T., & Shoman, M. (2014). MRI breast cancer diagnosis hybrid approach using adaptive ant-based segmentation and multilayer perceptron neural networks classifier. *Applied Soft Computing*, 14, 62–71.
83. Schaefer, G. (2014). ACO classification of thermogram symmetry features for breast cancer diagnosis. *Memetic Computing*, 6(3), 207–212.
84. Karnan, S. M. (2014). Medical image segmentation using firefly algorithm and enhanced bee colony optimization. *Bonfring International Journal of Advances in Image Processing*, 316–321.
85. Krawczyk, B., & Filipczuk, P. (2018). Cytological image analysis with firefly nuclei detection and hybrid one class classification decomposition. *Engineering Applications of Artificial Intelligence*, 31, 126–135.
86. Nazarian, M., Dezfouli, M. A., & Haronabadi, A. (2013). Classification of breast cancer samples using the artificial bee colony algorithm. *International Journal of Computer Applications Technology and Research*, 2(5), 522–525.
87. Sharma, A., & Mishra, P. K. (2022). Performance analysis of machine learning based optimized feature selection approaches for breast cancer diagnosis. *International Journal of Information Technology*, 14(4), 1949–1960.
88. Kavitha, T., Mathai, P. P., Karthikeyan, C., Ashok, M., Kohar, R., Avanija, J., & Neelakandan, S. (2022). Deep learning based capsule neural network model for breast cancer diagnosis using mammogram images. *Interdisciplinary Sciences: Computational Life Sciences*, 14(1), 113–129.
89. Rehman, M. U., Shafique, A., Ghadi, Y. Y., Boulila, W., Jan, S. U., Gadekallu, T. R., . . . Ahmad, J. (2022). A novel chaos-based privacy-preserving deep learning model for cancer diagnosis. *IEEE Transactions on Network Science and Engineering*, 9(6), 4322–4337.
90. PramitaManna, Tapas Si. (2016). Brain MRI segmentation for lesion detection using clustering with the fire-fly algorithm. *Artificial Intelligence and Evolutionary Computations in Engineering Systems*, 394, 1347–1355.

91. Shukla, R., & Motwani, D. (2014). Cancer detection using frequency pattern ant colony optimization. *International Journal of Engineering Development and Research*, 2, 3922–3927.
92. Sunny, S., & Pratheba, M. (2014). Detection of breast cancer using the firefly algorithm. *International Journal of Emerging Technologies and Engineering*, 1(3), 84–86.
93. Shin, H. C., Tenenholtz, N. A., Rogers, J. K., Schwarz, C. G., Senjem, M. L., Gunter, J. L., . . . Michalski, M. (2018). Medical image synthesis for data augmentation and anonymization using generative adversarial networks. In *Simulation and synthesis in medical imaging: Third international workshop, SASHIMI 2018, held in conjunction with MICCAI 2018*, Granada, Spain, September 16, 2018, Proceedings 3, pp. 1–11. Springer International Publishing.
94. Wang, Q., Zhou, X., Wang, C., Liu, Z., Huang, J., Zhou, Y., . . . Cheng, J. Z. (2019). WGAN-based synthetic minority over-sampling technique: Improving semantic fine-grained classification for lung nodules in CT images. *IEEE Access*, 7, 18450–18463.
95. Liu, Y., Zhou, Y., Liu, X., Dong, F., Wang, C., & Wang, Z. (2019). Wasserstein GAN-based small-sample augmentation for new-generation artificial intelligence: A case study of cancer-staging data in biology. *Engineering*, 5(1), 156–163.
96. Srivishnu, M. V., Shreyas, S., Akash, S., Srikanth, A., & Patil, M. *Empowering early cancer detection through machine learning and generative models.*
97. Karimzadeh, M., Momen-Roknabadi, A., Cavazos, T. B., Fang, Y., Chen, N. C., Multhaup, M., . . . Goodarzi, H. (2024). Deep generative AI models analyzing circulating orphan non-coding RNAs enable accurate detection of early-stage non-small cell lung cancer. *medRxiv*, 2024-04.
98. Saeed, M., Naseer, A., Masood, H., Rehman, S. U., & Gruhn, V. (2023). The power of generative AI to augment for enhanced skin cancer classification: A deep learning approach. *IEEE Access*, 11, 130330–130344.
99. Levine, A. B., Peng, J., Farnell, D., Nursey, M., Wang, Y., Naso, J. R., . . . Bashashati, A. (2020). Synthesis of diagnostic quality cancer pathology images by generative adversarial networks. *The Journal of Pathology*, 252(2), 178–188.
100. Xiao, Y., Wu, J., & Lin, Z. (2021). Cancer diagnosis using generative adversarial networks based on deep learning from imbalanced data. *Computers in Biology and Medicine*, 135, 104540.
101. La Salvia, M., Torti, E., Leon, R., Fabelo, H., Ortega, S., Martinez-Vega, B., . . . Leporati, F. (2022). Deep convolutional generative adversarial networks to enhance artificial intelligence in healthcare: A skin cancer application. *Sensors*, 22(16), 6145.
102. Inan, M. S. K., Hossain, S., & Uddin, M. N. (2023). Data augmentation guided breast cancer diagnosis and prognosis using an integrated deep-generative framework based on breast tumor's morphological information. *Informatics in Medicine Unlocked*, 37, 101171.
103. Liu, Y., Zhou, Y., Liu, X., Dong, F., Wang, C., & Wang, Z. (2019). Wasserstein GAN-based small-sample augmentation for new-generation artificial intelligence: A case study of cancer-staging data in biology. *Engineering*, 5(1), 156–163.
104 .Salama, W. M., Shokry, A., & Aly, M. H. (2022). A generalized framework for lung Cancer classification based on deep generative models. *Multimedia Tools and Applications*, 81(23), 32705–32722.
105. Cascella, M., Scarpati, G., Bignami, E. G., Cuomo, A., Vittori, A., Di Gennaro, P., . . Coluccia, S. (2023). Utilizing an artificial intelligence framework (conditional generative adversarial network) to enhance telemedicine strategies for cancer pain management. *Journal of Anesthesia, Analgesia and Critical Care*, 3(1), 19.
106. Wei, K., Li, T., Huang, F., Chen, J., & He, Z. (2022). Cancer classification with data augmentation based on generative adversarial networks. *Frontiers of Computer Science*, 16, 1–11.

107. Moulaei, K., Yadegari, A., Baharestani, M., Farzanbakhsh, S., Sabet, B., & Afrash, M. R. (2024). Generative artificial intelligence in healthcare: A scoping review on benefits, challenges and applications. *International Journal of Medical Informatics*, 105474.
108. Gupta, R. K., Bharti, S., Kunhare, N., Sahu, Y., & Pathik, N. (2022). Brain tumor detection and classification using cycle generative adversarial networks. *Interdisciplinary Sciences: Computational Life Sciences*, 14(2), 485–502.
109. Zhang, F., Zhang, Y., Zhu, X., Chen, X., Du, H., & Zhang, X. (2022). PregGAN: A prognosis prediction model for breast cancer based on conditional generative adversarial networks. *Computer Methods and Programs in Biomedicine*, 224, 107026.
110. Maiti, A., Chatterjee, B., & Santosh, K. C. (2021). Skin cancer classification through quantized color features and generative adversarial network. *International Journal of Ambient Computing and Intelligence (IJACI)*, 12(3), 75–97.
111. Iqbal, M. J., Javed, Z., Sadia, H., Qureshi, I. A., Irshad, A., Ahmed, R., . . . Sharifi-Rad, J. (2021). Clinical applications of artificial intelligence and machine learning in cancer diagnosis: Looking into the future. *Cancer Cell International*, 21(1), 270.
112. Nooreldeen, R., & Bach, H. (2021). Current and future development in lung cancer diagnosis. *International Journal of Molecular Sciences*, 22(16), 8661.
113. Yang, J., Xu, R., Wang, C., Qiu, J., Ren, B., & You, L. (2021). Early screening and diagnosis strategies of pancreatic cancer: A comprehensive review. *Cancer Communications*, 41(12), 1257–1274.
114. Savage, N. (2020). How AI is improving cancer diagnostics. *Nature*, 579(7800), S14–S14.
115. Nugroho, H. A., Frannita, E. L., Ardiyanto, I., & Choridah, L. (2021). Computer aided diagnosis for thyroid cancer system based on internal and external characteristics. *Journal of King Saud University-Computer and Information Sciences*, 33(3), 329–339.
116. Kose, U., & Alzubi, J. (2021). *Deep learning for cancer diagnosis*. Singapore: Springer.
117. Sagdic, K., Eş, I., Sitti, M., & Inci, F. (2022). Smart materials: Rational design in biosystems via artificial intelligence. *Trends in Biotechnology*, 40(8), 987–1003.
118. Onasanya, A., & Elshakankiri, M. (2021). Smart integrated IoT healthcare system for cancer care. *Wireless Networks*, 27(6), 4297–4312.
119. Wu, J., Gou, F., & Tan, Y. (2021). A staging auxiliary diagnosis model for nonsmall cell lung cancer based on the intelligent medical system. *Computational and Mathematical Methods in Medicine*, 2021(1), 6654946.
120. Singh, R., Sharma, A., Saji, J., Umapathi, A., Kumar, S., & Daima, H. K. (2022). Smart nanomaterials for cancer diagnosis and treatment. *Nano Convergence*, 9(1), 21.
121. Ali, U., Ali, S., & Ali, M. T. (2024). Synergies of AI and smart technology: Transforming cancer medicine, vaccine development, and patient care. *International Journal of Multidisciplinary Research and Growth Evaluation.*
122. Gupta, U., Pranav, A., Kohli, A., Ghosh, S., & Singh, D. (2024). The contribution of artificial intelligence to drug discovery: Current progress and prospects for the future. *Microbial data intelligence and computational techniques for sustainable computing,* pp. 1–23.
123. Gupta, D., Gupta, U., & Sarma, H. J. (2024). Functional iterative approach for Universum-based primal twin bounded support vector machine to EEG classification (FUPTBSVM). *Multimedia Tools and Applications*, 83(8), 22119–22151.
124. Gupta, U., & Jain, V. (2024). Social neuroscience: Inferring mental states in social media. In *Emotional AI and human-AI interactions in social networking*, pp. 15–39. Elsevier.
125. Sharma, M., Deswal, S., Gupta, U., Tabassum, M., & Lawal, I. (eds.). (2023). *Soft computing techniques in connected healthcare systems*. CRC Press.
126. Malik, K., Sadawarti, H., Sharma, M., Gupta, U., & Tiwari, P. (eds.). (2023). *Computational techniques in neuroscience*. CRC Press.

127. Singh, D., Singh, D., Manju, & Gupta, U. (2023). Smart healthcare: A breakthrough in the growth of technologies. In *Artificial intelligence-based healthcare systems*, pp. 73–85. Cham: Springer Nature Switzerland.
128. Gupta, M., Srivastava, D., Pantola, D., & Gupta, U. (2022). Brain tumor detection using improved Otsu's thresholding method and supervised learning techniques at early stage. In *Proceedings of emerging trends and technologies on intelligent systems: ETTIS 2022*, pp. 271–281. Singapore: Springer Nature Singapore.
129. Gupta, U., Gupta, D., & Agarwal, U. (2022). Analysis of randomization-based approaches for autism spectrum disorder. In *Pattern recognition and data analysis with applications*, pp. 701–713. Singapore: Springer Nature Singapore.
130. Gupta, D., Choudhury, A., Gupta, U., Singh, P., & Prasad, M. (2021). Computational approach to clinical diagnosis of diabetes disease: A comparative study. *Multimedia Tools and Applications*, 1–26.

8 Revolutionizing Medicine
The Impact of Artificial Intelligence in Healthcare

Jaishree Jain and Updesh Kumar Jaiswal

8.1 INTRODUCTION

Informatics breakthroughs in the twenty-first century have significantly changed our perception of data processing as the century of technology advances. Access to information was once a major issue, but in the scientific community today, rapidly expanding datasets are always available, easily shared, and stored in databases [1]. Human capacities have grown thanks to innovations and new advancements, which have also accelerated scientific advancement [2]. Innovations in informatics have brought about a significant shift in our perception of data processing in the twenty-first century, changing a number of fields and opening the door for previously unheard-of technological breakthroughs and problem-solving abilities [3–5]. Artificial intelligence (AI) will transform medicine in the upcoming years. The field of AI includes techniques such as deep learning (DL), machine learning (ML), and other methods that use neural networks (NNs) to mimic human thought processes in computers. Since the earliest achievements, when algorithms exhibited expert-level disease identification from medical images, the field of medical AI has undergone substantial change. AI is changing a wide number of businesses and is developing quickly.

Particularly in the area of medical physics, research has increased dramatically due to the fascinating opportunities presented by AI. Large data sets and quick processors enable deep learning, which pushes remarkable advancements in neural solid network models and creative algorithmic modelling. AI is poised to revolutionize medical physics research and practices because of the accessibility of promising learning methodologies and a wealth of computational resources. Because of this, our community needs to be prepared for upcoming opportunities and challenges and take the initiative in this new fourth industrial revolution that is underway [6]. Despite these developments, the application is largely unexplored, yet vital. In order to ensure that this technology is translated safely and effectively, the medical AI community is presently facing numerous ethical, technological, and human-centered difficulties [7].

 DOI: 10.1201/9781003539483-8

The application of AI technology for real medical practice is limited, despite the fact that AI algorithms have often demonstrated their efficacy in retrospective clinical studies [8]. Critics argue that because AI systems are too complex or slow for real-world use in medical situations, their benefits might not be as strong as what past research indicates [9, 10]. In addition, problems could arise from human–AI system interactions [11]. Once again, extensive filtering and cleaning are applied to retrospective in silico datasets; this could make them less representative settings [7]. AI technology is a very fast-developing approach that is being used in contemporary biology [12]. Its primary aim is to simulate human intellect in computer systems so that self-aware intelligent systems can be created.

Natural language processing (NLP) and vision are among the fields that use AI [13, 14]. Similarly, as its influence over medical practice grows, AI technology has had a significant impact on clinical medicine. AI-powered solutions can also improve administrative task efficiency, enable tailored treatment methods, and help with early disease identification. Furthermore, AI is becoming a potent tool with the potential to completely transform a number of domains of the delivery of healthcare, including data analysis, pharmaceutical creation, diagnosis, treatment planning, and customized care. AI's sophisticated algorithms and ML skills enable it to evaluate vast amounts of medical data, draw insightful conclusions, and offer precise forecasts. This facilitates better decision-making, enhances patient outcomes, and maximizes resource allocation for healthcare practitioners [15].

Genomic information from whole genome sequencing (WGS) research, clinical information from biomedical research, digital pathology, magnetic resonance imaging (MRI), and ultrasound (US) investigations all contribute to the necessary data [15–20]. Due to AI's enormous potential, major health tech companies like Philips, Siemens, and GE as well as prestigious hospitals like the Cleveland Clinic and Mayo Clinic have invested in the technology [4]. Pharmaceutical companies like Takeda and biotech companies like BERG use AI for medicine development and biomarker detection [21, 22].

Other businesses that are investing in wearables with AI capabilities to evaluate lifestyle and health include Google and Apple [23]. Another such is Facebook's Preventive Health service, which links users to health information and examination recommendations [24]. With AI transforming healthcare, these patterns show the rise of "Big Tech" or "GAFAM" American companies in the sector. Numerous thorough analyses highlighting AI's transformative impact on healthcare and medicine have been published [4]. This chapter explores medication discovery, individualized treatment, diagnostic and treatment planning, and medical imaging.

Banking, healthcare, and transportation are just a few of the areas that AI is currently transforming. As AI develops, it is imperative to make sure it is created morally and for the good of society [25–28].

Discussions about AI, in which computers carry out activities typically thought to need human intelligence, are now taking place in almost all scientific fields renowned for their ability to identify both individuals and images.

AI has also enabled significant improvements in NLP and speech recognition [29]. Concerns are raised by these discoveries on how these abilities can enhance or even replace human decision-making in the healthcare and medical domains. The

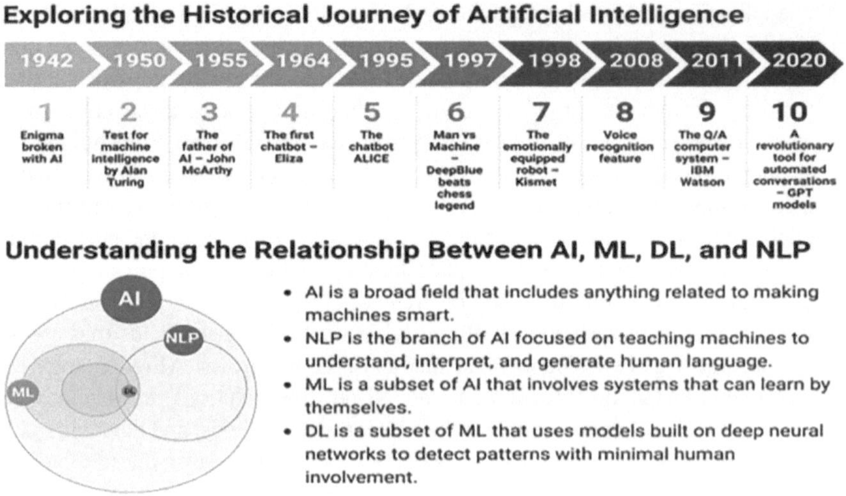

FIGURE 8.1 Development of AI via connections among AI, ML, DL, and NLP [25].

availability of pertinent data is a prerequisite for AI's potential [30]. There is a wealth of data in the health sectors [31]. But these resources' caliber and availability continue to be a substantial difficulty in the US.

Health data is more difficult to acquire and share than other forms of data since privacy concerns are linked to it. Furthermore, health data tends to be closely guarded after it is gathered since it can be expensive to obtain, especially in the case of clinical trials and longitudinal investigations. Furthermore, even the most basic computational techniques are hampered by the incompatibility of electronic health record systems [32, 33], and a crucial set of variables is absent from data streams related to an individual's health since these systems are unable to gather pertinent social and environmental data. Furthermore, there's a lot of curiosity in the corporate sector about AI in the gathering of health data and applications, as demonstrated by the several companies focusing on AI in health and healthcare [34]. Of the 106 listed startups, the majority have US headquarters. Fifteen different nations are home to startups. This research places a particular emphasis on the two most popular topics: patient data and risk analytics and medical imaging and diagnostics. The startup activity shown, however, does not fully demonstrate the impact of environmental factors—another major topic of this chapter.

8.2 RELATED WORK

Deep learning is a typical method for improving the effectiveness of the healthcare system aiding decision-making, decreasing errors, speeding up medical processes, and improving the efficiency and accuracy of diagnoses [35]. An important benefit of AI for medicine is the significant advancement in diagnosis that image analysis has made possible. In the 1970s, Stanford's blood-borne bacterial infection test was the first to use AI. They were not easily incorporated into workflows and medical record systems in the healthcare sector and their advantage over human diagnosticians was only marginally demonstrated. Therefore, when it became clear how difficult it would be to train treat integrate treatment methods, the initial enthusiasm subsided [36, 37].

AI has fundamentally altered the way that illnesses are identified and managed, offering vital assistance and new medical services. AI-powered solutions leverage cognitive technology, language processing, and autonomous reasoning to provide outstanding support for diagnosis and therapy. Using computer systems to intelligently support diagnosis and treatment is like having a machine brain that integrates data analysis and in-depth medical expertise. The system can recreate clinical reasoning and diagnostic thinking and generate a variety of diagnoses and related treatment options by combining examination results with patient histories. AI-assisted diagnosis and treatment technologies have advanced greatly thanks in large part to DL, greatly expanding access to healthcare. Patients are now able to witness firsthand the significance of AI.

Therefore, in order to increase trust in medical AI systems and show how they affect clinical outcomes, greater reporting transparency and validation standards must be developed [38]. For instance, AI systems have significantly improved the accuracy of radiology tasks, such as the interpretation of mammograms [39, 40], the evaluation of heart function [41, 42], and the screening of lung cancer, which addresses more than simply a diagnosis, in addition to risk assessment and treatment [43, 44]. For instance, radiologists' computed tomography (CT) readings and other clinical data were used to train an AI system to assess the diseases [45]. Subsequently, these predictions could be utilized to schedule CT scans for cancer patients as a follow-up, enhancing existing screening protocols. AI is getting closer to being used and having a useful impact on radiology thanks to the validation of such systems in numerous clinical settings and the expansion of prospective evaluations [46].

AI has significantly improved pathology, namely in tumor identification and the provision of new disease insights via whole-slide imaging [47]. The speed at which models identified regions of interest on slides could potentially expedite diagnostic procedures. Beyond this use, deep neural networks (DLNs) can identify structural differences and driving mutations, providing advantages beyond professional pathologist assessments. AI has also improved the accuracy of survival predictions for a variety of cancer types compared to histological subtyping and conventional grading [48]. Studies have demonstrated how AI may increase the effectiveness, accuracy, and value of pathology diagnoses [49]. In the field of gastroenterology, DL has made great strides, particularly in improving colonoscopy, an essential technique for the early detection of colorectal cancer. It has been possible to predict with more accuracy than experienced endoscopists whether colonic tumors are malignant by using DL algorithms [50]. AI algorithms have been created to help endoscopists diagnose colonoscopies because such polyps and other possible cancer indicators are frequently missed [51].

Furthermore, the projections generated by these methods may provide information to the public and authorities, as well as recommendations for control and prevention strategies. Principal component analysis (PCA) is one of the unsupervised learning techniques that can successfully reduce the dimensionality of data and help find important aspects linked to infectious diseases [52]. Similar to this, methods like K-means allow researchers to focus on particular medical cases by enabling the sorting of patients into subgroups and the detection of odd cases. For example, latent Dirichlet allocation models are topic models that extract relevant themes from documented medical records. The use of DL architectures has spread to a number of fields, including bioinformatics, social network filtering, prediction and classification, and more, offering useful tools for the analysis of infectious diseases [53]. The quick development of processing power, storage, ML, and biological data has accelerated the use of AI in scientific fields.

With the goals of minimizing human error, supporting decision-making, improving diagnosis accuracy, streamlining medical procedures, and boosting the effectiveness of the global health system, deep learning has become a prominent technique [54]. Medical diagnosis has been revolutionized by the surprising and useful application of AI in image analysis [55]. The application of AI has also greatly benefited dermatology, as research has repeatedly demonstrated how well AI can identify and categorize different kinds of skin lesions. These investigations have revealed an astounding degree of agreement between AI systems and knowledgeable dermatologists, highlighting AI's potential to improve dermatological procedures. Dermatologists may be able to speed up the diagnosis process, make better treatment decisions, and eventually improve patient outcomes by utilizing AI's analytical powers and large datasets [56].

Diagnostic and interpretation processes in cardiology have been expedited by the application of AI and ML. Faster measurements and assessments of heart function have made AI automation possible, which has improved cardiac MRI, echocardiography, SPECT imaging, cardiac CT angiography, and ECG readings [57]. Furthermore, it has been demonstrated that incorporating AI into electronic medical records (EMRs) can successfully reduce death rates and enable the early detection of heart failure. AI has also shown promise in identifying the optimal interventional approach for patients with angina.

AI and DL have been shown to be successful in ophthalmology in identifying diabetic retinopathy. High sensitivity and specificity rates have also been reported in investigations, suggesting the possibility of earlier diagnosis and better treatment [58, 59]. Nevertheless, more study in this area is still required [60, 61]. AI has demonstrated a lot of promise in the realm of oncology. AI applications have outperformed human readings. Watson and other ML algorithms have demonstrated strong concordance rates with multidisciplinary expert tumor boards, hence furnishing dependable therapy recommendations for breast cancer [62]. AI systems have outperformed human specialists in lung cancer detection, allowing for more accurate prognosis prediction and better patient treatment [63].

AI algorithms have shown exceptional diagnostic performance in pathology analysis as compared to pathologists, greatly cutting down on evaluation time [64]. Disease diagnosis is a key component of AI's application in biomedicine. Significant advancements in this sector have made it possible for medical practitioners to detect a variety of diseases early and with greater accuracy [65]. Using biosensors or biochips for in vitro diagnostics is an essential part of primary diagnosis. AI is crucial function in interpreting gene expression data from microarrays, enabling the classification and detection of abnormalities [66, 67]. Classifying cancer microarray data to assist in cancer detection is an emerging use [68]. Early detection of cardiovascular disorders may be possible with technologies and integrated AI systems [69]. AI is also able to forecast cancer patients' chances of survival, especially those with colon cancer [70]. Although there are known limitations to AI in biomedical diagnosis, researchers are currently trying to reduce these issues [71]. All things considered, AI has enormous promise for prognostics and diagnostics, opening the door to better healthcare outcomes. Diagnostic, therapeutic, and prognostic aspects of disease depend heavily on medical imaging and signal processing.

AI has been used to extract information from biomedical data, like EEG, EMG, and ECG, allowing advances in several domains, such as the prediction of epileptic seizures. As a dependable seizure prediction method, DL has shown promise and might be implemented on mobile platforms. AI has been applied to biomedical image processing for image segmentation, multidimensional imaging, thermal imaging, and even portable ultrasound equipment in underprivileged areas. Furthermore, AI can improve on current decision support systems, boosting their ability to accurately diagnose and manage conditions like cancer, tropical diseases, and cardiovascular disorders [72–75].

As AI advances, its potential for diagnosing illnesses comes to light more and more. With the introduction of AI into standard clinical practice, a new age in medicine is about to begin. AI shows great potential in the treatment of gastrointestinal issues. It can increase efficiency, improve endoscopic diagnostic capabilities, and provide patients with gastrointestinal bleeding and neoplasia with more precise risk classification. More investigation and verification of algorithms and their uses are required if we are to properly benefit from AI. In addition, in order to incorporate AI into their everyday clinical operations, affordable AI models and solutions must be created. Clinicians should view AI as a cooperative endeavor to enhance therapy results for gastrointestinal disorders rather than viewing it as a competition between humans and machines [75–80].

8.3 ARTIFICIAL INTELLIGENCE'S USE IN MEDICATION DEVELOPMENT

The growing chemical space makes it harder and more time consuming to find new medicinal molecules, which widens the gap between medication discovery and development [81]. Therefore, approaches based on the principles of AI are highly beneficial in many phases of drug discovery, including the identification and validation of therapeutic targets, the modeling of drugs, and the improvement of their attributes [82]. Furthermore, the development of patient-centered clinical trials is essential, as it enhances the decision-making process.

One of its applications is a new strategic program called Open Targets, which looks into the relationships between diseases, genes, and potential treatment targets. It provides a path that would lead to the identification of the target associated with the illness or the target-related disease. The drug-like molecule needs to abide by Lipinski's rule of five. Since then, 3N-MCTS (Monte Carlo Tree Search) has been developed. Neural network technology performs better than computer-aided retrosynthesis techniques [83].

An AI program called SPIDER is being used to assess how natural substances work and how to use them to find new medications. It was created mainly to predict targets for pharmaceutical substances like "Beta-Lapachone", and as a result, it was able to show that 5-lipoxygenase is allosterically and reversibly inhibited by "Lapa Chone" [84–86]. This innovative method is being developed to determine and identify the relationship between a molecule's structure and properties that can be hazardous. This is achieved with the aid of the chemical database [87–90].

A deep neural network (DNN) is a system that interacts with an artificially connected network of neurons to execute several types of data transformations [91, 92]. Pharmacological and toxicological data are used to establish the criteria for classifying medicines into the appropriate therapeutic groups. Newer-generation AI techniques, for instance, are built on top of generative adversarial networks (GANs). The basis of this field is the application of statistical attributes [93, 94].

8.4 ARTIFICIAL INTELLIGENCE'S PLACE IN CUSTOMIZED HEALTHCARE

8.4.1 Analyzing Data

Large AI systems are capable of easily analyzing a wide variety of medical data, including genetic data, biological literature, and patient information. Finding patterns, linkages, and interconnections using this research helps generate customized treatment plans [95].

8.4.2 Analytical Prediction

AI models are able to predict treatment and sickness outcomes based on specific patient characteristics such as genetic profiles, lifestyle conditions, and medical history. This enables medical providers to make more informed decisions about customized treatment options [96].

8.4.3 Accurate Diagnosis

AI-powered technology can increase the accuracy and speed of diagnostic operations by analyzing pathology slides, medical photos, and other diagnostic data. Systems using AI can spot subtle patterns and abnormalities that human observers might overlook, leading to earlier detection and more precise diagnosis.

8.4.4 Optimization of Treatment

The one of the characteristic of AI is optimization and customization of the treatment and diagnose provided by the AI.

8.4.5 Remote Observation and Assistance

Virtual assistants and monitoring technologies with AI capabilities can continuously track patient health data, provide tailored feedback, and alert medical personnel to any concerning changes. This improves the results for patients by permitting remote and proactive care of chronic illnesses [97, 98].

8.5 ARTIFICIAL INTELLIGENCE'S PLACE IN MEDICAL RESEARCH

Clinical investigations have shown that many drugs commonly fail. There are fewer drugs released onto the market each day. While some drug products do well in clinical trials, they face several challenges before entering the market. To solve such issues, a dedicated digital platform needs to be developed due to its significant impact on the following elements:

- Success or failure rate of drug products.
- Decrease in the absolute amounts of the costs associated with product development.

8.5.1 Objective of Clinical Research in Artificial Intelligence

This field contains a clearly organized list of references. These citations and the accompanying statistics prove to the superiority of AI over conventional medical practice approaches [99]. It is quite beneficial for examining the drugs, pathology data, and various lab results from physical examinations. This would make distinguishing the patient's condition from a normal one easier [100].

8.5.2 Education and Involvement of Patients

AI provides support and individualized answers to queries. Ultimately, because AI leverages data-driven techniques to provide patients with customized diagnoses, treatments, and care plans, it is critical to personalized medicine.

8.6 USING ARTIFICIAL INTELLIGENCE TO REPURPOSE DRUGS

A diagram illustrating the process of using AI to identify and evaluate existing drugs for new therapeutic uses, highlighting key steps such as data analysis, target identification, and validation of drug efficacy. Drugs approved by the Food and Drug Administration (FDA) for another ailment or symptom (see Figure 8.2).

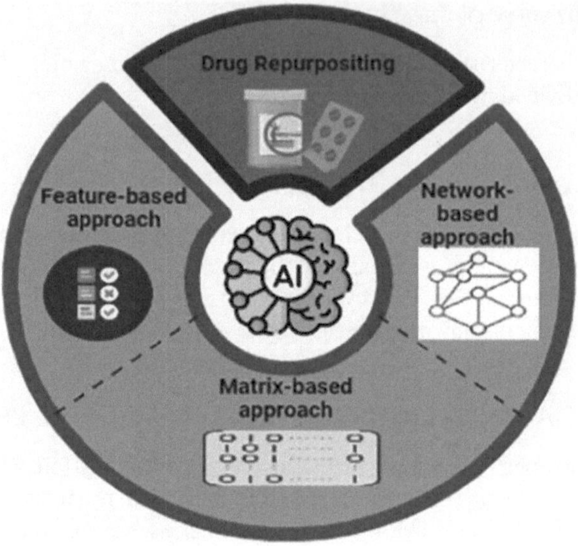

FIGURE 8.2 Using AI to repurpose drugs [101].

8.6.1 Network-Based Approach

The figure 8.3 provides the insights about various network-based techniques for reposition of drugs.

8.6.2 Feature-Based Approach

This approach begins with feature extraction, integrates them into databases, applies ML and predictive modeling to help anticipate repositioned medications, and then verifies and evaluates the results in a clinical setting (Figure 8.4).

8.6.3 Matrix-Based Approach

The drug repurposing depicted in Figure 8.5 employs a variety of techniques.

8.7 PHARMACOVIGILANCE AND MEDICATION SECURITY

Medication safety has a major positive impact on public health by enhancing patient safety, spotting safety problems early, and building confidence in the healthcare system. Furthermore, it helps manage concerns related to public confidence, regulatory compliance, and trust (see Figure 8.6).

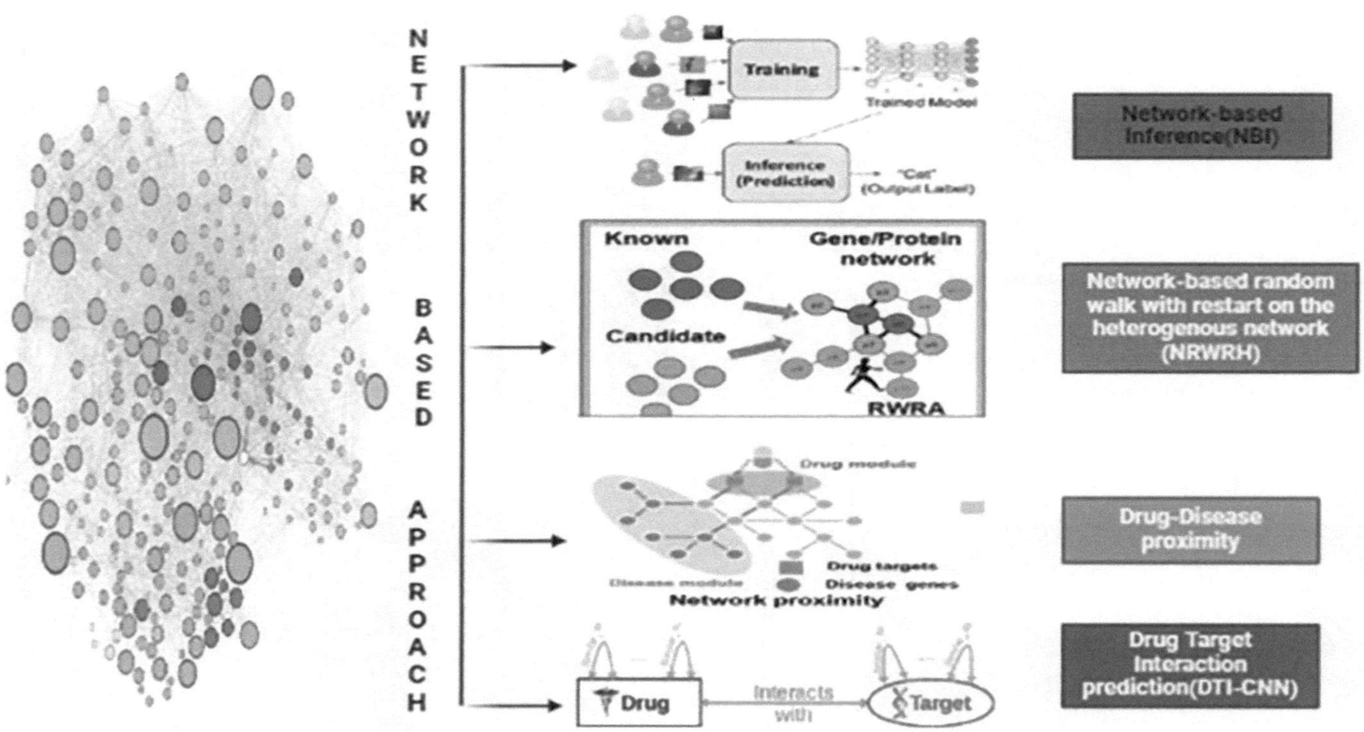

FIGURE 8.3 Various network-based techniques for repositioning drugs.

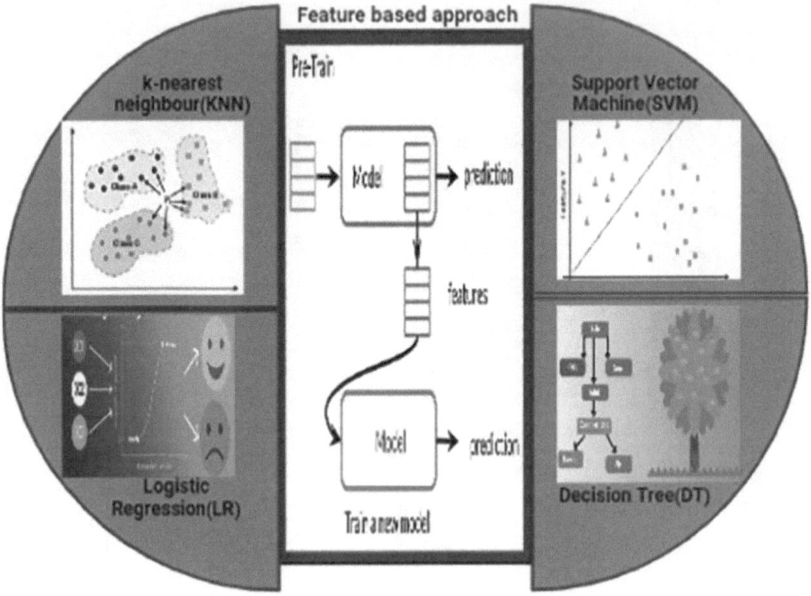

FIGURE 8.4 Distinct techniques for a feature-based strategy.

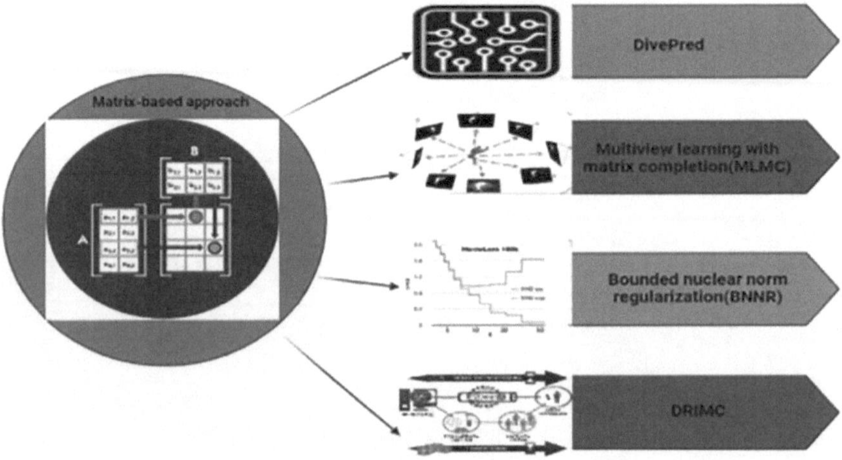

FIGURE 8.5 Distinct techniques for matrix-based methodologies.

8.7.1 Problems with Conventional Pharmacovigilance

Many obstacles stand in the way of the standard pharmacovigilance (PV) approach's ability to effectively monitor medication safety. These are a few issues that make medication safety difficult.

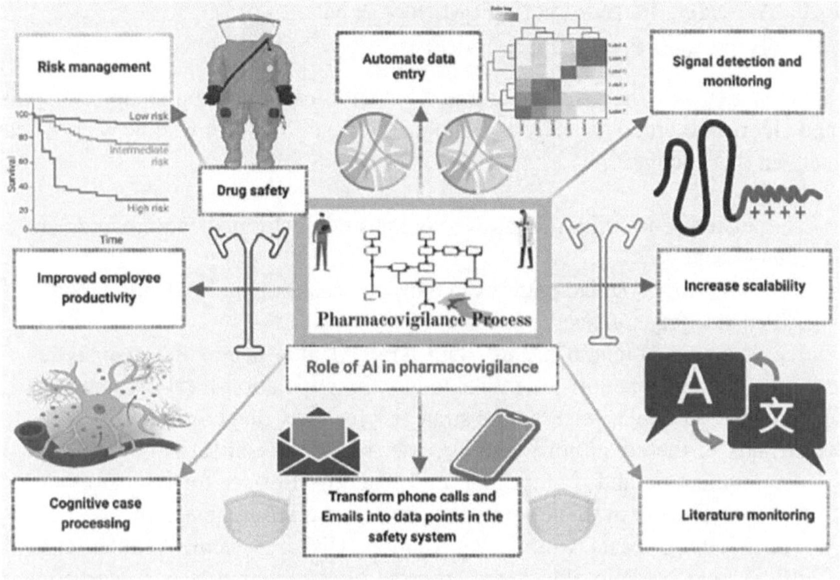

FIGURE 8.6 AI's place in pharmacovigilance.

8.7.1.1 Bias and Inadequate Reporting

Biases in the Adverse event can significantly affect the data, which can make it more difficult to uncover uncommon and unexpected AEs.

8.7.1.2 Vast Amounts of Intricate Data

Large data sets require a laborious manual review procedure that occasionally ignores safety alerts.

8.7.1.3 Risk Identification and Evaluation of Causation

Determining the exact cause of the drug-induced AEs and identifying the warning signs of possible risk issues are challenging tasks. Future safety risk assessment and causation evaluation cannot be adequately handled by the conventional approach.

8.7.1.4 Late Reporting

Decision-making and prompt intervention may suffer from AE reporting delays. Delays in the gathering and reporting of safety information may have arisen from the usage of manual reporting procedures in the past and the lack of established reporting schedules [102–105]. So, the pharmaceutical industry's continual change demands the development of more proactive and effective drug safety surveillance tools. Conventional methods cannot properly capture the overall safety profile of medications. Early detection of potential dangers and negative outcomes is crucial for facilitating prompt action and preserving patient safety.

8.7.2 Artificial Intelligence's Function in Medication Safety and Pharmacovigilance

AI technologies have the potential to transform PV through the application of sophisticated algorithms and data analysis techniques. The following are some ways AI can implement this change:

- Automated processing of massive volumes of electronic health records and related data.
- AI is able to recognize patterns in datasets, enabling early identification of AEs and safety signals.
- By detecting potential hazards and AEs, AI aids in predictive analytics. These studies function as a model to identify population-level risks and recommend particular intervention strategies for early diagnosis.
- AI aids in the creation of creative, user-friendly dashboards that enhance communication and prompt reporting, making it easier for regulators and PV specialists to evaluate safety data and take appropriate action.
- The WHO–Uppsala Monitoring Center (UMC) system, Venulet algorithms, and Naranjo algorithms are used by AI to support post-marketing surveillance.

8.7.3 Computer-Aided Drug Design for Drug Formulation

Every stage of the medication formulation process can benefit from the application of AI-based technology, which also helps to lower the health risks associated with pre-clinical studies and, in the end, lowers costs [106]. AI is regarded as an effective data mining technique for ML procedures and the massive volume of pharmaceutical data. Computer-aided drug design, or CADD, has supplanted conventional methods in drug design since it speeds up the process of finding new drugs while simultaneously improving design processes [107, 108]. Additionally, it is simple to identify the targeted molecules, increasing the likelihood that the intended medication will be successfully created. It can do this by streamlining important parameters, enhancing quality control (QC), and effortlessly increasing production levels [109, 110]. The following are some of the difficulties that traditional medication formulation and manufacturing techniques encounter which significantly affect quality control, productivity, and cost effectiveness:

- Limited real-time observation.
- Limited process optimization and manual QC operations.
- Decrease in predictive maintenance.
- Strict adherence to regulatory requirements.
- Ineffective supply chain oversight.
- Need for skilled and seasoned professionals.
- Difficulties in contacting medical professionals.
- Gathering and analyzing such a vast volume of data.

- Because of the increased transparency of the private information or method, there is a risk of loss.
- Opposition to modifications.
- Inadequate protection of data.

8.7.4 Artificial Intelligence's Function in Medication Development and Production

8.7.4.1 Accelerates Preformulating Research

By the use of computational techniques, it saves time and money by avoiding a higher level of ignorance and misinterpretation. It employs the Lipinski rule, often known as the rule of 5R, which is useful in predicting the likelihood of success or failure in drug research and development. Furthermore, it provides background knowledge on the chemical and physical properties, improved in vivo data, and a viable pharmacological target model [110–115].

When mainstreamed, AI-based processes can aid in optimizing output while reducing running expenses. In order to optimize formulations through the identification of the best composition, appropriate dosage form, and crucial manufacturing process parameters that enable error-free large-scale production, AI algorithms can assist in the analysis of vast volumes of data and IDs [116–120].

8.7.4.2 Process Scaling and Optimization

It facilitates the process of scaling up by forecasting how drug formulation will behave as it moves from small to large size. Temperature, speed, pressure, mixing time, and equipment settings are a few industrial processes or variables that can be optimized with ML to increase safety, quality, efficiency, and lower costs.

8.7.4.3 Adherence to Regulations

AI can be used to support adherence to regulatory body standards such as routine internal and external audits.

8.7.4.4 Inspection and Quality Control

AI systems that use image recognition and computer vision have the ability to improve, guarantee, and sustain the quality of products.

8.7.4.5 Supply Chain Optimization

During the pharmaceutical manufacturing process, AI helps with supply chain management by assessing certain production standards. Furthermore, it enhances the accuracy and efficiency of product manufacturing at the designated site, reducing expenses, waste, and inadvertent mistakes.

8.8 MEDICAL IMAGE ANALYSIS USING ARTIFICIAL INTELLIGENCE

For various issues in medical field, medical image analysis is very crucial.

8.8.1 Segmentation of Images

Three-dimensional data visualization and image segmentation for 3D printing have become essential components in many fields of medical research, education, and clinical work. For medical picture segmentation, sophisticated computational quantification and visualization techniques are needed. Recent developments in AI technology enable autonomous organ contouring from medical images and the quick and accurate identification of malignancies.

8.8.2 Lesion Identification and Classification

Using AI for classification demonstrated promising outcomes in a number of medical areas, including neurology, cardiology, dermatology, and the detection of head and neck cancer. Here, convolutional neural networks (CNNs) are an attractive approach to image classification from radiography, hyperspectral photography, confocal laser endo-microscopy, and classical histology.

8.8.3 Evaluation of Quality

AI facilitates image quality analysis and yields precise measurements of parameters with a quantitative foundation intended for illness diagnosis. It also facilitates the process of determining the disease's scope, intensity, and stage and enables more informed decision-making. AI algorithms facilitate the organization and fusion of various images, hence enhancing the ability to compare and understand medical images used for image-assisted procedures, treatment monitoring, and surgical planning.

8.8.4 Workflow Improvement and Automatic Reporting

AI-based technologies can automate the creation of radiology reports and provide structured templates. By reducing time and enhancing reporting uniformity, it increases workflow efficiency.

8.8.5 Phenotyping and Disease Prediction Using Medical Images

In addition to identifying risk factors before they may worsen, it analyzes and produces phenotypic data.

8.8.6 Radiomics Assessment and Texture Evaluation

Along with medical images, AI aids in the discovery of specific details such as texture patterns, shape, and intensity changes. All of these traits are influenced by radiomic analysis, which provides information on the prognosis assessment, therapy response, and heterogeneity of the disease.

8.9 ARTIFICIAL INTELLIGENCE AS NLP IN PHARMACY

It is important as an output is determined by NLP. NLP has an advantage over humans in that it can more thoroughly review a larger body of data.

It aids in diagnosis by coordinating patient admissions to emergency rooms and hospitals and enhancing clinical outcomes by accurately predicting the clinical reaction. Findings from clinical coding medical records contain a lot of patient data, but managing these records can be a challenge. NLP solves this problem by analyzing texts and providing examiners with information about patients' histories of treatment and assessments. This information is then transformed into structured data that is easily accessible and analyzed.

Conversational agents, such as chatbots or voice assistants, can be created utilizing NLP technology. In addition to scheduling appointments, answering questions from patients, and providing prescription information, these assistants are also capable of providing basic medical advice based on established guidelines.

8.10 ARTIFICIAL INTELLIGENCE AND THE SECURITY OF HEALTHCARE DATA

8.10.1 Identification and Mitigation of Threats

AI–based algorithms may search through massive amounts of data, including system activity logs, internet traffic, and user behavior, to identify anomalies and possible security risks.

ML models can identify and avoid dangers proactively by identifying trends that may indicate illegal conduct.

8.10.2 Patch Management and Vulnerability Assessment

AI can help with security assessments by evaluating networks, systems, and apps for potential flaws in order to ensure that security updates are implemented as soon as possible to protect against known vulnerabilities, AI algorithms have the ability to classify vulnerabilities based on their severity and offer patch management strategies [121].

8.10.3 Adherence to Oversight and Audit Assistance

AI can assist in monitoring legal compliance by evaluating and interpreting relevant regulations such as the Health Insurance Probability and Accountability Act (HIPAA) and the General Data Protection Regulation (GDPR).

AI algorithms can identify compliance holes, offer recommendations for how to close them, and support audit procedures by automatically generating compliance reports and keeping track of security-related events.

8.10.4 Privacy and Data Encryption

AI technology can assist in implementing efficient encryption techniques to protect sensitive health information, including patient data, intellectual property, and data from pharmaceutical research and development. By ensuring that the appropriate encryption methods are employed, AI algorithms can improve data privacy and maintain adherence to security requirements [122].

8.10.5 Adaptive Access Control

Adaptive access controls can be altered on the fly in response to user behavior, environmental factors, and risk assessments. By continuously monitoring user behavior and evaluating contextual data, AI may grant or deny access permissions in real time, reducing the risk of data leakage or unwanted access.

8.10.6 Behavioral Analytics and User Authentication

AI–enabled behavioral analytics can create user baselines and spot abnormal user behavior that can indicate misuse or illegal access to data. AI can also be used to enhance user authentication systems [123].

8.11 AI IN MEDICINE

AI has been used extensively in various sectors, including pharmacology, and has become more and more common in the healthcare industry in recent years. While supervised ML algorithms are used to identify potential pharmacological substances or relevant patient groups, they are also used to improve therapeutic drug monitoring.

8.11.1 Artificial Intelligence in the Pharmaceutical Sciences

It takes a lot of work to improve healthcare services. The most cutting-edge approach to improving the healthcare system is offered by AI. Numerous sources, including academic institutions, research and development teams, commercial facilities, and community and clinical pharmacies, produce data.

8.11.2 AI in Clinical Studies and Empirical Data

After the expensive preclinical development stage, a novel treatment enters the clinical trial phase. Clinical study recruitment and patient selection are two of the most challenging tasks. If insufficient participants are enrolled, the experiment could have to be ended. AI tools can help with patient recruiting by, for instance, sifting through enormous amounts of EHR data to find patients who meet the requirements and have the highest chance of enrolling. As a result, less time and money are lost on finding new patients.

Second, AI can support experimenter patient monitoring. Last but not least, AI methods can help gather empirical evidence by searching electronic health records for pertinent data and turning that data into outcomes that are clinically significant.

For instance, a variety of AI-based solutions have been discovered to be available for automated imaging data processing to deliver accuracy rates that are comparable to those of radiologists.

Real-world clinical data analysis is another application for AI. EHRs are a great resource for postmarked research because they provide a wealth of data regarding medication response and illness progression. The accuracy of automatic and human extractions in data mining in electronic health records was studied by Van Laar et al.

8.11.3 AI in Health Care Diagnostics

AI is effectively employed in the diagnosis of neurological conditions, strokes, and skin cancer. Infectious disorders are treated with NLP, the first reading tool that gave clinicians exceptional freedom to examine the descriptors of chest X-rays. Two years later, SVM was used to find imaging biomarkers for neurological and psychiatric illnesses. Alzheimer's disease early stages have been identified using a variety of SVM combinations.

A study using convolutional neural networks was conducted on diabetic patients who had referable diabetic retinopathy (RDR). It was suggested to use the naïve Bayes classifier to identify and eliminate severe stroke lesions from patients' T1-weighted MRI images. Congenital cataract diagnosis, classification, and treatment are other areas where CNN is used.

8.12 AI BENEFITS FOR HEALTHCARE

Healthcare AI has the potential to revolutionize medical research and provide a number of benefits to patients and healthcare providers alike. One of the primary advantages of AI for the healthcare sector is increased efficiency. Healthcare workers may focus on more challenging tasks by using AI to automate tedious tasks like data entry and appointment booking. This could lead to better patient satisfaction, reduced wait times, and higher output. Accuracy is enhanced, which is another benefit of AI in healthcare. Large volumes of data may be analyzed by AI algorithms, which can also spot patterns that humans might overlook. In the end, this may lead to more precise treatment suggestions and diagnoses, improving patient outcomes. AI systems, for instance, are able to analyze medical photos and recognize warning signals. of illnesses that would not be apparent to the unaided eye, such as cancer. AI may potentially be able to offer individualized medical treatment. AI algorithms may provide individualized treatment regimens that are specific to each patient's needs by analyzing patient data, including genetic and medical histories. This can lessen the possibility of pharmaceutical side effects and increase the efficacy of treatment.

Clinical decision-making, medication development, and medical imaging are just a few of the many uses of AI in healthcare. AI systems can evaluate enormous volumes of data in the drug discovery process to find promising medication candidates and forecast their efficacy. AI algorithms can help healthcare professionals make treatment recommendations in clinical decision-making by evaluating patient data and determining the best course of action. Numerous advantages of AI in healthcare include increased effectiveness, precision, and individualized treatment. Numerous AI applications in healthcare are exciting prospects for the field of medical science. We can transform healthcare delivery and enhance patient outcomes by utilizing AI technologies in the medical field.

8.13 CHALLENGES OF IMPLEMENTING AI IN HEALTHCARE

One of the main issues is data privacy. There is a chance of data breaches and unauthorized access to sensitive patient information because of the enormous volumes of healthcare data that AI algorithms gather and analyze. The lack of consistent laws pertaining to data privacy in the healthcare industry increases this danger in particular. A further difficulty is the ethical aspect. Certain populations may experience worse health outcomes and uneven access to healthcare as a result of biases and prejudice introduced by AI algorithms. Furthermore, using AI could make it harder to communicate with people and deliver empathetic care, which is essential to the healthcare industry. Concerns have also been raised about possible AI abuse, such as when facial recognition software is applied in medical environments. The use of AI in healthcare also presents regulatory challenges. To guarantee that AI is applied in healthcare in a safe and efficient manner, certain rules and regulations are required. For instance, regulatory supervision is required to guarantee that AI algorithms are created and approved in compliance with the necessary guidelines. These issues are being actively addressed by scholars and decision-makers. For instance, scientists are creating AI algorithms that are safe and respect patient privacy while delivering precise diagnosis and treatment suggestions. Additionally, legislators are attempting to address ethical issues surrounding data privacy in healthcare and develop uniform legislation surrounding them. Healthcare industry stakeholders must be involved in a diversified manner to address the issues posed by AI. Here are a few possible ways to deal with the issues:

1. **Data privacy:** Establishing robust data protection frameworks and policies that abide by current laws and regulations is one method to handle data privacy concerns. Encryption and secure data storage are two ways to do this while safeguarding private patient data. Healthcare institutions can also create a clear and simple consent procedure that explains to patients how their information will be utilized.
2. **Ethical considerations:** AI algorithms need to be created with bias and discrimination elimination in mind in order to solve ethical concerns. This can be accomplished by creating transparent and understandable algorithms and utilizing a variety of datasets.
3. **Concerns about regulations:** To tackle regulatory concerns, governments should endeavor to establish unambiguous protocols.

8.14 AI ASSISTANCE IN DIAGNOSTICS

8.14.1 Diagnosis Accuracy

AI technology has been used by researchers to many additional disease states, including the detection of diabetic retinopathy [115], abnormalities in electrocardiograms, and the prediction of illnesses [116, 117].

Furthermore, the sensitivity and specificity of deep learning algorithms for pneumonia from chest radiography are 96% and 64%, respectively [118]. The enhanced approach helps medical professionals detect and treat appendicitis with more knowledge. Moreover, the authors propose that such methods may be used for the analysis of appendicitis patients' photos or even in the use of blood specimens or images for the detection of infections like COVID-19 [119].

To cut down on needless ED visits, a trustworthy symptom assessment instrument might be introduced to rule out other disease causes. The patient can be questioned directly by a number of AI-enabled devices, and a thorough explanation is given at the conclusion to guarantee proper evaluation and treatment.

Furthermore, real-time recommendations from AI-powered decision support systems can help medical professionals make decisions about diagnosis and treatment. In the ED, patients are assessed with minimal information, and when risk-stratifying and making judgments, doctors usually have to consider probabilities. In the emergency department, it is critical to analyze clinical data more quickly in order to categorize the severity of the issue and the necessity for quick action. One of the biggest issues facing doctors and healthcare systems is the possibility of misdiagnosing patients. In the medical field, diagnostic errors can be costly and even deadly. According to one study, diagnostic mistakes are closely linked to higher death rates and longer hospital stays, especially in patients who visit the emergency department [120]. Thankfully, AI can help identify patients at an early stage of life-threatening illnesses and notify medical professionals quickly so that patients may get help right away. Finally, AI can assist in optimizing ED health care resources by forecasting patient demand, choosing the best course of treatment (drug, dosage, delivery method, and urgency of action), and recommending an extended stay in the emergency room. AI systems can provide insights into the best course of therapy selection, increasing productivity and decreasing congestion, by evaluating patient-specific data.

8.14.2 Artificial Intelligence in Genetic Medicine

We can aid in the early identification of possible epidemics by teaching ML algorithms to recognize these signals in real-time data. It is also possible to predict because of this combination.

The graph's X-axis shows the number, while the Y-axis shows the percentage chance of each. One particular area where AI and ML have shown promise is the discovery of genetic variations linked to certain characteristics or diseases, known as efficacy. By analyzing large genomic datasets, these methods can identify complex patterns that are difficult to find by manual examination. For example, a novel study that relied only on genomic data to predict the presence of autism spectrum disorder (ASD) identified genetic variations linked to ASD using a deep neural network [37].

Transcriptome profiling is a useful tool in oncology for classifying tumors into molecular subgroups that are clinically relevant. These molecular categories, which were initially created for breast cancer and subsequently expanded to include colorectal and ovarian cancer and sarcomas, have significant effects on diagnosis, prognosis, and choice of treatment [38, 39].

8.14.3 AI Support for Medical Care

AI has garnered respect for its ability to help doctors make treatment decisions, especially when it comes to predicting therapeutic response [49]. Huang and colleagues conducted research where the response to treatment was accurately predicted by the authors using the gene expression data from the patients to train. In order to reduce

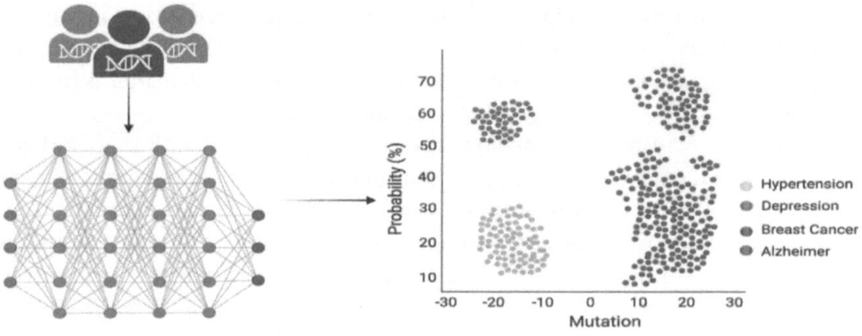

FIGURE 8.7 A schematic illustration of the procedure, which begins with DNA/RNA extraction and ends with sequencing.

confounding factors, the AI models took into account attributes that were predictive of treatment selection, and they performed well in predictions.

8.14.4 Monitoring of Drugs and Adjustment of Dosage

AI algorithms are designed to be specific to each patient and anticipate possible negative medication effects, lowering risks and enhancing treatment. Studies found that the algorithm performed better in predicting future PT/INRs than experienced doctors, with notable variances, and that the produced customized warfarin dosage was dependable.

In contrast, CURATE.AI, a revolutionary dose optimization system, is an AI-derived platform that allows for dynamic optimization of chemotherapy dosages based on the unique data of each patient [55]. An investigation was carried out in order to receive three distinct chemotherapy regimens for advanced solid tumors. Personalized dosages for the next cycle were created by CURATE.AI by using the association between tumor marker readouts and chemotherapy dose variation.

8.14.5 AI Support for Managing Population Health

Certain functions related to public health management, such as care coordination and patient outreach, can also be automated by AI [61, 62]. Furthermore, human oversight is essential to guarantee the suitability and efficacy of therapies for patients who are at risk. Population health is becoming more and more dependent on predictive analytics.

AI is also required to solve issues with vaccine manufacturing and bottlenecks in the supply chain. It might be difficult to test algorithms on live vaccination supply chains. To get around this, research and development spending is crucial in order to build reliable algorithms that can forecast vaccine supply chains with accuracy and optimize them. Edge analytics is also capable of forecasting.

To guarantee that patient treatments are appropriate and successful, predictive analytics implementation involves sophisticated technology, high-quality data, and human monitoring.

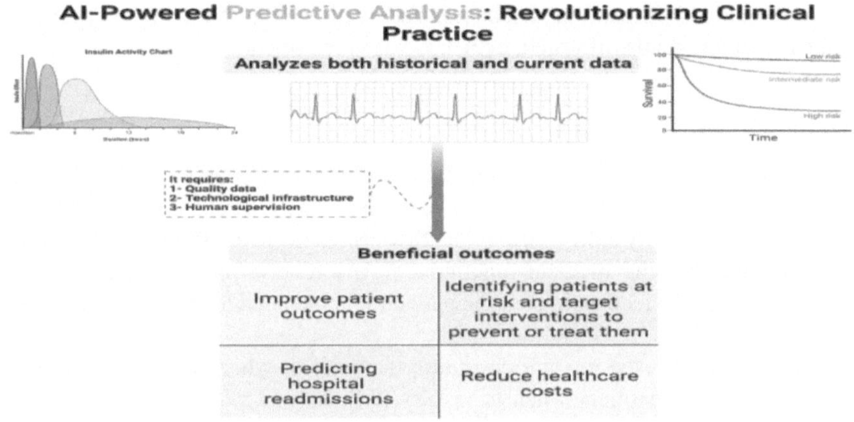

FIGURE 8.8 Unlocking the power of patient data with AI-driven predictive analytics.

8.14.6 Formation of Working Groups, Policies, and Structures

AI is changing the way that rules are made in a variety of industries. From identifying and distributing these recommendations, guidelines in the healthcare industry often take a long time.

Real-time, evidence-based suggestions that provide timely information exchange with clinicians—who are essential to clinical and ethical supervision—should direct the development of new products under the direction of scientists and subject matter experts [68–73]. Frameworks for resolving issues particular to creating, disclosing, and verifying AI in medicine have been created by a number of professional associations [69–73].

By providing principles for promoting with the therapeutic, these frameworks are largely aimed for educating the engineers that develop AI [69]. Furthermore, AI legislation is still in its early stages. Publications have been released by the US FDA. The goal of these legislative initiatives is to better position the healthcare industry to be a technology-driven industry in the future. But it's imperative to guarantee that AI-based rules are open, impartial, equitable, and founded on ethical and human knowledge [68].

8.14.7 AI for Medication Advice and Information

AI would suggest a fresh framework to help with sensible decision-making resources for medical professionals. AI greatly enhances the ability of healthcare practitioners to get accurate, current, and real-time information by incorporating cutting-edge technologies. According to researchers, these technologies improve decision-making; unleash creativity; boost clinical trial and research efficacy; and provide new tools that assist patients, insurers, regulators, and healthcare professionals [78].

AI makes it possible to get drug-related information quickly and thoroughly from a variety of sources by virtue of its capacity to evaluate the most recent clinical recommendations, medication databases, and medical literature in order to give healthcare professionals informed, evidence-based judgments.

8.14.8 Patient Care Enabled by AI

The global shortage of resources and the steadily rising demand for health care services make it imperative to develop answers to these problems [82]. A novel cutting-edge technology called virtual health assistants is revolutionizing the healthcare sector and helping medical practitioners. In order to provide individualized patient care based on feedback from the patient, it is intended to mimic human interaction [83].

Moreover, these resources are constantly accessible, which facilitates patients' access to medical treatment when necessary [84]. In general, virtual health aides have the ability to greatly enhance the caliber, effectiveness, and expense of healthcare delivery while simultaneously improving patient satisfaction and patient participation.

8.14.9 AI Assistance for Mental Health

Despite the fact that psychiatric professionals, more than other practitioners, rely on direct patient interaction and behavioral observation, AI-powered technologies can support their work in a number of ways. AI-powered mental health apps can offer individualized care and support in addition to helping with the early identification and treatment of mental health issues [88–91].

Recent findings on the most commonly studied use disease [88] support this claim. Additionally, AI-powered apps demonstrate significant advantages for people suffering from drug use disorders. According to this study, utilizing Woebot was substantially linked to improvements in drug usage, cravings, anxiety, and sadness [92]. While AI-powered mental health diagnosis has great potential, there are several important issues that need to be resolved. The primary constraint is the potential for bias in the algorithms and data used to fuel AI-based diagnoses. Results from AI systems may be skewed and erroneous if the data used to train them does not reflect a variety of populations. Furthermore, the intricacy of mental health disorders, which might manifest differently in various persons, may not be taken into consideration by AI-powered diagnosis. Last but not least, there's a chance that AI-powered diagnosis would result in less empathy and customization in mental health care, which is crucial for effective treatment [93]. As a result, even while AI-powered diagnosis has its uses in mental health care, professional diagnosis and therapy should always be utilized in conjunction with it rather than using it as a substitute.

8.14.10 Use of AI to Improve Patient Education and Lessen Burnout among Healthcare Professionals

Patient education is one of the newest uses of AI [94]. AI-driven chatbots are being used in a number of healthcare settings, including nutrition counselling [95, 96], help with quitting smoking [97], and cognitive-behavioral therapy [98]. In order to help people understand their medical diagnosis, available treatments, and preventative actions, patient education is essential to the delivery of healthcare [98]. By giving patients and their caregivers individualized, interactive information and assistance, AI has the potential to significantly contribute to patient education [100]. For instance, presenting a PROSCA chatbot to patients with prostate cancer resulted in a noticeable to modest improvement in participants' knowledge of the disease [101].

8.14.11 Artificial Intelligence to Human Healthcare Professionals

As well as the well-being of medical personnel. Patients in medicine frequently have unwavering trust in medical personnel and think that the placebo effect—a phenomena in medicine—will heal them of their ailments. Stated differently, trust between the patient and the physician plays a critical role in enhancing patient care and treatment efficacy [105]. Building a connection on trust is essential for the success of the patient-AI healthcare delivery system partnership [106].

According to some polls, most individuals are open to interacting with or using AI for health-related tasks, including monitoring, diagnosis, treatment, and decision support [108–110]. Still, other research indicates that individuals continue to choose receiving medical treatment from humans' practitioners regarding AI, particularly with regard to delicate or complicated matters like end-of-life care, chronic illnesses, or mental health [108, 111].

8.15 NEXT STEPS AND THINGS TO THINK ABOUT WHEN IMPLEMENTING AI IN CLINICAL SETTINGS

AI has the potential to completely transform clinical practice, but in order to do so, a number of issues need to be resolved. One of these issues is the dearth of reliable medical data, which might produce unreliable results. Achieving the intended results also depends on using the right approach and identifying pertinent clinical measures. The involvement of humans in the creation and utilization of AI tools is prone to prejudice, and, if not properly supervised, this may be enhanced by AI [113]. The data and/or analysis produced by AI may be realistic and compelling, but a serious problem that might arise is hallucination, which is the propensity to invent and create erroneous information that is not supported by available evidence [114]. Last, human experience and engagement are necessary to guarantee the suitable and useful deployment of AI to satisfy clinical demands; the practical application of AI may suffer from a lack of these resources of AI.

It would be feasible to develop technology that is useful, implementable, and successful if computer scientists and healthcare professionals collaborated appropriately.

Another recommendation is to offer suitable instruction and training that begins with the undergraduate degree for all health care professionals and continues with ongoing professional development and enhancement for those employed in practice to guarantee appropriate adaptation that prevents any ethical or legal problems or incorrect interpretation of the results without cross-checking the data [117]. It is advised that medical schools include lessons on AI in their curricula. According to research done among radiology residents, 86% of participants thought AI would transform and enhance their field, and up to 71% said medical schools should teach AI to increase comprehension and application [118–122]. Through this integration, core knowledge about AI and its applications is ensured for future healthcare professionals from the outset. AI in healthcare has a bright future ahead of it, with many opportunities for advancement that might completely transform the industry. The application of AI to remote patient monitoring and care is one area of focus. AI-powered monitoring systems may make it possible to watch patients' health more thoroughly and continuously, which might lead to early identification of possible problems and more focused therapies. Patients with chronic diseases or those who need continuous monitoring following surgery or other medical procedures may find this very helpful. Drug research and discovery represent yet another possible application of AI in healthcare. Through the utilization of AI to swiftly and precisely handle large volumes of data, scientists may discover novel therapeutic candidates and anticipate their possible effectiveness and adverse consequences far in advance of clinical trials. This may expedite the process of developing new drugs and speed up the effective and timely release of new therapies [123–127]. AI algorithms have the potential to assist physicians in making better-educated and individualized treatment decisions by analyzing patient data and medical histories. This might lower the likelihood of misdiagnosis and needless operations. Looking ahead, AI may contribute to the creation of cutting-edge medical technology like implanted devices and nanobots. By delivering medications and other therapies exactly where they are required, these technologies may be utilized to monitor and treat patients at the cellular level.

8.15.1 AI's Present and Potential Use in Healthcare

AI in the medium term, meaning the next five to ten years. Our prediction is that there will be substantial advancements in the medium term in the creation of potent algorithms that are effective (i.e., require less data to train); capable of utilizing unlabeled data; and able to integrate disparate structured and unstructured data, such as imaging, electronic health records, multi-omic data, behavioral data, and pharmaceutical data. Furthermore, medical practices and healthcare organizations will go beyond merely implementing AI platforms to collaborating with technology partners to create innovative AI-powered treatments systems.

Long-term (over a decade) AI with AI-augmented healthcare and linked care, AI systems will eventually grow more sophisticated, enabling AI healthcare systems to reach a level of precision medicine. The current one-size-fits-all approach to healthcare will give way to a personalized, data-driven, preventative disease management paradigm that improves patient outcomes (i.e., patient and clinician experiences of treatment) within a more economical delivery system of better healthcare that is connected [127–133, 134].

Wearable technology, such as smartwatches, may be used with AI chatbots to provide caregivers and patients advice into how to improve wellbeing, behavior, and sleep.

We also see that ambient sensing has emerged without the requirement for Emerald (www.emeraldinno.com): academics and researchers at the Massachusetts Institute of Technology established this wireless, touchless sensor, and ML platform for remote monitoring of respiration, sleep, and behavior. Google Nest claims to use motion and sound sensors to monitor sleep, including sleep disruptions like coughing. A recently released article investigated the possibility of contactless cardiac rhythm monitoring with smart speakers. Automation and ambient clinical intelligence: Automating administrative activities, such as entering patient visits into electronic health records, is possible with AI systems that leverage NLP technology. This would optimize clinical workflow and free up more time for clinicians to spend caring for patients. The most popular AI application at the moment is the automated classification of medical images for accurate diagnosis imaging. According to a recent study, 129 (58%) of the AI/ML-based medical devices that were approved in the United States and 126 (53%) of the devices that were approved in Europe between 2015 and 2020 received CE marks or were certified for use in radiology. The performance of the deep learning system was comparable to that of cardiologists [35–38]. While there are a few NHS exemplars in this field, such as the National Pathology Imaging Co-operative and the University of Leeds Virtual Pathology Project, we anticipate that AI-based diagnostic imaging will be widely adopted and scaled up in the medium future. We offer one example of how these technologies are used:

- *Screening for diabetic retinopathy:* Diabetic retinopathy screening and timely treatment are critical to lowering avoidable, diabetes-related visual loss globally. However, considering the large number of diabetic patients and the shortage of personnel for eye care globally, screening is expensive. Research on 40 automated AI systems for diabetic retinopathy in India, Thailand, Singapore, and the USA have all shown strong diagnostic performance at a reasonable cost [130–133, 134].

8.16 CONCLUSION

AI-powered predictive analytics can increase the accuracy, efficiency, and cost-effectiveness of clinical laboratory testing as well as disease diagnosis. By providing precise, up-to-date information and improving pharmaceutical selections, AI may also aid in the development of recommendations and the management of population health. There are several actions that need to be taken to ensure the efficient and moral use of AI in healthcare.

The most important thing is the safety of patient data. It is necessary to create and execute robust security protocols, cyber security plans, and healthcare initiatives. Working together, regulatory bodies, healthcare institutions, and AI researchers may develop guidelines and best practices. AI systems are able to continuously analyze a variety of factors, such as population demographics, sickness prevalence, and geographic dispersion. Views of the general public about AI differ in the healthcare industry; although some individuals are willing to use AI for medical purposes, others still prefer to see human physicians for complex issues. The successful use of AI in medical practice requires building patient education and confidence. It is imperative to address concerns around bias, privacy, data quality, and the need for human expertise in order to properly and successfully integrate AI. Collaboration among stakeholders is essential for ethical norms, robust AI systems, and patient-provider trust. More investigation, ingenuity, and interdisciplinary collaboration are needed to fully grasp AI's promise in healthcare. AI is expected to revolutionize healthcare through efficient integration, bettering patient outcomes, productivity, and accessibility of customized treatment and high-caliber therapy.

REFERENCES

1. Suleimenov IE, Vitulyova YS, Bakirov AS, Gabrielyan OA. Artificial intelligence: what is it? *Proc 2020 6th Int Conf Comput Technol Appl.* 2020;22–5. https://doi.org/10.1145/3397125.3397141.
2. Davenport T, Kalakota R. The potential for artificial intelligence in healthcare. *Future Healthc J.* 2019;6(2):94–8. https://doi.org/10.7861/futurehosp.6-2-94.
3. McCorduck P, Cfe C. *Machines Who Think: A Personal Inquiry into the History and Prospects of Artificial Intelligence.* AK Peters; 2004.
4. Jordan MI, Mitchell TM. Machine learning: Trends, perspectives, and prospects. *Science.* 2015;349(6245):255–60. https://doi.org/10.1126/science.aaa8415.
5. VanLehn K. The relative effectiveness of human tutoring, intelligent tutoring systems, and other tutoring systems. *Educational Psychol.* 2011;46(4):197–221. https://doi.org/10.1080/00461520.2011.611369.
6. Topol EJ. High-performance medicine: The convergence of human and artificial intelligence. *Nat Med.* 2019;25(1):44–56. https://doi.org/10.1038/s41591-018-0300-7.
7. Esteva A, Kuprel B, Novoa RA, Ko J, Swetter SM, Blau HM, et al. Dermatologist-level classification of skin cancer with deep neural networks. *Nature.* 2017;542(7639):115–8. https://doi.org/10.1038/nature21056.
8. Myszczynska MA, Ojamies PN, Lacoste AM, Neil D, Saffari A, Mead R, et al. Applications of machine learning to diagnosis and treatment of neurodegenerative diseases. *Nat Reviews Neurol.* 2020;16(8):440–56. https://doi.org/10.1038/s41582-020-0377-8.
9. Ahsan MM, Luna SA, Siddique Z. Machine-learning-based disease diagnosis: A comprehensive review. *Healthcare.* 2022;10(3):541. https://doi.org/10.3390/healthcare10030541.
10. McKinney SM, Sieniek M, Godbole V, Godwin J, Antropova N, Ashrafian H, et al. International evaluation of an AI system for breast cancer screening. *Nature.* 2020;577(7788):89–94. https://doi.org/10.1038/s41586-019-1799-6.
11. Kim H-E, Kim HH, Han B-K, Kim KH, Han K, Nam H, et al. Changes in cancer detection and false-positive recall in mammography using artificial intelligence: A retrospective, multireader study. *Lancet Digit Health.* 2020;2(3). https://doi.org/10.1016/s2589-7500(20)30003-0.
12. Han SS, Park I, Eun Chang S, Lim W, Kim MS, Park GH, et al. Augmented intelligence dermatology: Deep neural networks empower medical professionals in diagnosing skin cancer and predicting treatment options for 134 skin disorders. *J Invest Dermatol.* 2020;140(9):1753–61. https://doi.org/10.1016/j.jid.2020.01.019.
13. Haenssle HA, Fink C, Schneiderbauer R, Toberer F, Buhl T, Blum A, et al. Man against machine: Diagnostic performance of a deep learning convolutional neural network for dermoscopic melanoma recognition in comparison to 58 dermatologists. *Ann Oncol.* 2018;29(8):1836–42. https://doi.org/10.1093/annonc/mdy166.
14. Li S, Zhao R, Zou H. Artificial intelligence for diabetic retinopathy. *Chin Med J (Engl).* 2021;135(3):253–60. https://doi.org/10.1097/CM9.0000000000001816.
15. Alfaras M, Soriano MC, Ortín S. A fast machine learning model for ECG-based heartbeat classification and arrhythmia detection. *Front Phys.* 2019;7. https://doi.org/10.3389/fphy.2019.00103.

16. Raghunath S, Pfeifer JM, Ulloa-Cerna AE, Nemani A, Carbonati T, Jing L, et al. Deep neural networks can predict new-onset atrial fibrillation from the 12-lead ECG and help identify those at risk of atrial fibrillation–related stroke. *Circulation*. 2021;143(13):1287–98. https://doi.org/10.1161/circulationaha.120.047829.
17. Becker J, Decker JA, Römmele C, Kahn M, Messmann H, Wehler M, et al. Artificial intelligence-based detection of pneumonia in chest radiographs. *Diagnostics*. 2022;12(6):1465. https://doi.org/10.3390/diagnostics12061465.
18. Mijwil MM, Aggarwal K. A diagnostic testing for people with appendicitis using machine learning techniques. *Multimed Tools Appl*. 2022;81(5):7011–23. https://doi.org/10.1007/s11042-022-11939-8.
19. Undru TR, Uday U, Lakshmi JT, Kaliappan A, Mallamgunta S, Nikhat SS, et al. Integrating artificial intelligence for clinical and laboratory diagnosis—a review. *Maedica (Bucur)*. 2022;17(2):420–6. https://doi.org/10.26574/maedica.2022.17.2.420.
20. Peiffer-Smadja N, Dellière S, Rodriguez C, Birgand G, Lescure FX, Fourati S, et al. Machine learning in the clinical microbiology laboratory: Has the time come for routine practice? *Clin Microbiol Infect*. 2020;26(10):1300–9. https://doi.org/10.1016/j.cmi.2020.02.006.
21. Smith KP, Kang AD, Kirby JE. Automated interpretation of blood culture gram stains by use of a deep convolutional neural network. *J Clin Microbiol*. 2018;56(3):e01521–17. https://doi.org/10.1128/JCM.01521-17.
22. Weis CV, Jutzeler CR, Borgwardt K. Machine learning for microbial identification and antimicrobial susceptibility testing on MALDI-TOF mass spectra: A systematic review. *Clin Microbiol Infect*. 2020;26(10):1310–7. https://doi.org/10.1016/j.cmi.2020.03.014.
23. Go T, Kim JH, Byeon H, Lee SJ. Machine learning-based in-line holographic sensing of unstained malaria-infected red blood cells. *J Biophotonics*. 2018;11(9):e201800101. https://doi.org/10.1002/jbio.201800101.
24. Smith KP, Kirby JE. Image analysis and artificial intelligence in infectious disease diagnostics. *Clin Microbiol Infect*. 2020;26(10):1318–23. https://doi.org/10.1016/j.cmi.2020.03.012.
25. Vandenberg O, Durand G, Hallin M, Diefenbach A, Gant V, Murray P, et al. Consolidation of clinical microbiology laboratories and introduction of transformative technologies. *Clin Microbiol Rev*. 2020;33(2). https://doi.org/10.1128/cmr.00057-19.
26. Panch T, Szolovits P, Atun R. Artificial intelligence, machine learning and health systems. *J Global Health*. 2018;8(2). https://doi.org/10.7189/jogh.08.020303.
27. Berlyand Y, Raja AS, Dorner SC, Prabhakar AM, Sonis JD, Gottumukkala RV, et al. How artificial intelligence could transform emergency department operations. *Am J Emerg Med*. 2018;36(8):1515–7. https://doi.org/10.1016/j.ajem.2018.01.017.
28. Matheny ME, Whicher D, Thadaney Israni S. Artificial intelligence in health care: A report from the national academy of medicine. *JAMA*. 2020;323(6):509–10. https://doi.org/10.1001/jama.2019.21579.
29. Jiang F, Jiang Y, Zhi H, Dong Y, Li H, Ma S, et al. Artificial intelligence in healthcare: Past, present and future. *Stroke Vasc Neurol*. 2017;2(4):230–43. https://doi.org/10.1136/svn-2017-000101.
30. Gandhi SO, Sabik L. Emergency department visit classification using the NYU algorithm. *Am J Manag Care*. 2014;20(4):315–20.
31. Hautz WE, Kämmer JE, Hautz SC, Sauter TC, Zwaan L, Exadaktylos AK, et al. Diagnostic error increases mortality and length of hospital stay in patients presenting through the emergency room. *Scand J Trauma Resusc Emerg Med*. 2019;27(1):54. https://doi.org/10.1186/s13049-019-0629-z.
32. Haug CJ, Drazen JM. Artificial intelligence and machine learning in clinical medicine. *N Engl J Med*. 2023;388(13):1201–8. https://doi.org/10.1056/NEJMra2302038.

33. Abubaker Bagabir S, Ibrahim NK, Abubaker Bagabir H, Hashem Ateeq R. Covid-19 and artificial intelligence: Genome sequencing, drug development and vaccine discovery. *J Infect Public Health*. 2022;15(2):289–96. https://doi.org/10.1016/j.jiph.2022.01.011.
34. Pudjihartono N, Fadason T, Kempa-Liehr AW, O'Sullivan JM. A review of feature selection methods for machine learning-based disease risk prediction. *Front Bioinform*. 2022;2:927312. https://doi.org/10.3389/fbinf.2022.927312. Published 2022 Jun 27.
35. Widen E, Raben TG, Lello L, Hsu SDH. Machine learning prediction of biomarkers from SNPs and of disease risk from biomarkers in the UK biobank. *Genes (Basel)*. 2021;12(7):991. https://doi.org/10.3390/genes12070991. Published 2021 Jun 29.
36. Wang H, Avillach P. Diagnostic classification and prognostic prediction using common genetic variants in autism spectrum disorder: Genotype-based deep learning. *JMIR Med Inf*. 2021;9(4). https://doi.org/10.2196/24754.
37. Sorlie T, Perou CM, Tibshirani R, Aas T, Geisler S, Johnsen H, et al. Gene expression patterns of breast carcinomas distinguish tumor subclasses with clinical implications. *Proc Natl Acad Sci*. 2001;98:10869–74. https://doi.org/10.1073/pnas.191367098.
38. Yersal O. Biological subtypes of breast cancer: Prognostic and therapeutic implications. *World J Clin Oncol*. 2014;5(3):412–24. https://doi.org/10.5306/wjco.v5.i3.412.
39. Leek JT, Scharpf RB, Bravo HC, Simcha D, Langmead B, Johnson WE, et al. Tackling the widespread and critical impact of batch effects in high-throughput data. *Nat Rev Genet*. 2010;11:733–9. https://doi.org/10.1038/nrg2825.
40. Blanco-González A, Cabezón A, Seco-González A, Conde-Torres D, Antelo-Riveiro P, Piñeiro Á, et al. The role of AI in drug discovery: Challenges, opportunities, and strategies. *Pharmaceuticals*. 2023;16(6):891. https://doi.org/10.3390/ph16060891.
41. Tran TTV, Surya Wibowo A, Tayara H, Chong KT. Artificial intelligence in drug toxicity prediction: Recent advances, challenges, and future perspectives. *J Chem Inf Model*. 2023;63(9):2628–43. https://doi.org/10.1021/acs.jcim.3c00200.
42. Tran TTV, Tayara H, Chong KT. Artificial intelligence in drug metabolism and excretion prediction: Recent advances, challenges, and future perspectives. *Pharmaceutics*. 2023;15(4):1260. https://doi.org/10.3390/pharmaceutics15041260.
43. Guedj M, Swindle J, Hamon A, Hubert S, Desvaux E, Laplume J, et al. Industrializing AI-powered drug discovery: Lessons learned from the patrimony computing platform. *Expert Opin Drug Discov*. 2022;17(8):815–24. https://doi.org/10.1080/17460441.2022.2095368.
44. Ahmed F, Kang IS, Kim KH, Asif A, Rahim CS, Samantasinghar A, et al. Drug repurposing for viral cancers: A paradigm of machine learning, deep learning, and virtual screening-based approaches. *J Med Virol*. 2023;95(4). https://doi.org/10.1002/jmv.28693.
45. Singh DP, Kaushik B. A systematic literature review for the prediction of anticancer drug response using various machine-learning and deep-learning techniques. *Chem Biol Drug Des*. 2023;101(1):175–94. https://doi.org/10.1111/cbdd.14164.
46. Quazi S. Artificial intelligence and machine learning in precision and genomic medicine. *Med Oncol*. 2022;39(2):120. https://doi.org/10.1007/s12032-022-01711-1.
47. Subramanian M, Wojtusciszyn A, Favre L, Boughorbel S, Shan J, Letaief KB, et al. Precision medicine in the era of artificial intelligence: Implications in chronic disease management. *J Transl Med*. 2020;18(1):472. https://doi.org/10.1186/s12967-020-02658-5.
48. Johnson KB, Wei WQ, Weeraratne D, Frisse ME, Misulis K, Rhee K, et al. Precision medicine, AI, and the future of personalized health care. *Clin Transl Sci*. 2021;14(1):86–93. https://doi.org/10.1111/cts.12884.
49. Pulley JM, Denny JC, Peterson JF, Bernard GR, Vnencak-Jones CL, Ramirez AH, et al. Operational implementation of prospective genotyping for personalized medicine: The design of the vanderbilt PREDICT project. *Clin Pharmacol Ther*. 2012;92(1):87–95. https://doi.org/10.1038/clpt.2011.371.

50. Huang C, Clayton EA, Matyunina LV, McDonald LD, Benigno BB, Vannberg F, et al. Machine learning predicts individual cancer patient responses to therapeutic drugs with high accuracy. *Sci Rep*. 2018;8(1):16444. https://doi.org/10.1038/s41598-018-34753-5.
51. Sheu YH, Magdamo C, Miller M, Das S, Blacker D, Smoller JW. AI-assisted prediction of differential response to antidepressant classes using electronic health records. *NPJ Digit Med*. 2023;6:73. https://doi.org/10.1038/s41746-023-00817-8.
52. Martin GL, Jouganous J, Savidan R, Bellec A, Goehrs C, Benkebil M, et al. Validation of artificial intelligence to support the automatic coding of patient adverse drug reaction reports, using nationwide pharmacovigilance data. *Drug Saf*. 2022;45(5):535–48. https://doi.org/10.1007/s40264-022-01153-8.
53. Lee H, Kim HJ, Chang HW, Kim DJ, Mo J, Kim JE. Development of a system to support warfarin dose decisions using deep neural networks. *Sci Rep*. 2021;11(1):14745. Published 2021 Jul 20. https://doi.org/10.1038/s41598-021-94305-2.
54. Blasiak A, Truong A, Jeit W, Tan L, Kumar KS, Tan SB, et al. PRECISE CURATE.AI: A prospective feasibility trial to dynamically modulate personalized chemotherapy dose with artificial intelligence. *J Clin Oncol*. 2022;40(16suppl):1574–4. https://doi.org/10.1200/JCO.2022.40.16_suppl.1574.
55. Sjövall F, Lanckohr C, Bracht H. What's new in therapeutic drug monitoring of antimicrobials? *Intensive Care Med*. 2023. Published 2023 May 3. https://doi.org/10.1007/s00134-023-07060-5.
56. Partin A, Brettin TS, Zhu Y, Narykov O, Clyde A, Overbeek J, Stevens RL. Deep learning methods for drug response prediction in cancer: Predominant and emerging trends. *Front Med (Lausanne)*. 2023;10:1086097. https://doi.org/10.3389/fmed.2023.1086097.
57. Zhang H, Chen Y, Li F. Predicting anticancer drug response with deep learning constrained by signaling pathways. *Front Bioinform*. 2021;1:639349. https://doi.org/10.3389/fbinf.2021.639349.
58. Han K, Cao P, Wang Y, Xie F, Ma J, Yu M, Wang J, Xu Y, Zhang Y, Wan J. A review of approaches for predicting drug-drug interactions based on machine learning. *Front Pharmacol*. 2022;12:814858. https://doi.org/10.3389/fphar.2021.814858.
59. Liu JYH, Rudd JA. Predicting drug adverse effects using a new gastro-intestinal pacemaker activity drug database (GIPADD). *Sci Rep*. 2023;13(1):6935. https://doi.org/10.1038/s41598-023-33655-5.
60. Nelson KM, Chang ET, Zulman DM, Rubenstein LV, Kirkland FD, Fihn SD. Using PRedictive analytics to guide patient care and research in a national health system. *J Gen Intern Med*. 2019;34(8):1379–80. https://doi.org/10.1007/s11606-019-04961-4.
61. Amarasingham R, Patzer RE, Huesch M, Nguyen NQ, Xie B. Implementing electronic health care predictive analytics: Considerations and challenges. *Health Aff (Millwood)*. 2014;33(7):1148–54. https://doi.org/10.1377/hlthaff.2014.0352.
62. Ansari MS, Alok AK, Jain D, Rana S, Gupta S, Salwan R, et al. Predictive model based on health data analysis for risk of readmission in disease-specific cohorts. *Perspect Health Inf Manag*. 2021;18(Spring):1j. Published 2021 Mar 15.
63. Donzé J, Aujesky D, Williams D, Schnipper JL. Potentially avoidable 30-day hospital readmissions in medical patients: Derivation and validation of a prediction model. *JAMA Intern Med*. 2013;173:632–8.
64. Predictive Analytics in Healthcare | Reveal. https://www.revealbi.io/blog/predictive-analytics-in-healthcare. Accessed 6.20.2023.
65. Alotaibi S, Mehmood R, Katib I, Rana O, Albeshri A, Sehaa. A big data analytics tool for healthcare symptoms and diseases detection using Twitter, Apache spark, and machine learning. *Appl Sci*. 2020;10:1398. https://doi.org/10.3390/app10041398.
66. Crossnohere NL, Elsaid M, Paskett J, Bose-Brill S, Bridges JFP. Guidelines for artificial intelligence in medicine: Literature review and content analysis of frameworks. *J Med Internet Res*. 2022;24(8):e36823. https://doi.org/10.2196/36823.

67. Rivera SC, Liu X, Chan A, Denniston AK, Calvert MJ, SPIRIT-AICONSORT-AI. Working group guidelines for clinical trial protocols for interventions involving artificial intelligence: The SPIRIT-AI extension. *BMJ*. 2020;370:m3210. https://doi.org/10.1136/bmj.m3210.
68. Beam YK, Kohane AL. Artificial intelligence in healthcare. *Nat Biomed Eng*. 2018;2(10):719–31. https://doi.org/10.1038/s41551-018-0305-z.
69. Vollmer S, Mateen BA, Bohner G, Király FJ, Ghani R, Jonsson P, et al. Machine learning and artificial intelligence research for patient benefit: 20 critical questions on transparency, replicability, ethics, and effectiveness. *BMJ*. 2020;368:l6927. https://doi.org/10.1136/bmj.l6927.
70. Collins GS, Dhiman P, Andaur Navarro CL, Ma J, Hooft L, Reitsma JB, et al. Protocol for development of a reporting guideline (TRIPOD-AI) and risk of bias tool (PROBAST-AI) for diagnostic and prognostic prediction model studies based on artificial intelligence. *BMJ Open*. 2021;11(7):e048008. https://doi.org/10.1136/bmjopen-2020-048008.
71. Liu Y, Chen PC, Krause J, Peng L. How to read articles that use machine learning: Users' guides to the medical literature. *JAMA*. 2019;322(18):1806–16. https://doi.org/10.1001/jama.2019.16489.2754798.
72. Artificial Intelligence and Machine Learning in Software as a Medical Device. *US Food and Drug Administration*. FDA; 2021. https://www.fda.gov/medical-devices/software-medical-device-samd/artificial-intelligence-and-machine-learning-software-medical-device. Accessed 6.20.2023.
73. White Paper on Artificial Intelligence, European Commission. *A European Approach to Excellence and Trust*. 2020 Feb 19. https://ec.europa.eu/info/publications/white-paper-artificial-intelligence-european-approach-excellence-and-trust_en. Accessed 6.20.2023.
74. Radanliev P, De Roure D. Disease X vaccine production and supply chains: Risk assessing healthcare systems operating with artificial intelligence and industry 4.0. *Health Technol (Berl)*. 2023;13(1):11–5. https://doi.org/10.1007/s12553-022-00722-2.
75. Regulatory Science Strategy to 2025. *European Medicines Agency*. 2020. https://www.ema.europa.eu/en/about-us/how-we-work/regulatory-science-strategy#regulatory-science-strategy-to-2025-section. Accessed 6.20.2023.
76. Dasta J. Application of artificial intelligence to pharmacy and medicine. *Hosp Pharm*. 1992;27(4):312–5.
77. Pharma News Intelligence. https://pharmanewsintel.com/. Accessed 6.20.2023.
78. Chatbots. *Medicine Delivery*. https://hellotars.com/chatbot-templates/healthcare/Hk8N4h/medicine-ordering-chatbot. Accessed 6.20.2023.
79. Li LR, Du B, Liu HQ, Chen C. Artificial intelligence for personalized medicine in thyroid Cancer: Current status and future perspectives. *Front Oncol*. 2021;10:604051. https://doi.org/10.3389/fonc.2020.604051.
80. Davoudi A, Malhotra KR, Shickel B, Siegel S, Williams S, Ruppert M, et al. The intelligent ICU pilot study: Using artificial intelligence technology for autonomous patient monitoring. https://doi.org/10.48550/arXiv.1804.10201.
81. Buch VH, Ahmed I, Maruthappu M. Artificial intelligence in medicine: Current trends and future possibilities. *Br J Gen Pract*. 2018;68(668):143–4. https://doi.org/10.3399/bjgp18X695213.
82. Curtis RG, Bartel B, Ferguson T, Blake HT, Northcott C, Virgara R, et al. Improving user experience of virtual health assistants: Scoping review. *J Med Internet Res*. 2021;23(12):e31737. https://doi.org/10.2196/31737.
83. Ghosh PK, Jain P, Wankhede S, Preethi M, Kannan MK. Virtual nursing assistant. *J Geog Sci*. 2021;8:279–85. https://doi.org/20.18001.GSJ.2021.V8I3.21.36690.
84. Burgess M. The NHS is trialling an AI chatbot to answer your medical questions. *Wired*. 2017 Jan 5. http://www.wired.co.uk/article/babylon-nhs-chatbot-app. Accessed 20.06.2023.

85. Jiřík P. *Inspiring Applications of Digital Virtual Assistants in Healthcare*. 2022 Jul 22. https://www.phonexia.com/blog/inspiring-applications-of-digital-virtual-assistants-in-healthcare/. Accessed 20.06.2023.
86. Kim JW, Jones KL, D'Angelo E. How to prepare prospective psychiatrists in the era of artificial intelligence. *Acad Psychiatry*. 2019;43(3):337–9. https://doi.org/10.1007/s40596-019-01025-x.
87. Graham S, Depp C, Lee EE, Nebeker C, Tu X, Kim HC, et al. Artificial intelligence for mental health and mental illnesses: An overview. *Curr Psychiatry Rep*. 2019;21(11):116. https://doi.org/10.1007/s11920-019-1094-0.
88. Fitzpatrick KK, Darcy A, Vierhile M. Delivering cognitive behavior therapy to young adults with symptoms of depression and anxiety using a fully automated conversational agent (woebot): A randomized controlled trial. *JMIR Mental Health*. 2017;4(2):e19.
89. Williams AD, Andrews G. The effectiveness of internet cognitive behavioural therapy (iCBT) for depression in primary care: A quality assurance study. *PLoS ONE*. 2013;8(2):e57447.
90. Luxton DD. Artificial intelligence in psychological practice: Current and future applications and implications. *Prof Psychol Res Pract*. 2014;45(5):332–9. https://doi.org/10.1037/a0034559.
91. Prochaska J, Vogel E, Chieng A, Kendra M, Baiocchi M, Pajarito S, Robinson A. A therapeutic relational agent for reducing problematic substance use (woebot): Development and usability study. *J Med Internet Res*. 2021;23(3):e24850.
92. Lee EE, Torous J, De Choudhury M, Depp CA, Graham SA, Kim HC, et al. Artificial intelligence for mental health care: Clinical applications, barriers, facilitators, and artificial wisdom. Biol Psychiatry Cogn Neurosci Neuroimaging. 2021;6(9):856–64. https://doi.org/10.1016/j.bpsc.2021.02.001.
93. Artificial Intelligence in Healthcare. *39 Examples Improving the Future of Medicine*. Emerj; 2021. https://emerj.com/ai-sector-overviews/artificial-intelligence-in-healthcare-39-examples-improving-the-future-of-medicine/. Published 2021 Sep 21. Accessed 19.06.2023.
94. Chew HSJ. The use of artificial intelligence-based conversational agents (chatbots) for weight loss: Scoping review and practical recommendations. *JMIR Med Inform*. 2022;10(4):e32578. https://doi.org/10.2196/32578.
95. Zhang J, Oh YJ, Lange P, Yu Z, Fukuoka Y. Artificial intelligence chatbot behavior change model for designing artificial intelligence chatbots to promote physical activity and a healthy diet: Viewpoint. *J Med Internet Res*. 2020;22(9):e22845. https://doi.org/10.2196/22845.
96. Wang H, Zhang Z, Ip M, Lau J. T.F. Social media–based conversational agents for health management and interventions. *J Med Internet Res*. 2018;20(8):e261. https://doi.org/10.2196/jmir.9275.
97. Bombard Y, Baker GR, Orlando E, Fancott C, Bhatia P, Casalino S, et al. Engaging patients to improve quality of care: A systematic review. *Implement Sci*. 2018;13(1):98. https://doi.org/10.1186/s13012-018-0784-z.
98. Wong CK, Yeung DY, Ho HC, Tse KP, Lam CY. Chinese older adults' internet use for health information. *J Appl Gerontol*. 2014;33(3):316–35. https://doi.org/10.1177/0733464812463430.
99. Aggarwal A, Tam CC, Wu D, Li X, Qiao S. Artificial intelligence-based chatbots for promoting health behavioral changes: Systematic review. *J Med Internet Res*. 2023;25:e40789. https://doi.org/10.2196/40789.
100. Görtz M, Baumgärtner K, Schmid T, Muschko M, Woessner P, Gerlach A, et al. An artificial intelligence-based chatbot for prostate cancer education: Design and patient evaluation study. *Digit Health*. 2023;9:20552076231173304. https://doi.org/10.1177/20552076231173304.

101. Nakhleh A, Spitzer S, Shehadeh N. ChatGPT's response to the diabetes knowledge questionnaire: Implications for diabetes education. *Diabetes Technol Ther*. 2023. Published 2023 Apr 16. https://doi.org/10.1089/dia.2023.0134.
102. Kirchner GJ, Kim RY, Weddle JB, Bible JE. Can artificial intelligence improve the readability of patient education materials? *Clin Orthop Relat Res*. 2023. Published 2023 Apr 28. https://doi.org/10.1097/CORR.0000000000002668.
103. Lee D, Yoon SN. Application of artificial intelligence-based technologies in the healthcare industry: Opportunities and challenges. *Int J Environ Res Public Health*. 2021;18(1):271. https://doi.org/10.3390/ijerph18010271.
104. Kaptchuk TJ, Miller FG. Placebo effects in medicine. *N Engl J Med*. 2015;373(1):8–9. https://doi.org/10.1056/NEJMp1504023.
105. Lupton M. Some ethical and legal consequences of the application of artificial intelligence in the field of medicine. *Trends Med*. 2018;18(4). https://doi.org/10.15761/tim.1000147.
106. Pezzo MV, Beckstead JW. Patients prefer artificial intelligence to a human provider, provided the AI is better than the human: A commentary on Longoni, Bonezzi and Morewedge (2019). *Judgm Decis Mak*. 2020;15(3):443–5. Cambridge University Press. https://doi.org/10.1017/S1930297500007221.
107. How Americans View Use of AI in Health Care and Medical Research. https://www.pewresearch.org/science/2023/02/22/60-of-americans-would-be-uncomfortable-with-provider-relying-on-ai-in-their-own-health-care/. Accessed 19.06.2023.
108. Esmaeilzadeh P. Use of AI-based tools for healthcare purposes: A survey study from consumers' perspectives. *BMC Med Inform Decis Mak*. 2020;20(1):170. Published 2020 Jul 22. https://doi.org/10.1186/s12911-020-01191-1.
109. Khullar D, Casalino LP, Qian Y, Lu Y, Krumholz HM, Aneja S. Perspectives of patients about artificial intelligence in health care. *JAMA Netw Open*. 2022;5(5):e2210309. Published 2022 May 2. https://doi.org/10.1001/jamanetworkopen.2022.10309.
110. Russo S, Jongerius C, Faccio F, Pizzoli SF, Pinto CA, Veldwijk J, et al. Understanding patients' preferences: A systematic review of psychological instruments used in patients' preference and decision studies. *Value Health*. 2019;22(4):491–501. https://doi.org/10.1016/j.jval.2018.12.007.
111. Young AT, Amara D, Bhattacharya A, Wei ML. Patient and general public attitudes towards clinical artificial intelligence: A mixed methods systematic review. *Lancet Digit Health*. 2021;3(9):e599–e611. https://doi.org/10.1016/S2589-7500(21)00132-1.
112. West SM, Whittaker M, Crawford K. *Discriminating Systems: Gender, Race and Power in AI*. AI Now Institute; 2019.
113. Maynez J, Narayan S, Bohnet B, McDonald R. On faithfulness and factuality in abstractive summarization. *Proceedings of the 58th Annual Meeting of the Association for Computational Linguistics*. 2020. https://doi.org/10.18653/v1/2020.acl-main.173.
114. deBurca S. The learning health care organization. *Int J Qual Health Care*. 2000;12(6):457–8. https://doi.org/10.1093/intqhc/12.6.457.
115. IOM (Institute of Medicine). *Measuring the Impact of Interprofessional Education on Collaborative Practice and Patient Outcomes*. Washington, DC: The National Academies Press; 2015, p. 182.
116. Alqahtani T, Badreldin HA, Alrashed M, Alshaya AI, Alghamdi SS, bin Saleh K, et al. The emergent role of artificial intelligence, natural learning processing, and large language models in higher education and research. *Res Social Administrative Pharm*. 2023. https://doi.org/10.1016/j.sapharm.2023.05.016.
117. Pinto dos Santos D, Giese D, Brodehl S, Chon SH, Staab W, Kleinert R, et al. Medical students' attitude towards artificial intelligence: A multicentre survey. *Eur Radiol*. 2018;29(4):1640–6. https://doi.org/10.1007/s00330-018-5601-1.

118. Gerke S, Minssen T, Cohen G. Ethical and legal challenges of artificial intelligence-driven healthcare. *Artif Intell Healthc.* 2020;295–336. https://doi.org/10.1016/b978-0-12-818438-7.00012-5.
119. Cohen IG, Mello MM. HIPAA and protecting health information in the 21st century. *JAMA*. 2018;320(3):231. https://doi.org/10.1001/jama.2018.5630.
120. Yuan B, Li J. The policy effect of the general data protection regulation (GDPR) on the digital public health sector in the European union: An empirical investigation. *Int J Environ Res Public Health.* 2019;16(6):1070. https://doi.org/10.3390/ijerph16061070.
121. Al-Mistarehi AH, Mijwil MM, Filali Y, Bounabi M, Ali G, Abotaleb M. Artificial intelligence solutions for health 4.0: Overcoming challenges and surveying applications. *MJAIH*. 2023;15–20.
122. Radanliev P, De Roure D. Epistemological and bibliometric analysis of ethics and shared responsibility—health policy and IoT systems. *Sustainability*. 2021;13(15):8355.
123. Radanliev P, De Roure D, Ani U, Carvalho G. The ethics of shared Covid-19 risks: An epistemological framework for ethical health technology assessment of risk in vaccine supply chain infrastructures. *Health Technol (Berl).* 2021;11(5):1083–91.
124. Gupta U, Pranav A, Kohli A, Ghosh S, Singh D. *The Contribution of Artificial Intelligence to Drug Discovery: Current Progress and Prospects for the Future.* Microbial Data Intelligence and Computational Techniques for Sustainable Computing; 2024, pp. 1–23.
125. Gupta D, Gupta U, Sarma HJ. Functional iterative approach for Universum-based primal twin bounded support vector machine to EEG classification (FUPTBSVM). *Multimed Tools Appl.* 2024;83(8):22119–22151.
126. Gupta U, Jain V. *Social Neuroscience: Inferring Mental States in Social Media.* Emotional AI and Human-AI Interactions in Social Networking; 2024, pp. 15–39.
127. Sharma M, Deswal S, Gupta U, Tabassum M, Lawal I, eds. *Soft Computing Techniques in Connected Healthcare Systems.* CRC Press; 2023.
128. Malik K, Sadawarti H, Sharma M, Gupta U, Tiwari P, eds. *Computational Techniques in Neuroscience.* CRC Press; 2023.
129. Singh D, Singh D, Manju, Gupta U. Smart healthcare: A breakthrough in the growth of technologies. In *Artificial Intelligence-Based Healthcare Systems.* Cham: Springer Nature Switzerland; 2023, pp. 73–85.
130. Gupta M, Srivastava D, Pantola D, Gupta U. Brain tumor detection using improved Otsu's thresholding method and supervised learning techniques at early stage. In *Proceedings of Emerging Trends and Technologies on Intelligent Systems: ETTIS 2022.* Singapore: Springer Nature; 2022, pp. 271–281.
131. Gupta U, Gupta D, Agarwal U. Analysis of randomization-based approaches for autism spectrum disorder. In *Pattern Recognition and Data Analysis with Applications.* Singapore: Springer Nature; 2022, pp. 701–713.
132. Gupta D, Choudhury A, Gupta U, Singh P, Prasad M. Computational approach to clinical diagnosis of diabetes disease: A comparative study. *Multimed Tools Appl.* 2021; 1–26.
133. Gupta D., Gupta U. On robust asymmetric Lagrangian ν-twin support vector regression using pinball loss function. *Applied Soft Computing.* 2021;102:107099.

9 Deep Learning Innovations in Healthcare

Early Detection of Alzheimer's Disease

Sonali Deshpande and Nilima Kulkarni

9.1 INTRODUCTION

Alzheimer's is a major growing public health problem that needs help and attention right away. Over 80% of cases of dementia are caused by Alzheimer's disease (AD). This makes AD the main cause of dementia. There are changes in the brain that aren't normal up to 15–20 years before the first symptoms show up. This is called "preclinical AD," and it's possible to see the changes because of significant advances toward our understanding of how the disease starts over the last few decades. For this, a quick evaluation is very important. Deep learning algorithms are getting more attention these days because they might change how early Alzheimer's disease is found by looking at medical image data [1]. Alzheimer's disease is a gradual, irreversible neurological disease that affects thinking, memory, and behavior due to excessive neurofibrillary tangles and amyloid plaque buildup in the brain. The most prevalent type of dementia, AD, currently lacks a proven medication that modifies the condition. Deep neural network architectures are used in these ways to find subtle signs of Alzheimer's disease. The possibility is that this will lead to a more frequent and accurate diagnosis of a medical problem [2]. There are many deep learning methods that can be used to find Alzheimer's early. This chapter sorts them all into groups. It talks about how these methods might change professional practice, and a list of their pros and cons is given.

9.1.1 Importance of Early Detection in Alzheimer's Disease Management

Alzheimer's disease is a progressive brain illness that impairs thinking, memory, and daily functioning. It is the primary cause of dementia in older adults and affects a large number of people worldwide [3, 4]. As the sickness worsens, it becomes more difficult to remember things, think properly, and behave normally. To get the right medicine and help, it's important to get an evaluation as soon as possible. The quality

DOI: 10.1201/9781003539483-9

of life will get better, and the illness will get worse less quickly [5]. Because of this, it is very important to make early detection devices that work well. That way, Alzheimer's won't get worse, and its effects on people, their families, and healthcare systems will be lessened. People with Alzheimer's should be found as soon as possible so that they can get the best care. For better therapy and to stop the disease from spreading, it is important to find it early [6]. Families and patients can get the best care, get help, and get ready better when the truth is found early on. Early diagnosis also makes it easier for people to take part in clinical studies that test new medicines and treatments [7]. Finding Alzheimer's early is very important for better the quality of life for both the person who has it and the people who care for them.

9.1.2 Role of Deep Learning in Medical Imaging and Alzheimer's Detection

When it comes to healthcare, artificial intelligence (AI) has the power to totally change many areas, such as how neurological disorders are diagnosed and treated. As the name suggests, neurological illnesses are a group of diseases that affect the brain, spinal cord, and nerves. These include epilepsy, Multiple Sclerosis (MS), Alzheimer's, Parkinson's, and stroke. It is very hard to find these illnesses early, make a correct diagnosis, and plan a personalized treatment plan for each person. The name for computer systems that can see trends, make choices, and learn from their mistakes is artificial intelligence (AI) systems. DL and neural networks are the two main parts of ML, which makes it one of the most important areas of AI [8]. Deep learning's main goal is to teach the system from the dataset, user input, and past events. With the help of the feedback, the DL algorithm changes itself to be as good at a job as it can be. The end goal is for it to also work correctly with brand-new data sets that haven't been looked into before [9]. AI-assisted automatic diagnosis of medical imaging, especially in the area of DL, has successfully removed problems in medical imaging that were caused by mistakes made by humans who were not accurate enough or did not have enough experience [10].

9.1.3 Role of Generative AI in Medical

Utilizing cutting-edge technologies has become an important part of changing how healthcare is provided and experienced in this age of personalized medicine and digital progress. Generative artificial intelligence, a type of AI that has a lot of promise to change the patient journey, is one of these technologies that will change everything. Generative AI's combination with healthcare marks the start of a new age of patient empowerment, in which people are no longer passive receivers of care but active players in their own health. The journey of a patient can be changed by generative AI, which can offer personalized insights, predictive analytics, and virtual help at every step of the way, from evaluation to treatment and beyond.

Generative artificial intelligence tools and applications are referred to as GenAI. Systems learn these patterns and structures from the text entirely automatically. Images, sounds, animation, models, or other media inputs are used to generate new data with similar characteristics. In continuously changing healthcare, one aspect remains unchanged: the critical significance of the patient experience [11–13]. With the industry's transition towards a patient-centered care model, there is a significant emphasis on enabling individuals to engage actively in their health journeys. One of the most transformative technologies is generative artificial intelligence, a sector of artificial intelligence that possesses significant potential to transform the patient experience. By definition, generative AI is a very new type of artificial intelligence that can create new, customized content. For health care delivery, this means a paradigm shift. With the vastness of generative AI, it becomes more than evident how these technologies are specifically advancing the management of Alzheimer's disease in the creation of a revolutionized patient experience in healthcare. Figure 9.1 describes critical roles generative AI can play in identifying biomarkers, analyzing neuroimaging, predicting cognitive decline, and personalizing risk assessments. Each one of these components underscores that GenAI will enhance diagnostic accuracy, permitting interventions to be personalized and hence leading to a proactive, patient-centered approach to care for those suffering from Alzheimer's. It's a visualization not just of practical application but of sophisticated AI integration in the navigation of complex medical data toward more informed healthcare decisions.

9.1.4 Objective of the Comparative Analysis

To identify Alzheimer's early, a variety of deep learning techniques are employed. The chapter's primary objective is to thoroughly compare and contrast them. The aim of this research is to determine the effectiveness of several deep learning techniques, their ease of understanding, and their capacity for scaling. Some of these methods are autoencoders, convolutional neural networks (CNNs), and recurrent neural networks (RNNs). We must examine these approaches and detail the benefits and drawbacks. The comparison study aims to identify the most effective deep learning techniques for AD detection. Evaluation techniques, feature extraction, data

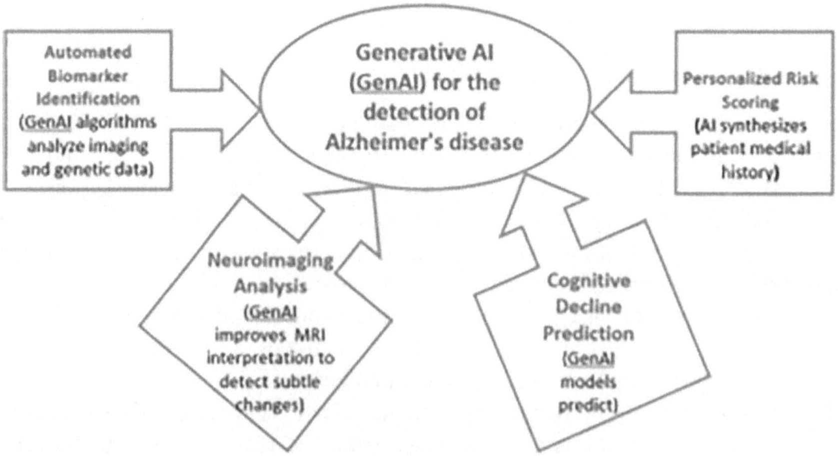

FIGURE 9.1 Generative AI in Alzheimer's disease detection framework.

TABLE 9.1
Details of Publications in Scopus Database

Keywords/Query	Documents Found
Alzheimer+ Deep learning	3854 documents
Alzheimer + Machine learning	5952 documents
Alzheimer + LLM	14 documents
Alzheimer + GenAI	1 document
Alzheimer + GAN	221 documents
Alzheimer + CNN	1342 documents
Alzheimer + RNN	97 documents

Source: www.scopus.com, accessed on 28 August 2024.

TABLE 9.2
Analysis by Document Type

Sr. No	Document Type	Publication
1	Journal article	1742
2	Conference paper	965
3	Review	219
4	Conference review	205
5	Book chapter	110

Source: http://www.scopus.com (accessed on 28 August 2024).

preparation, and model designs are few of the numerous aspects considered. When Alzheimer's disease is detected early, people can receive better care more quickly. This is made possible by deep learning. The intention here is to provide information about this to scientists, physicians, and decision-makers [14–16].

Researchers frequently rely on established research databases, such as Web of Science, ScienceDirect, Google Scholar, PubMed, Dimensions, Lens, and Sage Journals. These platforms provide a comprehensive array of publications. Notably, Scopus is recognized as a prominent database extensively employed for analytical purposes. A variety of keywords are used to locate documents within these databases, as illustrated in Table 9.1. There are no restrictions concerning country or source type, among other factors. Each publication encompasses information such as the abstract, literature, authors, keywords, country, and citation details. Table 9.2 shows the number of documents published in the years 2020 to 2024.

Data was gathered from the Scopus database covering the period from 2020 to 2024, incorporating various sources such as conference proceedings, journal articles, and book chapters. The accompanying table presents statistical information,

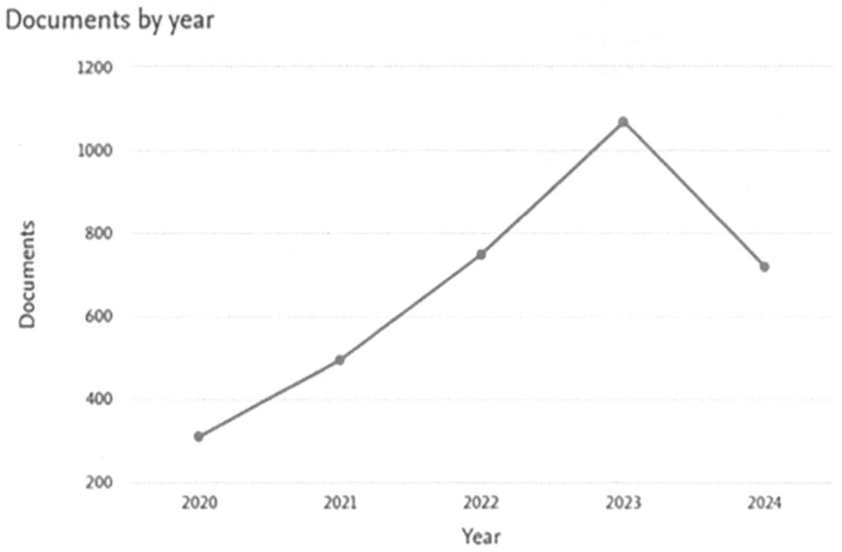

FIGURE 9.2 Year-wise paper publication related to Alzheimer's.

while the graphical representation is illustrated in Figure 9.2. The analysis reveals that the peak number of publications occurred in 2023, followed closely by 2022 and 2024. This indicates a promising opportunity for research in this field in the subsequent years.

9.1.4.1 Document Analysis by Sources

The database encompasses various sources, including conferences, journals, book chapters, notes, and reviews, among others. The table presents publication statistics categorized by different keywords. Additionally, Figure 9.3 illustrates a graphical representation of the various sources, along with the number of documents published each year.

9.1.4.2 Documents by Type

It is seen from the analysis that most of the publications are journal articles, followed by conference papers.

9.2 REVIEW OF DEEP LEARNING ALGORITHMS

A comprehensive search was undertaken to locate pertinent articles for this review. This search was executed across prominent scientific databases, including Scopus (https://scopus.com/), PubMed (https://pubmed.ncbi.nlm.nih.gov/), IEEE Xplore (https://ieeexplore.ieee.org/Xplore/home.jsp), ACM Digital Library (https://dl.acm.org/), and Google Scholar (https://scholar.google.com/). The search utilized various terms related to "Alzheimer's disease," "AD detection," "CNN," "Convolutional Neural Network," "RNN," "Recurrent Neural Network," "generative adversarial networks," "GANs," "Long Short-Term Memory Networks," and "LSTMs," along

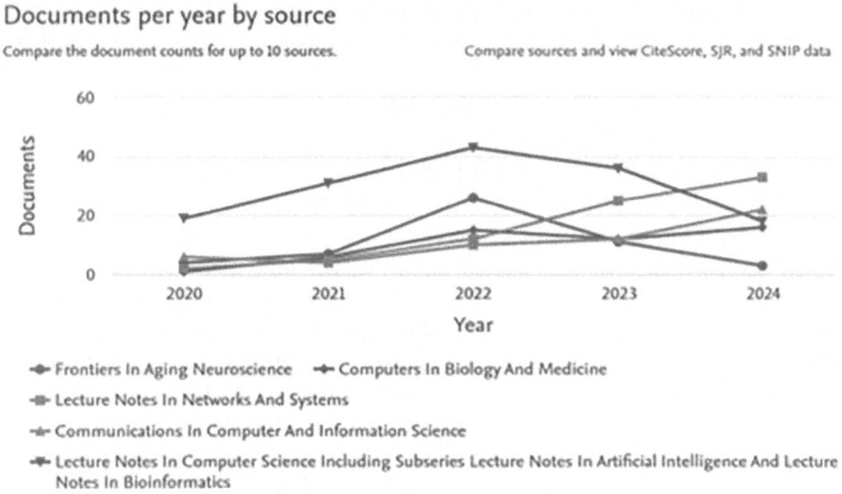

FIGURE 9.3 Analysis of documents by sources.

Source: http://www.scopus.com (accessed on 28 August 2024).

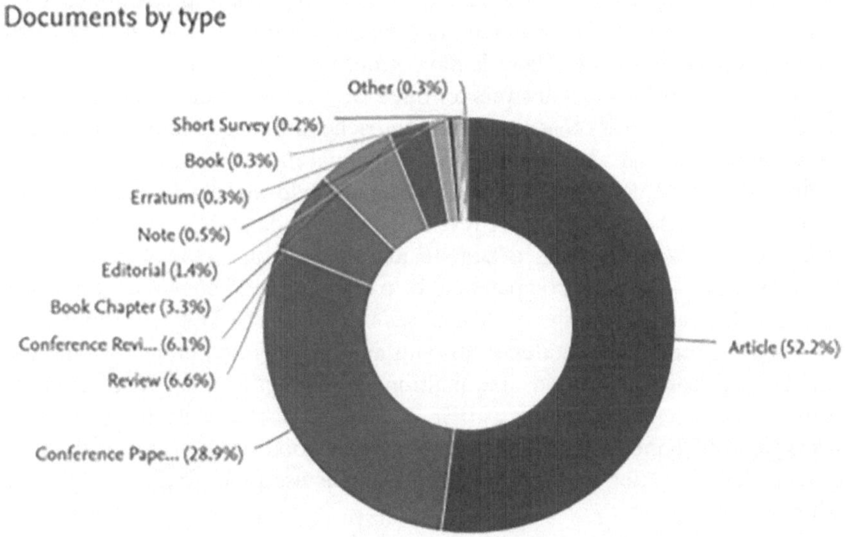

FIGURE 9.4 Analysis of publications by document type.

Source: http://www.scopus.com (accessed on 28 August 2024).

with their combinations. The search was restricted to articles published from 2020 through December 2024.

The selection procedure comprised two distinct phases: screening and eligibility evaluation. Screening involved independent review of titles and abstracts from the collected papers by two reviewers to ascertain their relevance to the review topic. Papers that evidently failed to satisfy the inclusion criteria were eliminated at this stage.

Eligibility Evaluation: The full texts of the papers that remained were acquired and assessed independently by two reviewers.

Data were extracted from selected papers using a standardized form. Extracted data included authors, year of publication, study objectives, characteristics of the dataset, CNN, RNN, or GAN, LSTM architectures employed, metrics used for performance evaluation, and key findings reported. The data extracted and thus synthesized provided an overview of methodologies, performances, and state of affairs regarding CNNs, RNNs, GAN, and LSTM on the detection of AD [17–21].

Alzheimer's disease is widespread and presents significant challenges for professionals in terms of diagnosis. This topic has been widely studied in the literature. This chapter investigates a range of research that utilizes artificial intelligence and machine learning to enhance comprehension, diagnosis, prediction, and treatment of Alzheimer's disease. Every study offers a distinct viewpoint on prediction models utilizing diverse data sets, prospective interventions, and ethical concerns associated with Alzheimer's care.

According to one study [22], an ensemble method based on deep learning can be used to find Alzheimer's disease early on using MRI scans. The study showed promising results by using ADNI data for dataset collection, preparation, model building, and evaluation. The accuracy rate ranged from 93.88% to 99.83% across several classification groups. There is more proof that the ensemble method works because it got 88.46% correct answers for three-way classification on a local dataset. Differential analysis shows that ensemble approaches still need more research, even if the ensemble method works better than individual models. These findings show that ensemble-based deep learning methods could help make AD detection more accurate and open the way for future research on bigger datasets.

The research [23] describes a dual fusion cluster graph convolution network (DFCGCN) model for using computers to help diagnose mild cognitive impairment (MCI), which is an early stage of Alzheimer's disease. The DFCGCN model can quickly pull out complex features from both non-imaging and brain imaging data thanks to deep learning methods and multi-modal data processing. With accuracy, sensitivity, and specificity of 90.7%, 91.1%, and 94.0%, respectively, the Alzheimer's Disease Neuroimaging Initiative sample gives very good results. This new way of diagnosing MCI is better, and it looks like it could be useful for finding and treating this illness early on.

Another study [24] addresses the need for scalable and actual-time Alzheimer's sickness detection the use of part devices, featuring a weighted ensemble community comprising fashions which include AlexNet, DenseNet-121, and InceptionV3. The model is applied on a Raspberry Pi four Model B and attains a remarkable 98.44% accuracy and sensitivity. Interestingly, the counseled ensemble network indicates a 6.5% development in sensitivity and exceeds associated studies by means of 5% in accuracy. This demonstrates how facet devices, which enable quicker inference times and decrease the threat of information breaches, connected with cloud-primarily based architectures, have the potential to absolutely rework the analysis of Alzheimer's disorder.

Using longitudinal MRI data from the OASIS Database, one study [25] shows a new way to find early signs of Alzheimer's disease in older people by using ensemble learning models. When you combine things like years of schooling and Mini-Mental State Examination (MMSE) results, you get a generalized classifier. The suggested model gives good results, with a 94.64% success rate and an 89.93% fivefold cross-validation AUC score. A comparison study also shows that the suggested model does better than the previous best research in terms of performance measures. This shows that it could be a useful tool for finding Alzheimer's disease early on [15, 25].

A study [26] shows how to use a multimodal image-fusion method that combines PET and MRI to find Alzheimer's disease. Using an ensemble classifier with this method, which identifies features based on a random forest, gives very good results: 91% for finding AD vs. MCI and 99% for AD vs. CN and MCI vs. CN binary classifications. Also, the multi-class categorization between AD, MCI, and CN is very good (96% accuracy). This data shows that the suggested fusion technique can find and classify different stages of Alzheimer's disease very well, which could lead to better diagnosis and treatment methods.

A paper [27] elaborates on the roles and potentials of generative AI in improving healthcare through better diagnostics and improved patient interaction. According to the authors, AI will be able to help in the administration of healthcare and outline that effective regulations will be required to deal with the various challenges thrown to privacy, trust, and ethics. While the shifting landscape brought by AI into medicine holds the promise of enormous gain, careful implementation will be required to maximize benefit while mitigating risk.

In another paper [28] Yasin Shokrollahi et al. elaborate on the incorporation of generative AI into several healthcare applications. This provides information regarding the tremendous progress and influence that AI technologies, such as transformers and diffusion models, have had on medical practices in areas like diagnostic imaging, protein structure prediction, and clinical documentation. The review also recommends directions for further research to be done in view of the present limitations so as to adapt to the changing healthcare needs. This review forms a platform by which the ever-increasing role of AI in improving diagnostic accuracy, treatment plan optimization, and health care delivery as a whole can be understood [13, 14, 28].

A study [29] provides a discussion on the extent of integration and the effectiveness of generative AI within healthcare settings. According to the report, while GenAI is primarily utilized in improving access to medical knowledge and diagnostic accuracy, its full potential in automating and guiding clinical services remains largely untapped. It also indicates that further studies were needed to really validate the capabilities of GenAI in real-world clinical environments and that more comprehensive evidence is required to underpin optimistic projections for a GenAI-transformed future in healthcare.

9.2.1 Convolutional Neural Networks

Convolutional neural networks have demonstrated significant success in clinical imaging tasks, including Alzheimer's disease detection. CNNs automatically extract hierarchical capabilities from neuroimaging statistics by way of utilizing convolutional layers [30]. This permits them to capture spatial correlations and styles which might be symptomatic of the course of an ailment. CNNs can accurately classify patients and healthy controls by learning discriminative features associated with Alzheimer's disease through training on large datasets of brain MRI scans. Convolutional neural networks demonstrate superior diagnostic accuracy when compared to conventional image analysis techniques, thereby decreasing the likelihood of misdiagnosis. They are capable of identifying Alzheimer's disease at earlier stages by recognizing subtle patterns in brain imaging that signal the initial onset of the condition. After training, convolutional neural networks are capable of swiftly analyzing new images on a large scale, thereby enabling extensive screening and monitoring of Alzheimer's disease.

9.2.2 Recurrent Neural Networks

They can represent sequential data very well, which makes recurrent neural networks ideal for looking at long-term neuroimaging data in Alzheimer's study [31]. Recurrent neural networks are valuable in identifying early indications of Alzheimer's disease because they can effectively demonstrate the temporal changes in brain structures and their dependence on time. RNNs can analyze brain imaging scan sequences to identify individuals who are susceptible to future cognitive impairment and detect subtle patterns that may indicate the progression of an illness. Because RNNs are able to model the temporal progression of cognitive and functional decline due to Alzheimer's disease, they show clearly how the disease is evolving in individual patients. This predicts the future state of cognitive and functional abilities of a patient to help in the planning of that care well in advance. RNNs are especially good at learning complex dependencies in sequential data, which is really important for a disease like Alzheimer's that involves several interacting biological and cognitive processes.

9.2.3 Autoencoders

A deep learning model that can work without being monitored is known as an autoencoder. It can put together random data again [32]. This means that they can be used to find Alzheimer's disease by getting rid of traits and cutting down on the number of dimensions. Images from brain scans can be turned into a latent space with fewer dimensions that autoencoders can use to figure out how brain areas connected to Alzheimer's disease are represented. It is also possible to teach autoencoders to make regular images of the brain. On the one hand, this lets you find habits that don't make sense and strange behaviors that could be signs of Alzheimer's. Autoencoders serve to decrease the dimensionality of data, thereby facilitating the storage and processing of extensive datasets of brain images. Denoising autoencoders improve the quality of medical images by eliminating extraneous noise, which aids clinicians in recognizing pathological characteristics more effectively.

9.2.4 Generative Adversarial Networks

Researchers have been able to create synthetic brain images that closely resemble actual brain scans by using generative adversarial networks (GANs). GANs have the

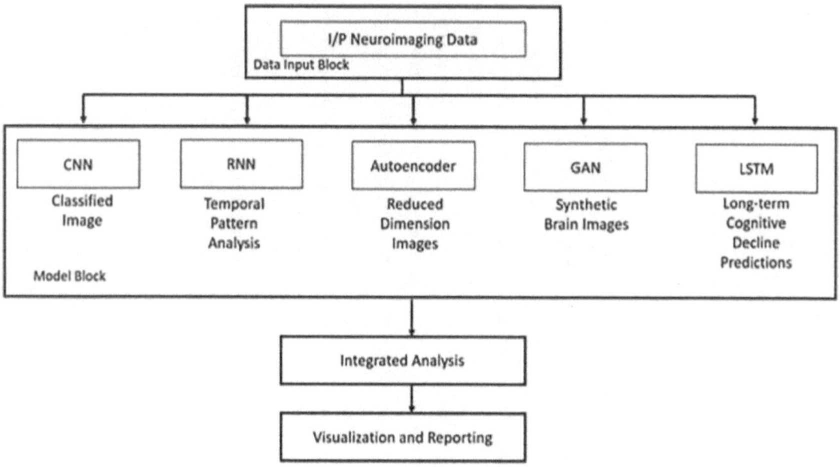

FIGURE 9.5 Deep learning models for Alzheimer's disease detection.

potential to detect Alzheimer's disease by producing a greater number of samples from smaller datasets. This improves the model's overall performance by making it stronger and more flexible [33]. Because GANs can also enhance data quality, it is simpler to employ specific brain imaging datasets to train deep learning models. Most importantly, GANs generate highly detailed and realistic images. These are very useful in overcoming limitations such as small or imbalanced datasets. By increasing the size of the dataset, GANs will make possible more accurate and robust diagnostic tools. GAN-generated synthetic data may enable researchers to investigate the potential disease patterns and time course of Alzheimer's disease in ways not possible with smaller data.

9.2.5 Long Short-Term Memory Networks

Long short-term memory (LSTM), a type of recurrent neural network, works like a list of long-distance dependent inputs. To find long-term patterns in brain data, LSTMs are used [34]. This makes it easier to spot Alzheimer's disease early. By combining data from several periods, LSTMs are able to determine who is most likely to get Alzheimer's disease and how their mental state will deteriorate over time. Long short-term memory networks are capable of analyzing and forecasting outcomes from extensive data sequences, effectively capturing temporal relationships that are essential for the early diagnosis and comprehension of Alzheimer's disease progression. By identifying patterns in cognitive and imaging data over time, LSTMs can facilitate the earlier detection of Alzheimer's, possibly even prior to the manifestation of notable symptoms. Figure 9.5 gives a detailed view of the discussed models used for Alzheimer's detection.

By identifying spatial correlations in the data, convolutional neural networks are skilled at interpreting brain MRI scans and PET pictures; nevertheless, during training, they frequently require large amounts of labelled data, as shown in Table 9.1.

TABLE 9.3
Summary of Deep Learning Approaches for Early Detection of Alzheimer's Disease

Algorithm	Description	Use Cases	Advantages	Disadvantages
Convolutional Neural Networks	Deep learning models designed for image analysis.	Analyzing brain MRI scans, PET images.	Captures spatial dependencies in data.	May require large amounts of labeled data for training.
Recurrent Neural Networks	Designed to handle sequential data with temporal dependencies.	Analyzing time-series data, EEG signals.	Captures temporal dynamics in data.	May suffer from vanishing/exploding gradient problem.
Autoencoders	Neural networks trained to reconstruct input data.	Dimensionality reduction, anomaly detection.	Unsupervised learning, good for feature extraction.	Performance may degrade with noisy or incomplete data.
Generative Adversarial Networks	Consist of two neural networks: generator and discriminator.	Generating synthetic medical images, data augmentation.	Produces realistic synthetic data.	Training instability, mode collapse.
Long Short-Term Memory Networks	Designed to model sequential data and handle long-term dependencies.	Analyzing time-series data, natural language processing.	Captures long-term dependencies in sequential data.	May require careful tuning of hyperparameters.
Attention Mechanisms	Mechanisms that allow neural networks to focus on specific parts of input data	Improving performance in sequence-to-sequence tasks, image captioning.	Enhances model interpretability and performance.	Additional computational overhead.

While recurrent neural networks are excellent at analyzing EEG signals and time-series data, they can have problems with vanishing or expanding gradients during training. Although their performance may suffer when dealing with noisy or imperfect data, autoencoders are useful for tasks such as dimensionality reduction and anomaly identification through unsupervised learning. While generative adversarial networks are a valuable tool for supplementing datasets and creating synthetic medical pictures, they can face challenges such mode collapse and training instability.

Out of all the algorithms mentioned in Table 9.4, for finding Alzheimer's disease early, the algorithm CNN-LSTM-with-Aug is the most accurate, with a score of 99.92%. This method uses techniques for adding more data and combines long short-term memory networks with convolutional neural networks. Because it can find temporal connections in image sequences, it is especially useful for looking at MRI scans over time, which is necessary to find small changes that are linked to Alzheimer's disease getting worse. Also, the fact that the algorithm CNN-LSTM-with-Aug is very accurate shows that it could be used to make accurate and reliable diagnoses in medical settings. However, the shallow convolutional neural network algorithm also does very well, with a success rate of 99.68%. Using 2D T1-weighted MR brain pictures, this method can classify both globally and locally, which makes it possible to find and group Alzheimer's disease stages early and without surgery. For professional uses, it works especially well because it is tough and resilient. Although CNN-LSTM-with-Aug is known for its ability to capture temporal dependencies in sequential data, the shallow convolutional neural network algorithm has the advantage of providing detailed local classification in specific diagnostic scenarios. In the end, the decision on which algorithms to use will rely on specific needs, such as the type of data and the level of classification detail desired.

As you look for the best deep learning way to find Alzheimer's early, there are many things to keep in mind. The type of data, the needs of the job, and the computer resources that are available are some of these factors. A lot of different things can be done with each program because they are all different and have their own pros and cons. CNNs are very popular because they can find Alzheimer's disease very well. Convolutional neural networks, which are types of artificial intelligence, are very good at finding links between data points. Because of this, they can be used to look at medical images like PET and MRI tests. These images are useful for convolutional neural networks to learn from and understand because they show a lot of spatial information about brain diseases and structure. People often use convolutional neural networks to separate and group parts of pictures, especially when they want to guess if someone has Alzheimer's. Always remember that the code you use can change based on the task at hand. This is because long short-term memory networks or recurrent neural networks are better at dealing with temporal interactions. They would work best with sequential or time-series data. Before making a final choice about which algorithm to use, it is important to perform a thorough analysis of the data types, task requirements, and pros and cons of each. Also, by looking at various methods and full tests, one can find the best way to find Alzheimer's disease early.

The summary in Table 9.5 enables the reader to understand how GenAI is being used within different healthcare contexts from a selection of scholarly articles: Key areas of application include improving accuracy in diagnoses, tailoring treatment

TABLE 9.4
Result-Based Summary of Deep Learning Approaches for Early Detection of Alzheimer's Disease

Algorithm	Use Cases	Dataset	Advantages	Accuracy	Inferences
[35] Shallow convolutional neural network	Early Alzheimer's disease detection and classification without invasive 2D T1-weighted MR brain imaging. Normal, MCI, AD global categorization Local MCI classification into VMD, MD, and MoD phases identifies prodromal AD	6400 brain MRIs were used for validation and testing	- Fast and accurate diagnosis of AD stages - Provides both global and local classification - Achieves high accuracy, sensitivity, specificity, and ROC values - Demonstrates resilience and robustness	99.68%	Combine different datasets using advanced data mining algorithms to improve AD prediction
[36] CNN-LSTM-with-Augmentation	Early diagnosis of Alzheimer's disease	MRI scans	Recognizes temporal relationships in image sequences, suitable for sequential data analysis	99.92%	Additional neuroimaging data could be incorporated into the model to improve it even more
[36] CNNs-with-Augmentation	Early diagnosis of Alzheimer's disease	MRI scans	Better generalization skills due to data augmentation	97.39%	
[36] VGG16-SVM-with-Augmentation	Early diagnosis of Alzheimer's disease	MRI scans	Utilizes transfer learning for improved performance	-	
[37] Deep ensemble learning (DEL) integrated with two-dimensional convolutional neural networks (2D-CNN)	Diagnosing and classifying Alzheimer's disease and healthy controls (HCs) using electroencephalography signals	Public EEG-based Alzheimer's datasets	- Integration of state-of-the-art supervised deep learning algorithms within an ensemble model architecture - Accurate diagnosis and classification of EEG signals of AD and HC subjects - High accuracy achieved without feature extraction, using 2D-CNN models directly - Utilization of five-fold cross-validation for evaluation	97.9%	Multimodal data such as EEG, fMRI, and MRI can be used

[38] Word2Vec-based	AD detection using spontaneous speech	Alzheimer's dementia recognition through spontaneous speech (ADReSS) challenge dataset	Straightforward and efficient model	92%	Consideration of larger dataset to get more robustness in the model
[39] BERT based	AD detection using contextualized models	ADReSS challenge dataset	Captures contextual information effectively	-	
[38] GPT based	AD detection using contextualized models	ADReSS challenge dataset	Effective in capturing context	-	
[39] Hybrid deep learning approach	Early detection of Alzheimer's disease	MRI and PET images	- Utilizes multimodal imaging and convolutional neural network with long short-term memory algorithm - Incorporates MRI, PET, and neuropsychological test scores	98.5%	Use of deep CNN with transfer learning
[39] Automatic early detection of AD	Early detection of Alzheimer's disease	MRI images	- Utilizes DL for automated detection of AD based on MRI images - Utilizes ACO for noise reduction and MFCM for picture segmentation - Employs CNN and LSTM for training - Enhances accuracy using Adam's optimization	98.5%	
[40] VGG-TSwinformer (combination of VGG-16 CNN and transformer)	Short-term longitudinal study of mild cognitive impairment progression prediction	ADNI dataset (Alzheimer's Disease Neuroimaging Initiative)	- Utilizes VGG-16 CNN for extracting low-level spatial features from longitudinal sMRI images, capturing detailed structural information - Employs transformer-based architecture for fine-grained fusion of spatially adjacent feature representations, allowing for better integration of spatial information	77.2%	Multimodal cross-sectional and longitudinal biomarkers will be used together in future studies; this work only uses sMRI

(*Continued*)

TABLE 9.4 *(Continued)*
Result-Based Summary of Deep Learning Approaches for Early Detection of Alzheimer's Disease

Algorithm	Use Cases	Dataset	Advantages	Accuracy	Inferences
[41] MultiAzNet (multi-modal ensemble-based deep neural network)	Diagnosis of Alzheimer's disease	Alzheimer Neuroimaging Dataset (publicly available)	- Incorporates heterogeneous information from PET and MRI images for more accurate diagnosis - Automates the process of predicting the onset of Alzheimer's disease at an early stage - Utilizes image fusion, feature extraction, and classification steps to enhance diagnostic accuracy - Employs the multi-objective grasshopper optimization algorithm (MOGOA) to optimize model layers.	92.3%	Additional neuroimaging data could be incorporated into the model to improve it even more
[42] Hybrid model combining a deep neural network and a multi-layer feed-forward neural network	Early detection and classification of Alzheimer's disease stages (AD, MCI, CN)	MRI dataset collected from ADNI and Kaggle datasets	- Accurate feature extraction and classification - Achieves high accuracy, AUC, sensitivity, and specificity	93.38%	Use of additional promising modalities like PET

TABLE 9.5
Summary of Various Studies on Deployments in Healthcare with Generative AI

Ref	GenAI Utility in Healthcare	Identified Obstacles	Proposed Advancements
[43]	Enhances diagnostic precision, manages patient care, and facilitates drug repurposing.	Concerns over data privacy, bias in algorithms, and system integration challenges.	Advocate for robust AI model development and better integration techniques.
[44]	Specializes in enhancing treatment personalization and predictive healthcare analytics.	Requires diverse, high-quality data sets and faces ethical dilemmas.	Push for advancements in data management and ethical AI practices.
[45]	Focuses on identifying and validating drug repurposing candidates using clinical data.	Struggles with data validation and the necessity of real-world efficacy testing.	Improve AI-driven drug validation mechanisms.
[46]	Applied to improve diagnostic accuracy and enhance healthcare operational efficiencies.	Encounters regulatory challenges and issues with technology adaptation.	Encourage regulatory improvements and acceptance of new technologies.
[47]	Aids in clinical decision-making and optimizes healthcare delivery mechanisms.	Faces privacy and ethical concerns, reliant on high-quality data.	Tackle ethical considerations and enhance data quality and access.
[48]	Utilized for automating medical imaging processes and identifying biomarkers.	Issues with algorithm transparency and interpretability.	Refine algorithms for enhanced clarity and precision.
[49]	Boosts patient interaction and supports the use of virtual health assistants.	Difficulties in managing patient data and refining AI interaction models.	Develop AI systems that ensure patient privacy and interaction quality.
[50]	Streamlines administrative healthcare functions and supports expansive data analyses.	Incurs high computational demands and requires specific expertise.	Work on reducing AI operational costs and improving user interfaces.

solutions for individuals, and making the processes more efficient in health care. It also displays the most relevant challenges, such as guaranteeing patients' data privacy and the need to address biases in AI algorithms. Additionally, it gives suggestions of prospective improvements to foster responsible use and development of GenAI technologies in medical settings. In view of this comparative review, it serves to shed light on the continuous advancement of GenAI into healthcare and the necessary considerations for it, as shown by contemporary research.

9.3 PROPOSED METHODOLOGY

To detect Alzheimer's disease at an early stage using deep learning approaches, a generalized architecture could include the following components:

Data Preprocessing Module: Responsible for handling raw medical imaging data, including MRI and PET scans [51]. Operations are implemented to enhance the quantity and quality of the input data, including resizing, normalization, and data augmentation.

Feature Extraction Module: Utilizes convolutional neural networks as an illustration of a deep learning model for extracting valuable features from pre-processed medical images. May involve networks specifically designed for analyzing medical imaging data or pre-trained CNN architectures like VGG or ResNet.

Classifier Module: Sorts the features that were collected into groups, like Alzheimer's disease stages (AD, MCI, CN) and uses those groups as input. Can be made up of fully connected layers, recurrent neural networks, or other classification models like random forests or support vector machines (SVMs).

Evaluation and Validation Module: Checks the accuracy, sensitivity, and precision of the deep learning model to see how well it is working. To make sure the model can be used in many cases, different test sets are used for validation and cross-validation.

Deployment and Integration Module: Makes it easier for the learned model to be used in healthcare systems or clinical settings. Simple integration with current diagnostic equipment and electronic health record (EHR) systems makes it easy to add to the healthcare workflow.

Monitoring and Maintenance Module: Keeps track of the deployed model's performance in practical environments. Employs techniques for updating and retraining models to adjust to changing clinical procedures and data distributions.

The essential elements and workflow of deep learning techniques for Alzheimer's disease early diagnosis are depicted in Figure 9.6. The data preprocessing module, which is the first step in the process, preprocesses and augments raw medical imaging data to improve both its quantity and quality. Then, from pre-processed data, the feature extraction module uses deep learning models to extract relevant features. The classifier module receives these features, after which it classifies them into various illness stages. The evaluation and validation module uses different measurements and validation methods to check how well the model works. If you do well on the test, the deployment and integration module will help you use the model you learned in real medical situations. Last, the monitoring and maintenance module makes sure that models are always up to date and retrained and that their work is always being checked to make sure they can adapt to new clinical data and processes. In the end, our way gives you a solid and well-organized foundation for making useful deep learning systems that can find Alzheimer's disease.

To detect Alzheimer's disease at an early stage using GenAI approaches, a generalized framework could include the following components:

Data Collection and Management:

Objective: Collect diverse, high-quality healthcare data.

Activities: This relates to the sources from which data is collected on patients, diversification and quality of data, and the privacy of the data is guaranteed.

Result: Create a robust and analytically ready dataset that is privacy-compliant.

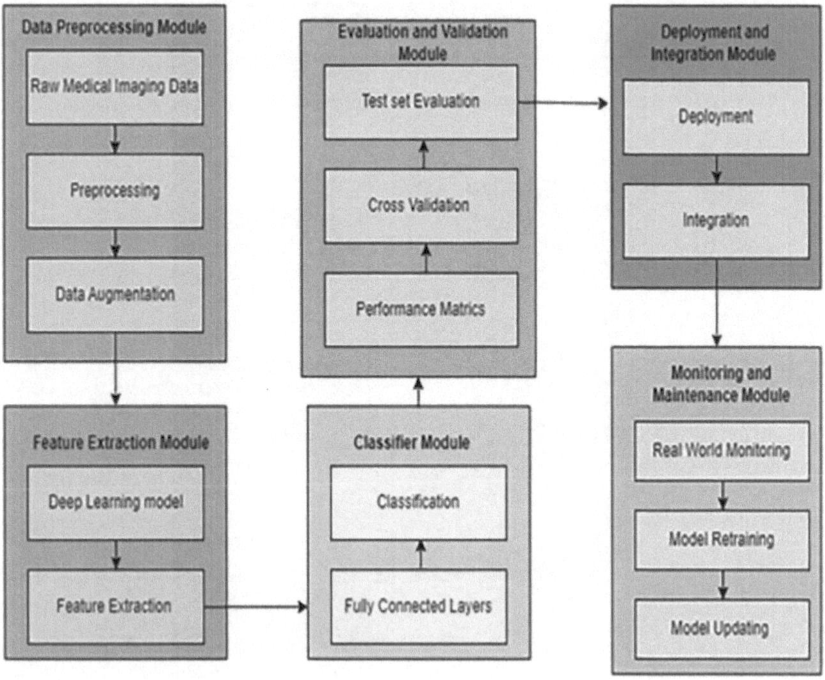

FIGURE 9.6 Architecture for the early detection of Alzheimer's disease using a deep learning approach.

GenAI Model Development:

Purpose: Designing and refining AI algorithms for applications in healthcare.
Activity: Construct models for diagnostics, drug repositioning, and patient management. Address algorithm bias and enhance transparency.
Result: Effective AI models in healthcare are those that are ethical.

Integration into Healthcare Systems:

Objective: To enable existing health care workflows to seamlessly integrate AI models.
Activities: Tailor AI tools to clinical and administrative processes and ensure that they augment, but do not duplicate, existing technologies.
Result: AI-driven improvement of diagnostic accuracy and operational efficiency of healthcare settings.

Validation and Testing:

Purpose: There was a need to validate the effectiveness of AI models using real-world data and measure their reliability.
Activities: Run trials for testing AI predictions and decisions against clinical outcomes and patient data.
Result: Validated AI tools ready for wider deployment.

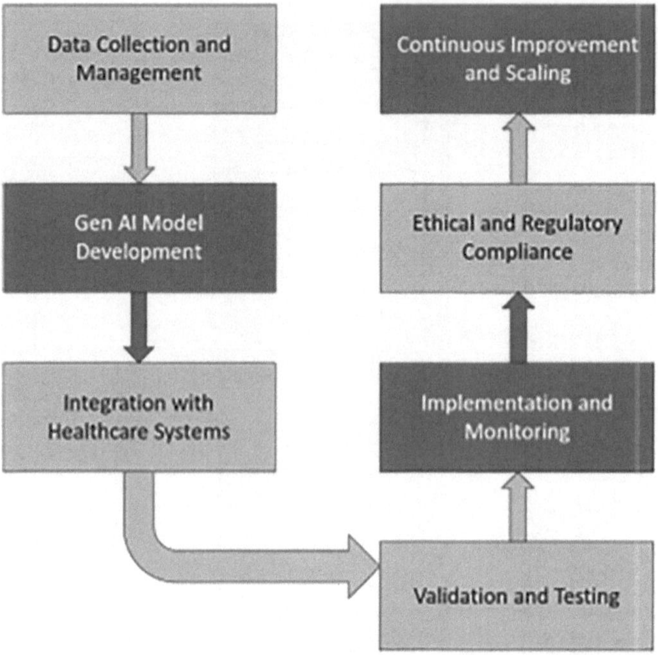

FIGURE 9.7 Strategic framework for integrating generative AI into healthcare systems.

Implementation and Monitoring:

Purpose: Implementation of AI solutions in healthcare settings and observing their impact.
Activities: Carry out the implementation of health artificial intelligence tools and technologies into clinical settings, follow up on their performance, and get feedback from health workers and patients.
Results: Continuous improvements in patient care and healthcare operations

Ethical and Regulatory Compliance:

Objective: AI implementations will be ethical and regulatory-compliant.
Activities: Provide for regular checking of AI's impact, update privacy safeguards, maintain data security, and make AI decisions transparent.
Results: When artificial intelligence is used ethically, it will sustain public trust while adhering to the rule of law. Figure 9.7 shows the framework of merging GenAI with healthcare system.

Continuous Improvement and Scaling:

Aim: Advance and expand health AI capabilities.
Activities: Use insights learned from the implementation to improve models of AI, reproduce applications across other parts of health care, and scale solutions to benefit all constituent parts of the population.

Results: Advanced, scalable AI solutions that never stop learning from the advances in healthcare.

9.4 CHALLENGES AND FUTURE DIRECTIONS

9.4.1 Challenges Encountered in Deep Learning-Based Alzheimer's Detection: Data

Quantity and Quality: There isn't enough high-quality labeled medical image data to teach deep learning models correctly.

Interpretability and Explainability: You can't easily use complicated deep learning models in clinical situations where being open is important.

Robustness and Generalization: We can see that deep learning models might not work as well in real life when we use them with different kinds of patients and imaging tools.

Regulatory and Ethical Considerations: People worry about privacy, morals, and following the rules, which makes it hard to gather, share, and use private patient information.

9.4.2 Potential Solutions and Areas for Improvement

Data Augmentation and Synthesis: There are ways to fix problems with not having enough data and make models more useful in the real world. These include adding to existing data and making new data.

Model Interpretability: Making it easier to understand and trust the clinical choices made by deep learning models is one way to make things more open and certain.

Transfer Learning and Domain Adaptation: You can make this better by using models that have already been trained and domain adaptation methods on a lot of different datasets and communities. It's called area adaptation and transfer learning.

Techniques for Preserving Privacy: You can make this better by using models that have already been trained and domain adaptation methods on a lot of different datasets and communities. It's called area adaptation and transfer learning.

9.4.3 Future Research Directions in Deep Learning for Alzheimer's Detection

Multimodal Fusion and Integration: It would be better and faster to identify people if biomarkers, clinical data, and different types of images could all be used together.

Advanced Architectures and Model Optimization: Looking at cutting-edge regularization strategies, optimization algorithms, and deep learning structures that are made to handle the problems that come with being diagnosed with Alzheimer's.

Therapeutic Translation and Validation: Evaluating the diagnostic and treatment usefulness of deep learning-based tools in the real world by conducting large-scale clinical studies and validation trials.

9.4.4 Integration with Other Diagnostic Modalities and Clinical Applications

Collaborative Research and Data Sharing: Collaborative study and data sharing means getting researchers, doctors, and healthcare organizations to work together to share resources, talk about their findings, and test deep learning models in a range of settings and with different groups of people.

Clinical Decision Support Systems: Adding deep learning-based diagnosis tools to clinical decision support systems will help doctors figure out risks, find problems early, and plan personalized treatments.

Telemedicine and Remote Monitoring: People who live in poor or rural places may find it easier to get checked for and diagnosed with Alzheimer's if they use telemedicine, mobile health apps, and online tracking that use deep learning.

Multidisciplinary Approaches: Brain scientists, computer scientists, doctors, and ethicists need to work together to figure out how to use deep learning to find Alzheimer's. This is because using deep learning to find Alzheimer's comes with a lot of hard problems and moral questions.

9.5 CONCLUSION

The primary objective of this chapter and comparison is to demonstrate the significance of early detection of Alzheimer's disease and the potential benefits of employing deep learning techniques in achieving this goal. Generative adversarial networks, recurrent neural networks, and convolutional neural networks are utilized to detect Alzheimer's disease. This chapter offers insightful information about the effectiveness of various techniques, such as the usage of generative AI in the medical field, for diagnosing Alzheimer's disease. The chapter also addresses the problems that require solutions and proposes potential areas for future study in this field. This chapter examines the present condition of using deep learning for diagnosing Alzheimer's disease and emphasizes the necessity for further research and enhancement in this crucial healthcare domain via the comparison and analysis of previous studies.

REFERENCES

1. A. A. Khan, O. Chaudhari, and R. Chandra, "A review of ensemble learning and data augmentation models for class imbalanced problems: Combination, implementation and evaluation," *Expert Systems with Applications*, vol. 244, p. 122778, (2024), https://doi.org/10.1016/j.eswa.2023.122778.
2. Q. Chen, and Y. Hong, "Longformer: Longitudinal transformer for Alzheimer's disease classification with structural MRIs," pp. 3575–3584, (2023), https://doi.org/10.48550/arXiv.2302.00901.

3. S. Sharma, K. Guleria, S. Tiwari, and S. Kumar, "A deep learning based convolutional neural network model with VGG16 feature extractor for the detection of Alzheimer disease using MRI scans," *MEAS Sensors*, vol. 24, no. October, p. 100506, (2022), https://doi.org/10.1016/j.measen.2022.100506.
4. H. M. Chong, X. Y. Yap, and K. S. Chia, "Effects of different pretrained deep learning algorithms as feature extractor in tomato plant health classification," *Pattern Recognition and Image Analysis*, vol. 33, pp. 39–46, (2023), https://doi.org/10.1134/S1054661823010017.
5. C. M. Chabib, L. J. Hadjileontiadis, and A. Al Shehhi, "DeepCurvMRI: Deep convolutional curvelet transform-based MRI approach for early detection of Alzheimer's disease," *IEEE Access*, vol. 11, no. April, pp. 44650–44659, (2023), https://doi.org/10.1109/ACCESS.2023.3272482.
6. A. Mishra, P. Arora, A. Jaiswal, and B. Mazumdar, "Deep learning and extreme learning machine for the diagnosis of Alzheimer's disease," (2024), https://doi.org/10.22541/au.170664821.18176002/v1.
7. N. Goenka *et al.*, "A regularized volumetric ConvNet based Alzheimer detection using T1-weighted MRI images," *Cogent Engineering*, vol. 11, no. 1, (2024), https://doi.org/10.1080/23311916.2024.2314872.
8. R. Shi *et al.*, "Generative adversarial network constrained multiple loss autoencoder: A deep learning-based individual atrophy detection for Alzheimer's disease and mild cognitive impairment," *Human Brain Mapping*, vol. 44, no. 3, pp. 1129–1146, (2023), https://doi.org/10.1002/hbm.26146.
9. M. Al Olaimat, J. Martinez, F. Saeed, and S. Bozdag, "PPAD: A deep learning architecture to predict progression of Alzheimer's disease," *Bioinformatics*, vol. 39, no. 1, pp. I149–I157, (2023), https://doi.org/10.1093/bioinformatics/btad249.
10. U. Gupta, A. Pranav, A. Kohli, S. Ghosh, and D. Singh, "The contribution of artificial intelligence to drug discovery: Current progress and prospects for the future," *Microbial Data Intelligence and Computational Techniques for Sustainable Computing*, pp. 1–23, (2024).
11. D. Gupta, U. Gupta, and H. J. Sarma, "Functional iterative approach for Universum-based primal twin bounded support vector machine to EEG classification (FUPTBSVM)," *Multimedia Tools and Applications*, vol. 83, no. 8, pp. 22119–22151, (2024).
12. U. Gupta, and V. Jain, "Social neuroscience: Inferring mental states in social media," *Emotional AI and Human-AI Interactions in Social Networking*, pp. 15–39 (2024).
13. M. Sharma, S. Deswal, U. Gupta, M. Tabassum, and I. Lawal eds., *Soft Computing Techniques in Connected Healthcare Systems*. CRC Press, (2023).
14. K. Malik, H. Sadawarti, M. Sharma, U. Gupta, and P. Tiwari eds., *Computational Techniques in Neuroscience*. CRC Press, (2023).
15. D. Singh, D. Singh, Manju, and U. Gupta, "Smart healthcare: A breakthrough in the growth of technologies," in *Artificial Intelligence-Based Healthcare Systems*. Cham, Switzerland: Springer Nature, pp. 73–85, (2023).
16. M. Gupta, D. Srivastava, D. Pantola, and U. Gupta, "Brain tumor detection using improved Otsu's thresholding method and supervised learning techniques at early stage," in *Proceedings of Emerging Trends and Technologies on Intelligent Systems: ETTIS 2022*. Singapore: Springer Nature, pp. 271–281, (2022).
17. U. Gupta, D. Gupta, and U. Agarwal, "Analysis of randomization-based approaches for autism spectrum disorder," in *Pattern Recognition and Data Analysis with Applications*. Singapore: Springer Nature Singapore, pp. 701–713, (2022).
18. D. Gupta, A. Choudhury, U. Gupta, P. Singh, and M. Prasad, "Computational approach to clinical diagnosis of diabetes disease: A comparative study," *Multimedia Tools and Applications*, pp. 1–26, (2021).

19. D. Gupta, and U. Gupta, "On robust asymmetric Lagrangian ν-twin support vector regression using pinball loss function," *Applied Soft Computing*, vol. 102, p. 107099, (2021).
20. B. A. Kobrinskii, "Artificial intelligence: Problems, solutions, and prospects," *Pattern Recognition and Image Analysis,* vol. 33, pp. 217–220, (2023), https://doi.org/10.1134/S1054661823030203.
21. N. A. Andriyanov, "Combining text and image analysis methods for solving multimodal classification problems," *Pattern Recognition and Image Analysis*, vol. 32, pp. 489–494, (2022), https://doi.org/10.1134/S1054661822030026.
22. S. Fathi, A. Ahmadi, A. Dehnad, M. Almasi-Dooghaee, and M. Sadegh, "A deep learning-based ensemble method for early diagnosis of Alzheimer's disease using MRI images," *Neuroinformatics*, pp. 1–18, (2023), https://doi.org/10.1007/s12021-023-09646-2.
23. L. Meng, and Q. Zhang, "Research on early diagnosis of Alzheimer's disease based on dual fusion cluster graph convolutional network," *Biomedical Signal Processing and Control*, vol. 86, no. PA, p. 105212, (2023), https://doi.org/10.1016/j.bspc.2023.105212.
24. V. Nagarajan, L. Venkataramana, V. Prasad, V. Narasimhan, and S. Santhanakrishnan, "Deployable and weighted ensemble-based deep learning model for Alzheimer's disease detection," pp. 1–21, (2023), https://doi.org/10.21203/rs.3.rs-2594226/v1.
25. S. Tripathi, A. Augustin, and E. Kim, "Longitudinal neuroimaging data classification for early detection of Alzheimer's disease using ensemble learning models," *Authorea Preprint*, (2023), https://doi.org/10.36227/techrxiv.19295120.
26. A. Shukla, R. Tiwari, and S. Tiwari, "Alzheimer's disease detection from fused PET and MRI modalities using an ensemble classifier," *Machine Learning and Knowledge Extraction*, vol. 5, no. 2, pp. 512–538, (2023), https://doi.org/10.3390/make5020031.
27. P. Zhang, and M. N. Kamel Boulos, "Generative AI in medicine and healthcare: Promises, opportunities and challenges," *Future Internet*, vol. 15, p. 286, (2023), https://doi.org/10.3390/fi15090286.
28. Y. Shokrollahi, S. Yarmohammadtoosky, M. M. Nikahd, P. Dong, X. Li, and L. Gu, "A comprehensive review of generative AI in healthcare," (2023), arXiv/abs/2310.00795(2023).
29. D. Yim, J. Khuntia, V. Parameswaran, and A. Meyers, "Preliminary evidence of the use of generative AI in health care clinical services: Systematic narrative review," *JMIR Medical Informatics*, vol. 12, no. March 20, p. e52073, (2024), https://doi.org/10.2196/52073.
30. T. K. K. Ho *et al.*, "Deep learning-based multilevel classification of Alzheimer's disease using non-invasive functional near-infrared spectroscopy," *Frontiers in Aging Neuroscience*, vol. 14, no. April, pp. 1–16, (2022), https://doi.org/10.3389/fnagi.2022.810125.
31. M. Raju, M. Thirupalani, S. Vidhyabharathi, and S. Thilagavathi, "Deep learning based multilevel classification of Alzheimer's disease using MRI scans," *IOP Conference Series: Materials Science and Engineering*, vol. 1084, no. 1, p. 012017, (2021), https://doi.org/10.1088/1757-899x/1084/1/012017.
32. U. Khatri, and G. Kwon, "RMTnet: Recurrence meet transformer for Alzheimer's disease diagnosis RMTnet: Recurrence meet Transformer for Alzheimer's disease diagnosis using FDG-PET," no. January, (2024), https://doi.org/10.36227/techrxiv.170594596.62106929/v1.
33. D. A. Arafa, H. E. D. Moustafa, H. A. Ali, A. M. T. Ali-Eldin, and S. F. Saraya, *A Deep Learning Framework for Early Diagnosis of Alzheimer's Disease on MRI Images*, vol. 83, no. 2. Springer US, pp. 3767–3799, (2024), https://doi.org/10.1007/s11042-023-15738-7.
34. C. Wang, H. Tachimori, H. Yamaguchi, A. Sekiguchi, Y. Li, and Y. Yamashita, "A multimodal deep learning approach for the prediction of cognitive decline and its effectiveness in clinical trials for Alzheimer's disease," *Translational Psychiatry*, vol. 14, no. 1, p. 105, (2024), https://doi.org/10.1038/s41398-024-02819-w.

35. M. EL-Geneedy, H. E. D. Moustafa, F. Khalifa, H. Khater, and E. AbdElhalim, "An MRI-based deep learning approach for accurate detection of Alzheimer's disease," *Alexandria Engineering Journal*, vol. 63, pp. 211–221, (2023), https://doi.org/10.1016/j.aej.2022.07.062.
36. S. E. Sorour, A. A. A. El-Mageed, K. M. Albarrak, A. K. Alnaim, A. A. Wafa, and E. El-Shafeiy, "Classification of Alzheimer's disease using MRI data based on deep learning techniques," *Journal of King Saud University—Computer and Information Science*, vol. 36, no. 2, p. 101940, (2024), https://doi.org/10.1016/j.jksuci.(2024).101940.
37. M. Nour, U. Senturk, and K. Polat, "A novel hybrid model in the diagnosis and classification of Alzheimer's disease using EEG signals: Deep ensemble learning (DEL) approach," *Biomedical Signal Processing and Control*, vol. 89, no. June 2023, p. 105751, (2024), https://doi.org/10.1016/j.bspc.(2023).105751.
38. B. TaghiBeyglou, and F. Rudzicz, "Context is not key: Detecting Alzheimer's disease with both classical and transformer-based neural language models," *Natural Language Processing Journal*, vol. 6, no. December 2023, p. 100046, (2024), https://doi.org/10.1016/j.nlp.(2023).100046.
39. P. Balaji, M. A. Chaurasia, S. M. Bilfaqih, A. Muniasamy, and L. E. G. Alsid, "Hybridized deep learning approach for detecting Alzheimer's disease," *Biomedicines*, vol. 11, no. 1, (2023), https://doi.org/10.3390/biomedicines11010149.
40. Z. Hu, Z. Wang, Y. Jin, and W. Hou, "VGG-TSwinformer: Transformer-based deep learning model for early Alzheimer's disease prediction," *Computer Methods and Programs in Biomedicine*, vol. 229, p. 107291, (2023), https://doi.org/10.1016/j.cmpb.(2022).107291.
41. W. N. Ismail, F. R. Fathimathul, and M. A. S. Ali, "A meta-heuristic multi-objective optimization method for Alzheimer's disease detection based on multi-modal data," *Mathematics*, vol. 11, no. 4, pp. 1–22, (2023), https://doi.org/10.3390/math11040957.
42. C. R. Nagarathna, M. Kusuma, and K. Seemanthini, "Classifying the stages of Alzheimer's disease by using multi layer feed forward neural network," *Procedia Computer Science*, vol. 218, pp. 1845–1856, (2022), https://doi.org/10.1016/j.procs.2023.01.162.
43. "Empowering the patient journey: The role of generative AI in healthcare," *IJSDAI*, vol. 2, no. 2, pp. 1–18, (July 2023), accessed: August 16 (2024), https://ijsdai.com/index.php/IJSDAI/article/view/43.
44. U. Hwang, S. W. Kim, D. Jung, S. Kim, H. Lee, S. W. Seo, J. K. Seong, S. Yoon, "Alzheimer's disease neuroimaging initiative. Real-world prediction of preclinical Alzheimer's disease with a deep generative model," *Artificial Intelligence in Medicine,* vol. 144, no. October, p. 102654, (2023), https://doi.org/10.1016/j.artmed.2023.102654.
45. C. Yan *et al.*, "Leveraging generative AI to prioritize drug repurposing candidates for Alzheimer's disease with real-world clinical validation," *NPJ Digital Medicine*, vol. 7, p. 46, (2024), https://doi.org/10.1038/s41746-024-01038-3.
46. G. P. Suja, and P. Raajan, "Early diagnosis of Alzheimer's disease with generative adversarial networks," *ICTACT Journal on Image and Video Processing*, vol. 14, no. 3, (February 2024), https://doi.org/10.21917/ijivp.2024.0454.
47. CE-GAN: Community Evolutionary Generative Adversarial Network for Alzheimer's Disease Risk Prediction Xia-An Bi, Member, IEEE, Zicheng Yang, Yangjun Huang, Ke Chen, Zhaoxu Xing, Luyun Xu, Zihao Wu, Zhengliang Liu, Xiang Li, and Tianming Liu, Senior Member, IEEE.
48. J. Jiang, R. Shi, J. Lu, M. Wang, Q. Zhang, S. Zhang, L. Wang, I. Alberts, A. Rominger, C. Zuo, and K. Shi, "Detection of individual brain tau deposition in Alzheimer's disease based on latent feature-enhanced generative adversarial network," *NeuroImage*, vol. 291, p. 120593, (2024), ISSN 1053-8119, https://doi.org/10.1016/j.neuroimage.2024.120593.

49. Q. Zuo, L. Chen, Y. Shen, M. K.-P. Ng, B. Lei, and S. Wang, "BDHT: Generative AI enables causality analysis for mild cognitive impairment," *IEEE Transactions on Automation Science and Engineering*, (2024), https://doi.org/10.1109/TASE.2024.3425949.
50. P. C. Wong, S. S. Abdullah, and M. I. Shapiai, "Exceptional performance with minimal data using a generative adversarial network for Alzheimer's disease classification," *Scientific Reports,* vol. 14, p. 17037, (2024), https://doi.org/10.1038/s41598-024-66874-5.
51. B. J. Shivaprasad, and M. Ravikumar, "Enhancement of brain magnetic resonance images using cascade of notch filter and linear transformation methods," *Pattern Recognition and Image Analysis*, vol. 33, pp. 66–79, (2023), https://doi.org/10.1134/S1054661822040137.

10 Generative AI in Personalized Medicine

Enhancing Data Privacy and Precision Treatment

Sreedeep Dey

10.1 INTRODUCTION

The field of personalized medicine has seen a breakthrough in healthcare sectors. As each and every individual has a unique genetic and molecular makeup, as well as a clinical profile, personalized medicine will be very useful to provide treatment to different people. Previously, one-size-fits-all treatment was well established in the market, which means that a product is suitable for everyone or every person. But now personalized medicine uses a large amount of data for tailoring treatment procedures, increasing drug efficacy, and improving overall patient outcomes. However, despite this possibility and opportunity, sometimes it poses some substantial difficulties. Unique technology, noteworthy resources, and, perhaps most importantly, careful consideration of data privacy issues are needed during the sensitive process of acquisition, analysis, and application of individualized data. We know personalized medicine as N-of-1 medicine. Interventions are identified using patients' own clinical data. This approach is different from traditional medicine. The basis of traditional medicine was population-derived guidelines. Genomic and phenotypic data derived from genomic profiling and phenotypic-driven approaches are the target of these recent personalized strategies (You et al. 2022). Patient-derived models can overcome some of the obstacles existing in traditional vitro/vivo practices. With the help of patient-derived xenografts (PDX) and patient-derived organoid (PDO) models, we can closely evaluate the disease condition of a patient. How much data we have to acquire depends upon the personalized strategy we are going to utilize. To build comprehensive databases we can use available clinical platforms. Molecular profiling can guide us in selecting the regimen. By predicting how a patient is responding against certain treatments molecular profiling provides personalized regimens. We can obtain PDX samples from tumors that have been removed surgically or via biopsies. Whereas, to obtain PDO samples we need adult stem cells. These stem cells can be obtained invasively. We can obtain them from blood circulation or bone marrow. These strategies are prevalent in clinically relevant settings. With those strategies, we can identify potential treatment strategies and target each patient (Liu et al. 2023). Further improvement of data about molecular alteration which drives drug selection

DOI: 10.1201/9781003539483-10

can be leveraged to personalize treatment by harnessing drug dosing which strongly correlates with the composition of drug regimens. More specifically, dose optimization can be acquired with additional data pertaining. This sustains the practice of N-of-1 medicine longitudinally. Utilizing their own clinical data CURATE.AI platform performed dynamical optimization of combination therapy in the context of multiple prospective clinical trials (Blasiak et al. 2020). The frequency and approach for data collection depend upon what type of personalized strategy is being utilized. The approach for accessing data should be carefully derived while considering a patient's quality of life. Moreover, if there is a possibility of using non-invasive or minimally-invasive approaches it should be utilized. Digital platforms are already employed for scaling the deployment of personalized medicine. To access personalized medicine in a better way we have to link personalized strategies with digital medicine. There are always some patients who don't respond to already standardized care. For them, we can apply QPOP, a digital platform (Toh et al. 2024). This platform can be useful for providing more tailored and personalized treatment strategies for them. AI has evaded the healthcare sector, particularly generative AI, which provides a viable solution to many of these challenges. Predictive analytics, data management, and decision-making become more handy with the use of AI, which in turn enables physicians to use enlightened models based on large datasets to make more precise diagnosis and treatment decisions. However, generative AI opens a new path by creating synthetic data, modeling medical outcomes, and producing precise insights that may be used without sacrificing the privacy of patients (Goetz and Schork 2018).

10.1.1 Challenges in Personalized Medicine

Data scarcity, particularly for rare diseases or ailments that are underrepresented in clinical trials, is one of the most significant difficulties in personalized medicine. Furthermore, sometimes it becomes very difficult to maintain data privacy while dealing with sensitive patient information. Infringement of data security could have negative consequences for patients, healthcare providers, and the medical research community as a whole.

The price of collecting, maintaining, and evaluating such large datasets can be restrictive. Given the difficulties of merging genomic, proteomic, transcriptomic, and clinical data, it is critical to build solutions that may give the necessary insights without incurring additional expenses or demanding vast resources (Green et al. 2023).

10.1.2 The Role of AI in Overcoming Challenges

Generative AI, particularly deep generative models (DGMs), offers the ability to address many of the most pressing issues in personalized medicine. These models generate synthetic data that closely resembles real patient data. It provides a mechanism to strengthen research, improve diagnostic tools, and further develop predictive modeling while reducing privacy problems. However, this ability to generate high-quality, realistic data has long-term consequences for tailored treatment planning and patient care. There are a variety of healthcare industries that use DGMs, such as generative adversarial networks (GANs) and variational autoencoders

(VAEs). These are used for many purposes and range from generating realistic medical images that are used for training diagnostic models to developing synthetic datasets mainly for rare diseases. This chapter deals with the various applications of DGMs in personalized medicine. It provides a perception of their role in overcoming some of the important existing obstacles. These obstacles include data privacy, scarcity, and the complexities of integrating multi-omic data (Templin et al. 2024).

10.1.3 Generative AI: Bridging the Gap between Data Privacy and Precision

Therapeutic precision is the foundation of personalized medicine. The combination of a variety of data sources, ranging from every individual's genetic profiles to lifestyle factors, is very important in the case of therapeutic precision. However, integrating these datasets has frequent challenges relating to patient privacy, particularly in terms of obedience to rules such as the General Data Protection Regulation (GDPR) and the Health Insurance Portability and Accountability Act (HIPAA). Generative AI can be a precise solution to these issues because it has the ability to generate privacy-preserving synthetic data. Healthcare practitioners can improve precision therapy by using synthetic data created by DGMs without exposing sensitive patient information (Johnson et al. 2021). Furthermore, researchers can use these models to estimate the effects of alternative treatment options without depending on potentially sensitive real-world data.

In one sentence, two of the most urgent issues of personalized medicine, the complexities of combining various datasets and data privacy, can be transformed by generative AI.

10.2 DEEP GENERATIVE MODELS IN HEALTHCARE

Nowadays, deep generative models are appearing as a very efficient tool used in healthcare. In numerous ways, they produce data for a variety of real-world applications. DGMs represent complex data distributions with the help of neural networks, and they are particularly crucial in healthcare for activities such as developing medical imaging, creating synthetic data, and clinical decision-making. New data instances can be created by learning the underlying structure of existing data and thus resolving crucial challenges (Ghebrehiwet et al. 2024). This section describes the numerous types of DGMs that are routinely used in healthcare, as well as their principles and applications in various medical areas.

10.2.1 Types of DGMs

There are two frequently used efficient DGMs in healthcare sectors. The first one is generative adversarial networks, and the other is variational autoencoders. These two models have emerged as the main characters that create synthetic data. They have medical applications because they show the capacity to learn complex data distributions and produce realistic, high-quality samples according to them.

10.2.1.1 Generative Adversarial Networks

A generator and a discriminator—these are the two neural networks that work together in GANs. The generator produces synthetic data. On the other hand, the discriminator determines the legality of the data. A feedback loop is formed by the two networks in which the generator speeds up its output, while the discriminator improves its detection abilities. This process is repeated again and again. As a result, we get synthetic data. It closely resembles real-life data. Therefore, GANs are considered ideal for producing patient datasets and protecting privacy.

10.2.1.2 Variational Autoencoders

At first, data is incorporated in VAEs. Then, it encodes input data into a latent and then decodes it back into the original space. New data samples can be generated by VAEs that are comparable to the original. Feature extraction and dimensionality reduction can be done using VAEs, but they are also useful to generate synthetic datasets and improve patient-specific models. Therefore, the most frequent concerns in healthcare systems, including medical imaging, development of drugs, and synthesis of clinical data, can be solved by using GANs as well as VAEs.

10.2.2 Applications of DGMs in Healthcare

10.2.2.1 Clinical Informatics and Bioinformatics

Clinical informatics and bioinformatics can be transformed using DGMs by generating synthetic data. This can be used to train machine learning models besides protecting the privacy of patients. Benefits of these models include providing realistic electronic health records (EHRs) that can be used to train prediction models, improve clinical decision-making, and replicate treatment outcomes. In bioinformatics, novel biological sequences such as proteins and DNA can be created by using DGMs in order to detect probable mutations or test new medicines (Chen et al. 2021). By augmenting limited datasets with synthetic data, it becomes easier for the researchers to investigate a greater variety of options, rushing the development of individualized treatments. A framework for USP7 putative inhibitors was developed by Pereira et al. (2022). More than 90% of compounds that have drug-like properties and are potentially active groups were generated by them. With the help of deep generative techniques, Hess et al. (2020) were able to extract patterns from omics data. To do that, they used log-linear models. RELATION is a 3D-based generative model proposed by Wang et al. (2022). BiTL algorithm is used by this model while extracting geometric features of large arrays of complexes of proteins and ligands. Inhibitor of AKT1 and CDK2 was designed with this progressive model. This experiment demonstrated how much efficiency generating novel molecules shows when they are equipped with favorable binding affinities and pharmacophore features.

10.2.2.2 Medical Imaging

Realistic synthetic images can be generated using DGMs, which are particularly effective for training diagnostic algorithms. For example, GANs can generate synthetic MRI or CT scan images that look like real-world patient scans, allowing radiologists and AI models to learn on a more diversified dataset. This is especially useful in disciplines like oncology, where early diagnosis of malignancies using imaging is important for better patient outcomes. Furthermore, DGMs can improve existing imaging datasets by creating variations of medical images, simulating different illness phases, or supplementing unusual examples. Thus, exposure of AI algorithms to a diverse set of imaging data significantly increases diagnosis accuracy and model validity (Kazuhiro et al. 2018). Bashyam et al. (2022) conducted a retrospective study on a deep learning-based image harmonization method. Cross-site generalizability of deep learning age prediction was improved by this method. In this study, 88,000 subjects from six sites, with age prediction models were involved by them. Ultimately the models were trained with the help of 2739 subjects from a single site and 6137 subjects from multiple. A substantial improvement was observed while predicting the age in out-of-sample data. An improvement in overall mean absolute error (MAE) from 15.81 to 11.86 years was also observed. Latent space projection and style mixing were the main focus of the study by Hong et al. (2021). For this purpose, they used the StyleGAN2 model that synthesized 3D image synthesis. The model was found applicable to any kind of 3D volumetric image. They showed excellent performance with approximately 12,000 full-brain MR T1 images.

10.2.2.3 Drug Discovery and Development

DGMs help to generate unique molecular structures, which speeds up the hunt for new therapeutic molecules and, in turn, accelerates the drug discovery process. GANs, for example, can be trained on existing chemical compounds to generate new molecules with the appropriate pharmacological characteristics. On the other hand, the latent space of molecular structures can be investigated by VAEs. It also helps to recognize innovative compounds that could treat specific diseases or conditions. DGMs enable pharmaceutical researchers to fasten the discovery process and lower the cost associated with the early-stage drug development (Blanchard et al. 2021). By imitating clinical trial scenarios with synthetic data, patient responses and potential side effects can be detected using DGMs. Zhavoronkov et al. (2019) used generative tensorial reinforcement learning (GENTRL) to design small molecules, identifying potent inhibitors of discoidin domain receptor 1 (DDR1) in 21 days. When biochemical assays were performed four compounds were found to be active. Whereas, when cell-based assays were performed two compounds were validated, and one showed favorable pharmacokinetics in mice.

10.2.2.4 Significance of DGMs in Precision Medicine

Synthetic patient data can be generated by DGMs that mimic actual data. It helps to train machine learning for individualized treatment. As a very small number of individuals are affected by uncommon diseases, datasets for training AI models are frequently stilted. DGMs are used to produce synthetic data. This synthetic data can also be used to model clinical trials, providing information on how different individuals react to specific treatments.

Patient-specific treatment plans can also be improved using DGMs (Ho et al. 2020). This allows for the creation of a more tailored, advanced, compact, and data-driven treatment protocol. This will improve patient outcomes while resolving the ethical and legal considerations associated with handling real patient data. Unsupervised Deep Fuzzy C-Means clustering Network (UDFCMN) is a new deep learning as well as clustering model called. This model was proposed by Zhao et al. (2020). Lung cancer patients were treated with clustered CT images. This model helped the clustering process. Winner-Take-All (WTA) idea helps this model to improve the traditional DBN structure. FCM produces initial cluster labels. They tested the algorithm on both public and private datasets. In each case, this showed superior performance in comparison to other already existing unsupervised classification methods. A whole new methodology and software implementation was created by Lenz et al. (2021) that could create artificial data. These software preserved complex patterns from the distribution of individual patient data. Aggregated data from participating sites was analyzed by DataSHIELD software. They used Deep Boltzmann machines (DBMs) as generative models. Testing of this approach was done on a synthetic data set that showcased genetic variant data. Several generative approaches like DBMs, VAEs, GANs, and multivariate imputation were compared in this study. An exploration of their utility and disclosure in distributed settings (with relatively smaller sample sizes) was revealed.

10.3 SYNTHETIC DATA GENERATION FOR PERSONALIZED MEDICINE

Day by day, healthcare sectors are becoming dependent on data-driven approaches. Personalized medicine faces many challenges in balancing data privacy and access to large databases. Synthetic data production, powered by deep generative models, produces synthetic data that closely resembles genuine patient information while preserving privacy and thus providing a solution to the problem.

10.3.1 How DGMs Generate Synthetic Data

Generative adversarial networks and variational autoencoders play a crucial role in generating synthetic data (Alsafadi and Wu 2023).

10.3.1.1 Generative Adversarial Networks

In the previous section, we saw that GANs basically consist of two networks: a generator and a discriminator. First, the generator generates synthetic data. Then the discriminator determines how authentic the synthetic data is. In this way, they gradually improve the quality of synthetic data. This type of data gathers genuine patient information. While training AI, they do not disclose actual information about the patient. Poudevigne-Durance et al. (2022) introduce MaWGAN, a novel generative adversarial network (GAN) that generates synthetic data from missing datasets. The method compares the generator output with the original data without discarding incomplete observations. Numerical experiments show that MaWGAN outperforms discarding incomplete observations and imputing missing values. Torfi & Fox (2020) propose CorGAN, a novel framework for generating synthetic healthcare records. It uses convolutional neural networks (CNNs) to capture medical features' correlations.

Similarly, real data in classification and prediction settings are performed by CorGAN. CorGAN is also helpful for assessing privacy and analyzing statistically.

10.3.1.2 Variational Autoencoders

The other type of DGM—VAEs—encodes patient data in a latent space. They do this by capturing key properties. They sample from this area, which helps them to generate fresh synthetic data. This fresh synthetic data is then used for continuous datasets that include physiological or genomic data. In this way, for personalized medicine models, improvement of dataset training occurs. Gootjes-Dreesbach et al. (2020) propose a new ML approach named Variational Autoencoder Modular Bayesian Network (VAMBN). VAMBN simulates realistic virtual patients in longitudinal clinical study data. VAMBN ensures data privacy, allows simulation of counterfactual scenarios, and facilitates data sharing and clinical trial design, addressing the gap in existing methods. Biswal et al. (2021) propose an EHR Variational Autoencoder (EVA) that synthesizes discrete EHR encounters and encounter features. EVA produces realistic EHR sequences, and accounts for individual differences. We can utilize them according to specific disease conditions. The method's utility is assessed on a large amount of real-world EHR repositories with more than 2.5 lakh patients. Augmenting real data with synthetic EHRs improves predictive performance.

10.3.2 Benefits of Synthetic Data in Personalized Medicine

10.3.2.1 Privacy-Preserving Solutions

One of the benefits of using synthetic data is that it protects patient privacy, as it simulates real data. This process allows healthcare organizations in several ways. Without disclosing any sensitive information, these organizations can exchange datasets with worldwide researchers and AI developers. As this process also complies with data protection rules made by GDPR and HIPAA, it becomes safer to test protocols of treatments that maintain a more controlled setting that protects privacy to a greater extent.

10.3.2.2 Addressing Data Scarcity

Data scarcity is a prevalent problem, especially with rare disorders. DGMs can produce synthetic data for underrepresented communities, thereby addressing gaps in real-world datasets. This ensures that AI models developed for personalized treatment are varied and unbiased, including ailments and demographics that are underrepresented in real data.

10.3.2.3 Cost-Effective Data Generation

The process of collecting patient data with higher accuracy is very costly, labor intensive, and time consuming. But with synthetic data, researchers can readily obtain large amounts of data without worrying about expenses related to clinical studies. Synthetic data allows pharmaceutical companies, in a cost-effective way, to recreate these costly trials and drug efficacy assessment processes and fasten research and development.

10.3.2.4 Enhancing Model Performance

With the help of these synthetic data AI models, they get enhancements in their performance. These synthetic datasets supplement the models real-world datasets. They also expose the algorithms in front of a relatively big set of data points. This process helps AI systems in two ways. First, they can generalize, and second, they can forecast with more accuracy than before across a larger, more varied population (Pezoulas et al. 2024). Not only that, synthetic data can imitate occurrences that are generally rare or severe. It improves the capacity of the model so that they can manage outliers proceeding with unusual circumstances.

10.3.3 Challenges of Synthetic Data Generation

Now let's see what the challenges are in synthetic data generation when we go for personalized medicine.

10.3.3.1 Data Bias

Synthetic data can include the biases from real-world datasets. This occasionally occurs when the training data is overrepresented due to certain types of demographics. These consequences cause AI models to be less effective for certain underrepresented populations. In an attempt to limit this risk, we have to focus on collecting training data that is diverse and representative in nature. Additionally, we must conduct continuous review processes.

10.3.3.2 Ensuring Accuracy and Realism

DGMs generate data that closely resembles real data. However, they may overlook nuances of patient information. In cases of clinical forecasts or treatment recommendations, it decreases the effectiveness of AI models. To ensure that synthetic data is of high quality for clinical use, we have to follow rigorous validation approaches per the need.

10.3.3.3 Ethical and Legal Considerations

Synthetic data improves privacy. But unfortunately, some ethical and legal concerns still exist, particularly when we apply them in therapeutic judgments. For addressing these challenges, transparency and accountability in the creation and use of synthetic data might be studied as two critical parameters (Miletic and Sariyar 2024).

10.4 GENERATIVE AI IN MEDICAL IMAGING AND DIAGNOSTICS

We can get crucial health profiles and insights from medical imaging. But these traditional analysis methods sometimes fail to manage MRIs, CT scans, and X-ray data. The data is generally massive in amount. Traditional techniques seem inefficient to handle it and lead to missed diagnoses. For this, there are generative AI models, particularly deep generative models, such as generative adversarial networks. These networks are able to diagnose accurately. They increase streamlining workflows. In this way, they become superior, providing dramatic benefits in medical imaging (Pinto-Coelho 2023).

10.4.1 Role of Generative AI in Medical Imaging

In the area of medical imaging, generative AI enhances data quality, provides information that has been missed, and detects underlying anomalies (Khalifa and Albadawy 2024).

10.4.1.1 Image Augmentation and Enhancement

GANs generate synthetic medical pictures. After that, they supplement these pictures with datasets. This eliminates further patient scans. We know that in the case of cancer, to increase early-stage tumor diagnosis, we need datasets in large numbers. In that view, GANs are crucial in these cases. Sometimes, just because of lower image quality, restrictions occur in imaging technology. GANs can increase resolution, contrast, and diagnostic value. This improves low-quality photos. In image segmentation, the Segment Anything Model (SAM) is becoming popular but has underperformed in medical image segmentation due to a lack of medical-specific knowledge. Domain-specific medical knowledge gets incorporated into the Medical SAM Adapter (Med-SA). This includes a light adaptation technique. Wu et al. (2023) evaluated 17 medical image segmentation tasks using this model. Med-SA outperformed several renowned state-of-the-art methods. They were able to update only 2% of the parameters.

10.4.1.2 Data Imputation and Missing Information Recovery

Sometimes some variables are unavoidable. For example, because of patient movement or device restrictions, medical imaging may be affected and result in insufficient data. Especially in the case of volumetric imaging, missing elements of medical images can be credited by generative AI. Hence, doctors get a complete dataset to diagnose correctly. On the other hand, DGMs can lower expenses. They reduce or eliminate our need for repetitive scans. Between two neighboring slices, they fill the gaps by incorporating missing information. These processes increase overall patient comfort. Liu et al. (2023) used deep learning (DL)-based imputation techniques that handled missing values in high-stakes fields of clinical trials. They searched five databases and examined articles. The articles were from four perspectives including types of data, imputation strategies, backbones of the respective model, and comparisons with other methods that are not based on DL. The study found a pattern in model backbones and data types. Autoencoder and recurrent neural networks dominated tabular temporal data. For tabular temporal and multi-modal data, the "integrated" imputation strategy is more popular than other methods.

10.4.1.3 Image Segmentation and Anomaly Detection

Types of tissues, organs, and anomalies are identified automatically by generative AI models. In this way, they segment medical images. With an example, we can understand it better. Regions of a tumor in CT or MRI scans can be segmented by these AI models. These models measure the size of the tumor more precisely. They also tell us where the tumor is located. And how do they detect the anomalies? GANs and VAEs generally compare fresh data with patterns that have already been learned. This helps them to be aware of normal anatomy. Afterwards, they detect anomalies. This whole sequential process results in early diagnosis of cancer and many other fatal diseases. With the help of deep spatial autoencoding models normal anatomical variability of entire 2D brain MR slices was captured by Baur et al. (2019). Experiments on real MR data with MS lesions confirmed this, with constraints on latent space and adversarial training improving segmentation performance. Outlier detection is a growing field in ML, with deep learning-based methods outperforming handcrafted techniques. VAE is used by this method which uniformly distributes while separating inliers from outliers. The model's generative and adversarial parts generate three main losses, wrapped with a one-class SVM for predictions. The method outperforms common outlier detection techniques like DBSCAN, GMM, K-means, and one-class SVM on all datasets, demonstrating its effectiveness (Ibrahim et al. 2021).

10.4.1.4 Cross-Modality Image Synthesis

Completing all scans becomes drastic and labor intensive when it comes to performing too many imaging modalities with CT, MRI, or PET. AI models equipped with cross-modality synthesis functions can synthesize one sort of medical image from another one. Without going for additional procedures, clinicians can get comprehensive insights with them. Relatively complicated diseases like brain abnormalities and cardiovascular problems can be diagnosed by combining anatomical as well as functional data. A computational image translation technique was proposed by Wei et al. (2023). This technique used deep learning which enabled bright-field microscopy contrast. For this purpose snapshots of Stokes images of stained slides of pathological tissue were taken. Co-registered image pairs in training were possible to be avoided as they adopted a translation model named CycleGAN. They tested the method on pathological slices of liver, breast, and lung tissues. Different staining protocols were used in each case. Evaluation of the output results was done through four image quality assessment methods.

10.4.2 Early Diagnosis and Treatment Planning

With generative AI, now we can identify diseases at their early stage and customize therapy accordingly (Hunter et al. 2022).

10.4.2.1 Detecting Diseases in Early Stages

To apply effective therapy, particularly in cases of cancer and neurological diseases, detecting the disease at an early stage is critical. Unfortunately, if the symptoms are mild or modest, it becomes difficult to diagnose it in an early stage. Generative AI enhances diagnostic accuracy as it is able to detect some of the patterns that are generally unseen to the human eye. DGMs have been proven to detect early-stage cancers in breast cancer screenings. In MRI scans, they have also identified structural changes occurring in the brain before the appearance of symptoms. This helps them to forecast Alzheimer's disease. Hwang et al. (2023) used a deep generative model in their study. Amyloid positivity in cognitively normal individuals was predicted by this study. Proxy measures like MRI scans and cognitive scores were used in their study procedure. The model surprisingly eliminated the previously equipped methods and was proven to be adaptable even in a diverse range of clinical scenarios. Regions and variables of the brain were identified by this model. This identification helped the researcher to classify the disease and provide more accurate and non-invasive diagnostics for preclinical Alzheimer's disease. With this study, they meet the requirements for real-world clinical translation.

10.4.2.2 Personalized Treatment Strategies

Generative AI studies patient data and forecasts the outcomes so that they can create specialized, individualized treatment strategies. During cancer therapy, physicians can apply GANs to personalize medicines, as it can help to predict the phases when the growth of a tumor occurs. Similarly, in cardiology, AI can generate a 3D replica model of a patient's heart. Surgical procedures can be stimulated, or stents can be placed with these models. We can predict how the heart of a patient will react, improve precision in therapy, and make the right decision.

10.4.3 Challenges and Future Directions in Medical Imaging with Generative AI

We have discussed the promising advances generative AI contributes to clinical practice. Now let us explore what the major barriers are (Koohi-Moghadam and Bae 2023).

10.4.3.1 Model Interpretability and Trust

DGM deep learning models sometimes appear to be "black boxes." Physicians get confused when they try to analyze how the results have been achieved. Radiologists encode intrinsic representations of fat and fluid in their brains, storing them as bright on T1 and dark on T2, raising questions about deep neural networks. Therefore, it is necessary to develop confidence in healthcare workers for using them. As a solution model, interpretability could be improved. Further continuation of research is needed that will allow clinicians to comprehend better and create trust in AI-driven diagnostics with proper explanation and visualization of AI insights.

10.4.3.2 Regulatory and Ethical Concerns

Ethical and regulatory concerns are the most prominent concerns that arise when we try to apply generative AI for medical imaging purposes. Medical images can be misused in many ways. They can give rise to fake data that ultimately changes the whole diagnostic results. Especially when we are using AI for critical diagnosis purposes, we have to be careful about the fact that AI-generated images should be of higher resolution and are maintaining their accuracy. Regulatory authorities like the FDA and EMA are already working on bringing recommendations for AI models to be used in medical imaging. We can hope that this will ensure the safety and efficacy of treatment procedures.

10.5 GENERATIVE AI FOR DRUG DISCOVERY AND DEVELOPMENT

From discovery to commercialization, the process of drug discovery is typically a lengthy and costly process, and it takes 12–15 years on average (Hughes et al. 2011). Generative AI technology, particularly deep generative models, is able to synthesize novel drug compounds rapidly, predict interactions between a drug and its target, and improve chemical structures. Therefore, it is able to accelerate drug development. In this section, we describe how generative AI is transforming drug discoveries in every area, starting from the generation of drug molecules and ending with preclinical testing (Gangwal et al. 2024).

10.5.1 Applications of Generative AI in Drug Discovery

As we mentioned, drug discovery is being transformed by generative AI at all phases of the drug discovery, starting from finding new compounds and ending with predicting their interaction with biological targets. Now we shall explore the process in detail.

10.5.1.1 De-Novo Molecular Design

Two of the most promising generative AI models, variational autoencoders and generative adversarial networks, are useful to create novel chemical structures from scratch. De-Novo molecular design uses these models. Traditional approaches required an enormous number of databases of chemicals, whereas nowadays it is possible to develop drug-like molecules with the desired qualities, like higher efficacy and lower toxicity, with the use of AI models that usually learn the underlying chemical patterns while building. With an example, we can clearly understand that. In contrast to recurrent neural networks (RNNs), which generally design molecules as forms of atomic sequences, GANs try to construct molecular architectures in three dimensions while considering chemical composition as well as their spatial arrangements (Meyers et al. 2021). Wang et al. (2022) developed a deep molecular generative framework that could be able to generate novel drug-likeness molecules from seed compounds. The framework uses key features of PPI inhibitors as input and demonstrates comparable performance to other models. The generated molecules share chemical space with iPPI-DB inhibitors and can be used for peptide characterization-oriented and ligand-based design of PPI inhibitors. Merk et al. (2018) trained a recurrent neural network to recognize bioactive compounds as SMILES strings. They synthesized five top-ranking compounds, four of which showed receptor-modulatory activity in cell-based assays. The study suggests generative AI for molecular design and medicinal chemistry. The study by Grisoni et al. (2021) demonstrates the potential of a design-make-test-analyze framework for automated drug design using AI and miniaturized bench-top synthesis. The framework was used to generate liver X receptor (LXR) agonists from scratch. The computational pipeline explored the chemical space of known LXRα agonists and novel molecular candidates were generated.

10.5.1.2 Predicting Drug Target Interactions

Needless to say, prior to drug development, we need to predict how a potent medicine interacts with its target. By anticipating binding affinities, possible interactions, and probable side effects, generative AI models deal with pharmacological compounds and their biological targets that are likely proteins or enzymes in nature. We can train AI models on interactions of drug targets that are already known to us. The positive interactions can be helpful to identify new drugs. Some precision medicine efforts, along with targeted cancer therapy, can be supported with these initiatives (Paul et al. 2021). A comprehensive network was constructed using curated drug-protein/protein-protein interaction data and SARS-CoV-2 protein interaction data. The network was used to predict missing links. To do that it used variational graph autoencoders (VGAEs). Any existence of unknown links between drugs and human proteins was the main focus. This led to novel host-directed therapy options (Ray et al. 2022). A graph convolutional autoencoder and Gaussian ANN were used to learn drug-target node networks. A LightGBM classifier was developed to estimate drug-target interaction propensities, outperforming existing methods. The classifier also demonstrated the ability to discover potential drug targets, outperforming several state-of-the-art methods (Sun et al. 2022).

10.5.1.3 Molecular Optimization

When ultimately we are able to discover a potential medication candidate, we need to optimize that candidate in an attempt to improve its efficacy and reduce its toxicity. In this area, generative AI models seem to be helpful. They suggest changes that can improve the chemical structure of the candidates per our desirable qualities. For example, besides maintaining therapeutic potential, GANs make minor modifications and ultimately optimize medicinal compounds. In this way, prior to clinical trials, refining drug molecules helps us to obtain a more safe and effective type of therapeutic approach. For molecular optimization, Chen et al. (2021) developed Modof, a deep generative model. Modof predicts disconnection sites and removes or adds fragments. Modof-pipe, a pipeline of identical Modof models, can modify input molecules at multiple disconnection sites. It outperforms state-of-the-art methods on benchmark datasets, achieving an 81.2% improvement in the octanol-water partition coefficient. Mol-CycleGAN is a CycleGAN-based model that optimizes compounds that show a higher extent of structural similarity with the original ones. It outperforms previous results in optimizing penalized logP of drug-like molecules, demonstrating its effectiveness in compound design (Maziarka et al. 2020).

10.5.2 Generative AI in Preclinical Testing and Toxicology

The need for animal models for testing is minimized, as generative AI already predicts the safety and toxicity profile of drug candidates in the development stage prior to preclinical testing.

10.5.2.1 Predicting Toxicity and Side Effects

In both preclinical and clinical trials, a drug fails because of its toxic effects. Researchers can eliminate potentially hazardous drug candidates with the use of VAEs, a generational AI model. These generative AI models examine synthetic molecular structures with the help of already-known toxicological data. These examinations reveal the toxicity profile to them. Not only that, with the use of these models, we can also get insights about drug metabolism in the human body. On the basis of interactions with drug-metabolizing enzymes, probable side effects can also be determined simultaneously (Kapustina et al. 2024). From over 1,000 unique chemicals in the ToxCast library, a study used embryonic zebrafish and examined the morphological and mortality endpoints. For effective prediction of toxic outcomes of untested chemicals, conditional generative adversarial networks (cGAN) or deep neural networks (DNN) were aimed to be used in this study. The study found that Go-ZT outperformed other models in cross-validation and external test datasets. SP, SE, PPV, and Kappa were improved when GAN-ZT and Go-ZT were combined. The consensus model resulted in an AUROC of 0.837. These models could provide in vivo toxicity predictions and prioritize compounds for HT testing (Green et al. 2021). A deep generative adversarial network (GAN)-based framework was proposed by Chen et al. (2022) that generated new animal results from previous existing studies. Pre-existing rat liver TGx data derived from the Open Toxicogenomics Project-Genomics-Assisted Toxicity Evaluation System (Open TG-GATES) was used by them to generate transcriptomic profiles with high similarity to actual gene expression profiles. The Tox-GAN model showed outstanding performance in two critical TGx applications, gaining molecular understanding of toxicological mechanisms and gene expression-based biomarker development. It also demonstrated potential utility in chemical-based read-across.

10.5.2.2 Generating Synthetic Data for Preclinical Models

The unavailability of high-quality data, especially for cases of rare diseases or relatively new or novel therapeutic targets, is a major problem of preclinical trials in drug discovery processes. Much synthetic biological data, including profiles of gene expression and/or networks of protein interactions, is used by generative AI to supplement real-world data. As this improves model performance in terms of prediction, researchers can readily find promising drug candidates (Pezoulas et al. 2024). Synthetic patient profiles generated by AI replicate genuine patient data and assist us in discovering drugs for rare diseases. Studying animal models is essential for chemical and drug safety evaluation. GANs can be utilized to generate animal data synthetically from legacy studies, potentially assessing chemicals that are not still tested. AnimalGAN, a GAN method, simulates clinical pathology measures of 38 rats and outperforms conventional quantitative structure-activity relationship approaches. It represents a significant step toward the global effort in replacing, reducing, and refining animal use (Chen et al. 2023).

10.5.2.3 Improving Animal Testing Models

Besides reducing the need for animal testing, generative AI models mimic the behavior of drugs in specific populations, thus helping in the improvement of animal model design. Researchers can choose the best animal model for testing, as AI helps them predict how a drug would react on diverse types of animals. We discussed that generative AI provides synthetic data. This synthetic data represents the behavior of a drug in animal populations. These insights lower the number of animals required for testing. Not only that, the ethical considerations of preclinical research are simultaneously considered (Vora et al. 2023). The study by Cao et al. (2024) investigates the potential of generative AI to produce high-fidelity human embryo images. These images were utilized for improving embryo selection models that were based on AI. The researchers used time-lapse microscopy (TLM) videos to train generative models. They fine-tuned a style-based GAN (generative model) and a residual network (morphokinetic classification model). The models were tested for synthetic image quality using Fréchet Inception Distance (FID) and Kernel Inception Distance (KID) metrics. Among the three groups, the AUG+Pretrained-R model ensured the highest performance. They showed significant differences in accuracy and sensitivity. Using real data solely, the embryonic stage classification model was integrated with generated data. This integration outperformed the model. Validation accuracy was increased by 18% from 72.6% to 90.6%. The study suggests that generative AI is a potent candidate for generating high-fidelity human embryo images. They address class imbalances for robust AI-based methods. Ultimately, embryo selection and IVF outcomes get transformed. A set of 5,000 generated images at each embryonic developmental stage was deposited in open-source that can help future AI studies.

10.5.3 Challenges and Future Directions in Drug Discovery with Generative AI

No doubt, generative AI has immense promise in the drug discovery process. However, before implementing it completely in the drug discovery process, we have to overcome several obstacles related to it.

10.5.3.1 Data Quality and Availability

Generative AI models are basically dependent upon high-quality data. But sometimes insufficient, skewed, or noisy data gives rise to errors and ultimately promotes faulty drug candidates. To explore AI's full promise in drug development, we have to be careful in collecting data and annotation.

10.5.3.2 Model Validation and Regulatory Approval

While working with AI-driven drug development, another challenge arises when regulatory bodies try to approve AI models, as they are confused by the fact that they cannot test these models before giving approval based on universal parameters. AI models develop novel compounds and forecast drug interactions. That's why they demand reliable validation processes so that their safety profiles and effectiveness can be verified. Reputed regulatory organizations worldwide, including the FDA, are still creating standards so that AI can be integrated into drug research and development. Therefore, it is high time researchers, pharmaceutical businesses, and regulators collaborate to take us to the future of AI adoption.

10.5.3.3 Ethical and Safety Concerns

Regarding privacy in data, intellectual property, and overall safety, generative AI models bring some serious ethical concerns. Synthetic data that is generated by artificial intelligence, in the wrong hands, could be used to create fake or inappropriate drug candidates and novel compounds. These compounds could pose unknown hazards. In an attempt to mitigate these hazards, we have to be aware of transparency, accountability, and ethical norms.

Until now, we have understood that generative AI has clear potential in drug discovery and development. It has the ability to generate novel compounds, anticipate interactions, optimize structures, and streamline preclinical testing

(Blanco-González et al. 2023). However, to enable safe and effective incorporation of AI into the pharmaceutical and clinical sectors, we have to manage the hurdles of data quality, regulatory validation, and ethical issues.

10.6 ETHICAL, LEGAL, AND REGULATORY CONSIDERATIONS IN GENERATIVE AI FOR PERSONALIZED MEDICINE

As generative AI is integrated into customized medicine, it presents substantial ethical, legal, and regulatory difficulties. While AI has made advances in diagnosis, treatment, and drug discovery, its use with sensitive medical data and life-changing decisions necessitates careful consideration of privacy, fairness, safety, and governance. This section looks at the main problems around responsible AI use in healthcare (Naik et al. 2022).

10.6.1 Ethical Considerations in AI-Driven Personalized Medicine

10.6.1.1 Data Privacy and Patient Consent

Generative AI models require larger types of datasets. We have to keep in mind that patient health data is extremely sensitive. Privacy is maintained through differential privacy and federated learning techniques. Yet some issues appear while ensuring data protection when we rely on AI. First of all, we have to make patients understand how AI models will use their data to synthesize drug molecules. Therefore, we have to get informed consent from them.

10.6.1.2 Algorithmic Bias and Fairness

If biases are found in training data, AI algorithms will result in inequality in healthcare systems. When we are dealing with customized medicine for an underrepresented group, these kinds of biases ultimately cause ineffective therapies. Addressing this requires us to ensure that, regardless of demographics, each and every citizen gets the benefit of AI, and we can focus more on diversified datasets and validating models. Besides that, we have to be careful to affirm equal performance across all of the populations.

10.6.1.3 Ethical Use of Synthetic Data

In the previous section, we saw that generative AI can generate synthetic data to protect patient privacy. But when it comes to the extent of accurately representing real populations, we have to test it thoroughly. For commercial goals, misusing synthetic data raises ethical considerations (Farhud and Zokaei 2021). Therefore, transparency is essential. There should be clear criteria on which synthetic data is generated and consequently is going to be used in decision-making in clinical approaches.

10.6.2 Legal Challenges in AI-Driven Personalized Medicine

10.6.2.1 Data Protection Laws

There are data protection rules, such as GDPR and HIPAA. Generative AI must adhere to these rules. It is clear that synthetic data provides privacy protection.

However, it can still be reverse-engineered. Fatal hazards may be posed from this. These difficulties would be handled through legal frameworks. While maintaining data protection rules, these frameworks have to be sufficient for providing direction to use synthetic data.

10.6.2.2 Liability in AI-Driven Medical Decisions

If an injury is caused while continuing AI-generated treatment, it is unclear who bears responsibility: the AI developer, the healthcare provider, or the institution. When we are taking benefits of AI decisions that are ultimately influencing patient outcomes, to safeguard patients and clarify accountability, clear legal criteria must be established.

10.6.2.3 Intellectual Property in AI-Generated Solutions

Researchers face problems about intellectual property (IP) when, in drug discovery and other medical applications, they use generative AI. In some circumstances, when AI is employed to develop novel pharmaceuticals or implemented in medical insights, the ownership of these breakthroughs becomes ambiguous. Thereafter, it is necessary to focus on ongoing disputes about AI-generated IP. Not only that, these protocols would have to be able to define how rights are being awarded to developers, researchers, and the AI model itself (Gerke et al. 2020).

10.6.3 Regulatory Considerations for Generative AI in Healthcare

10.6.3.1 AI Model Validation and Approval

AI models are basically dynamic in nature, which means they constantly learn from fresh data. This dynamic nature raises some concerning issues when regulating AI in healthcare. Relevant validation frameworks should be established by the FDA and EMA. These frameworks should be used to examine the safety and efficacy of AI models. Transparency, interpretability, and continuous monitoring of AI models in therapeutic settings should be a matter of priority for these frameworks.

10.6.3.2 Addressing Bias and Disparities

To avoid incidents like inequities in matters of health, AI models have to be evaluated on a diverse population. Data accumulation and validation should be based on universal guidelines. These guidelines will make sure that AI models are able to show good performance regardless of demographics. While using synthetic data in clinical studies and processes of decision-making, it should be done ethically and should be scrutinized closely.

10.6.3.3 Regulatory Framework for AI-Generated Therapies

It is being observed that AI is continuously developing breakthrough therapeutics. Therefore, it is the responsibility of the authorities to provide frameworks that will evaluate and approve pharmaceutical products generated by AI and treatment programs and protocols. Here again comes an occasion where AI developers, healthcare providers, and regulatory bodies must emerge and work together to guarantee that new therapies will satisfy the same safety and efficacy standards as traditional treatments were delivering previously (Palaniappan et al. 2024).

10.7 FUTURE DIRECTIONS AND CHALLENGES IN GENERATIVE AI FOR PERSONALIZED MEDICINE

Generative AI is all set to transform the field of personalized medicine. But we know that with advancement come hurdles. This also applies to generative AI. Before we can achieve its full potential, we must overcome these hurdles. In this section, we discuss the future directions of AI-powered healthcare, popular technological trends, and challenges associated with them.

10.7.1 Emerging Trends and Technological Advancements

10.7.1.1 Foundation Models in Healthcare

Trained on large medical datasets, GPT and BERT are two widely used foundation models in customized medicine. With them, we can go for process medical languages, improve accuracy of diagnosis, and get assistance in clinical decision-making. These models are called models of the future, as they are meant to predict diseases, identify biomarkers, and model overall patient outcomes in cases of individualized treatments.

10.7.1.2 Federated Learning for Decentralized Data Sharing

We have come to know about federated learning. These models are valuable, as they offer a privacy-preserving alternative for training AI models and do not rely on sharing sensitive patient information. Besides following GDPR and HIPAA rules, this decentralized model allows healthcare sectors to collaborate with one another. On the other hand, federated learning enables worldwide AI models to incorporate data from multiple healthcare providers. The accuracy of individualized therapies increases this way.

10.7.1.3 Reinforcement Learning for Personalized Treatment Plans

For managing chronic diseases like diabetes or cancer, reinforcement learning (RL) models rely on continuous improvement strategies. They leverage real-time data from devices or electronic health records. Patient outcomes and treatment adherence are enhanced by this strategy.

10.7.1.4 AI-Driven Drug Discovery and Repurposing

By creating new molecules and/or repurposing current ones based on specific biological objectives, generative AI speeds up the process of drug development. In the case of rare or complex diseases, AI-driven therapeutic plans tailor to a molecular profile of the particular patient and design personalized medicine based on that (Moor et al. 2023).

10.7.2 Challenges for Widespread Adoption

10.7.2.1 Model Interpretability and Trust

As AI models such as generative adversarial networks sometimes create trust concerns among healthcare providers, they are frequently perceived as "black boxes." To make clinicians understand and to build their trust on AI-powered advice, explainable AI (XAI) tools would be developed.

10.7.2.2 Data Scarcity and Quality

The scarcity of diversified, high-quality medical data restricts practitioners from using generative AI in personalized medicine. Moreover, privacy concerns and scattered healthcare systems complicate these problems. Federated learning and synthetic data production may be found reliable to close these gaps to some extents. However, there will remain significant difficulty while it comes to the matter of providing representative training datasets.

10.7.2.3 Ethical Concerns and Bias Mitigation

If biases are not addressed appropriately in AI models, they can create health disparities. Being trained on homogeneous datasets, generative AI models may appear to underperform ones in underrepresented groups. As already discussed, to bring fairness to the creation of AI models, researchers must validate those models across diverse demographic groups. Moreover, to ensure fairness norms, universal regulatory guidelines have to be applied.

10.7.2.4 Integration with Existing Healthcare Systems

While integrating AI models into healthcare systems, we face obstacles not only technologically but also operationally. To perform a seamless work through with EHRs and clinical workflows, we need significant investment and cooperative help. To develop confidence in patients and to ensure safety, we need to employ humans to oversee the overall AI decision-making process (Yadav et al. 2024).

10.7.3 Promising Areas for Future Research

The most prominent research areas for generative AI in personalized medicine are:

- **Model Generalization:** Improving model performance across multiple populations of patients.
- **Data Privacy:** Enabling large-scale data exchange and developing strategies like federated learning that preserve privacy.
- **Real-Time AI Integration:** Using data from wearable devices and EHRs and applying them in real time for modifying therapies and protocols.
- **AI-Driven Drug Discovery:** Expanding the emerging role of AI in the discovery of tailored medicines.
- **Hybrid AI Models:** Using reinforcement learning and GANs that can enhance accuracy and adaptability

Last but not least, generative AI has great potential for personalized medicine. Continuous innovation and collaboration among researchers, doctors, and regulatory agencies are needed to overcome the discussed obstacles (Reddy 2024).

10.8 CONCLUSION

Generative AI models speed up drug development processes, as they provide data-driven treatment plans more precisely and also protect patient privacy. In this way, these models transform personalized medicine. Although there are some hurdles present, the future of AI-driven healthcare looks bright. Advancements in foundation models, federated learning, and reinforcement learning show their potential to alter the viewpoint by which healthcare practitioners were previously relied on for individualized care. To successfully integrate generative AI with personalized medicine, there is an obvious need for cross-disciplinary collaboration in fields of AI research and development, clinical medicine, ethical guidelines, and legislation. Data privacy, bias, model interpretability, and regulatory compliance are the obstacles that burden healthcare systems from realizing the transformational promise of generative AI. Overcoming these hurdles is crucial in these areas. Needless to say, the use of generative AI in customized medicine does not appear without risks, but this initiative has the potential to become a cornerstone of twenty-first–century healthcare with more careful planning, strong foundations of ethics, and a dedication to fairness.

REFERENCES

Alsafadi, Farah, and Xu Wu. 2023. "Deep Generative Modeling-Based Data Augmentation with Demonstration Using the BFBT Benchmark Void Fraction Datasets." *Nuclear Engineering and Design* 415: 112712. https://doi.org/10.1016/j.nucengdes.2023.112712.

Bashyam, Vishnu M., Jimit Doshi, Guray Erus, Dhivya Srinivasan, Ahmed Abdulkadir, Ashish Singh, Mohamad Habes, et al. 2022. "Deep Generative Medical Image Harmonization for Improving Cross-Site Generalization in Deep Learning Predictors." *Journal of Magnetic Resonance Imaging* 55 (3): 908–16. https://doi.org/10.1002/jmri.27908.

Baur, Christoph, Benedikt Wiestler, Shadi Albarqouni, and Nassir Navab. 2019. "Deep Autoencoding Models for Unsupervised Anomaly Segmentation in Brain MR Images." In, 161–69. https://doi.org/10.1007/978-3-030-11723-8_16.

Biswal, Siddharth, Soumya Ghosh, Jon Duke, Bradley Malin, Walter Stewart, and Jimeng Sun. 2020. "EVA: Generating Longitudinal Electronic Health Records Using Conditional Variational Autoencoders," December.

Blanchard, A. E., C. Stanley, and D. Bhowmik. 2021. "Using GANs with Adaptive Training Data to Search for New Molecules." *Journal of Cheminformatics* 13: 14. https://doi.org/10.1186/s13321-021-00494-3.

Blanco-González, A., A. Cabezón, A. Seco-González, D. Conde-Torres, P. Antelo-Riveiro, Á. Piñeiro, and R. Garcia-Fandino. 2023. "The Role of AI in Drug Discovery: Challenges, Opportunities, and Strategies." *Pharmaceuticals* 16, no. 6: 891. https://doi.org/10.3390/ph16060891.

Blasiak, Agata, Jeffrey Khong, and Theodore Kee. 2020. "CURATE.AI: Optimizing Personalized Medicine with Artificial Intelligence." *SLAS Technology* 25 (2): 95–105. https://doi.org/10.1177/2472630319890316.

Chen, R. J., M. Y. Lu, T. Y. Chen, D. F. K. Williamson, and F. Mahmood. 2021. "Synthetic Data in Machine Learning for Medicine and Healthcare." *Nature Biomedical Engineering* 5, no. 6: 493–497. https://doi.org/10.1038/s41551-021-00751-8.

Chen, Xi, Ruth Roberts, Weida Tong, and Zhichao Liu. 2022. "Tox-GAN: An Artificial Intelligence Approach Alternative to Animal Studies—A Case Study WithToxicogenomics." *Toxicological Sciences* 186 (2): 242–59. https://doi.org/10.1093/toxsci/kfab157.

Chen, Xi, Ruth Roberts, Zhichao Liu, and Weida Tong. 2023. "A Generative Adversarial Network Model Alternative to Animal Studies for Clinical Pathology Assessment." *Nature Communications* 14 (1): 7141. https://doi.org/10.1038/s41467-023-42933-9.

Chen, Ziqi, Martin Renqiang Min, Srinivasan Parthasarathy, and Xia Ning. 2021. "A Deep Generative Model for Molecule Optimization via One Fragment Modification." *Nature Machine Intelligence* 3 (12): 1040–49. https://doi.org/10.1038/s42256-021-00410-2.

Farhud, D. D., and S. Zokaei. 2021. "Ethical Issues of Artificial Intelligence in Medicine and Healthcare." *Iranian Journal of Public Health* 50, no. 11: i–v. https://doi.org/10.18502/ijph.v50i11.7600.

Gangwal, A., A. Ansari, I. Ahmad, A. K. Azad, V. Kumarasamy, V. Subramaniyan, and L. S. Wong. 2024. "Generative Artificial Intelligence in Drug Discovery: Basic Framework, Recent Advances, Challenges, and Opportunities." *Frontiers in Pharmacology* 15: 1331062. https://doi.org/10.3389/fphar.2024.1331062.

Generative Artificial Intelligence Substantially Enhances the Accuracy of Embryo Selection Models." Cao, P, J Derhaag, E Coonen, H Brunner, G Acharya, A Salumets, and M Zamani Esteki1. 2024. "O-251 *Human Reproduction* 39 (Supplement_1). https://doi.org/10.1093/humrep/deae108.298.

Gerke, S., T. Minssen, and G. Cohen. 2020. "Ethical and Legal Challenges of Artificial Intelligence-Driven Healthcare." *Artificial Intelligence in Healthcare*: 295–336. https://doi.org/10.1016/B978-0-12-818438-7.00012-5.

Ghebrehiwet, I., N. Zaki, R. Damseh, et al. 2024. "Revolutionizing Personalized Medicine with Generative AI: A Systematic Review." *Artificial Intelligence Review* 57: 128. https://doi.org/10.1007/s10462-024-10768-5.

Goetz, L. H., and N. J. Schork. 2018. "Personalized Medicine: Motivation, Challenges, and Progress." *Fertility and Sterility* 109, no. 6: 952–963. https://doi.org/10.1016/j.fertnstert.2018.05.006.

Gootjes-Dreesbach, Luise, Meemansa Sood, Akrishta Sahay, Martin Hofmann-Apitius, and Holger Fröhlich. 2020. "Variational Autoencoder Modular Bayesian Networks for Simulation of Heterogeneous Clinical Study Data." *Frontiers in Big Data* 3 (May). https://doi.org/10.3389/fdata.2020.00016.

Green, Adrian J., Martin J. Mohlenkamp, Jhuma Das, Meenal Chaudhari, Lisa Truong, Robyn L. Tanguay, and David M. Reif. 2021. "Leveraging High-Throughput Screening Data, Deep Neural Networks, and Conditional Generative Adversarial Networks to Advance Predictive Toxicology." *PLOS Computational Biology* 17 (7): e1009135. https://doi.org/10.1371/journal.pcbi.1009135.

Green, S., B. Prainsack, and M. Sabatello. 2023. "Precision Medicine and the Problem of Structural Injustice." *Medicine, Health Care, and Philosophy* 26, no. 3: 433–450. https://doi.org/10.1007/s11019-023-10158-8.

Grisoni, Francesca, Berend J. H. Huisman, Alexander L. Button, Michael Moret, Kenneth Atz, Daniel Merk, and Gisbert Schneider. 2021. "Combining Generative Artificial Intelligence and On-Chip Synthesis for de Novo Drug Design." *Science Advances* 7 (24). https://doi.org/10.1126/sciadv.abg3338.

Hess, Moritz, Maren Hackenberg, and Harald Binder. 2020. "Exploring Generative Deep Learning for Omics Data Using Log-Linear Models." *Bioinformatics* 36 (20): 5045–53. https://doi.org/10.1093/bioinformatics/btaa623.

Ho, D., S. R. Quake, E. R. B. McCabe, W. J. Chng, E. K. Chow, X. Ding, B. D. Gelb, G. S. Ginsburg, J. Hassenstab, C. M. Ho, W. C. Mobley, G. P. Nolan, S. T. Rosen, P. Tan, Y. Yen, and A. Zarrinpar. 2020. "Enabling Technologies for Personalized and Precision Medicine." *Trends in Biotechnology* 38, no. 5: 497–518. https://doi.org/10.1016/j.tibtech.2019.12.021.

Hong, Sungmin, Razvan Marinescu, Adrian v. Dalca, Anna K. Bonkhoff, Martin Bretzner, Natalia S. Rost, and Polina Golland. 2021. "3D-StyleGAN: A Style-Based Generative Adversarial Network for Generative Modeling of Three-Dimensional Medical Images." In, 24–34. https://doi.org/10.1007/978-3-030-88210-5_3.

Hughes, J. P., S. Rees, S. B. Kalindjian, and K. L. Philpott. 2011. "Principles of Early Drug Discovery." *British Journal of Pharmacology* 162, no. 6: 1239–1249. https://doi.org/10.1111/j.1476-5381.2010.01127.x.

Hunter, B., S. Hindocha, and R. W. Lee. 2022. "The Role of Artificial Intelligence in Early Cancer Diagnosis." *Cancers* 14, no. 6: 1524. https://doi.org/10.3390/cancers 14061524.

Hwang, Uiwon, Sung-Woo Kim, Dahuin Jung, SeungWook Kim, Hyejoo Lee, Sang Won Seo, Joon-Kyung Seong, and Sungroh Yoon. 2023. "Real-World Prediction of Preclinical Alzheimer's Disease with a Deep Generative Model." *Artificial Intelligence in Medicine* 144 (October): 102654. https://doi.org/10.1016/j.artmed.2023.102654.

Ibrahim, Bekkouch Imad, Dragoş Constantin Nicolae, Adil Khan, Syed Imran Ali, and Asad Khattak. 2020. "VAE-GAN Based Zero-Shot Outlier Detection." In *Proceedings of the 2020 4th International Symposium on Computer Science and Intelligent Control*, 1–5. New York, NY, USA: ACM. https://doi.org/10.1145/3440084.3441180.

Johnson, K. B., W. Q. Wei, D. Weeraratne, M. E. Frisse, K. Misulis, K. Rhee, J. Zhao, and J. L. Snowdon. 2021. "Precision Medicine, AI, and the Future of Personalized Health Care." *Clinical and Translational Science* 14, no. 1: 86–93. https://doi.org/10.1111/cts.12884.

Kapustina, Olga, Polina Burmakina, Nina Gubina, Nikita Serov, and Vladimir Vinogradov. 2024. "User-Friendly and Industry-Integrated AI for Medicinal Chemists and Pharmaceuticals." *Artificial Intelligence Chemistry* 2, no. 2: 100072. https://doi.org/10.1016/j.aichem.2024.100072.

Kazuhiro, K., R. A. Werner, F. Toriumi, M. S. Javadi, M. G. Pomper, L. B. Solnes, F. Verde, T. Higuchi, and S. P. Rowe. 2018. "Generative Adversarial Networks for the Creation of Realistic Artificial Brain Magnetic Resonance Images." *Tomography* 4, no. 4: 159–163. https://doi.org/10.18383/j.tom.2018.00042.

Khalifa, Mohamed, and Mona Albadawy. 2024. "AI in Diagnostic Imaging: Revolutionising Accuracy and Efficiency." *Computer Methods and Programs in Biomedicine Update* 5: 100146. https://doi.org/10.1016/j.cmpbup.2024.100146.

Koohi-Moghadam, M., and K. T. Bae. 2023. "Generative AI in Medical Imaging: Applications, Challenges, and Ethics." *Journal of Medical Systems* 47, no. 1: 94. https://doi.org/10.1007/s10916-023-01987-4.

Lenz, Stefan, Moritz Hess, and Harald Binder. 2021. "Deep Generative Models in DataSHIELD." *BMC Medical Research Methodology* 21 (1): 64. https://doi.org/10.1186/s12874-021-01237-6.

Li, Dun, Dezhi Han, Tien-Hsiung Weng, Zibin Zheng, Hongzhi Li, Han Liu, Arcangelo Castiglione, and Kuan-Ching Li. 2022. "Blockchain for Federated Learning toward Secure Distributed Machine Learning Systems: A Systemic Survey." *Soft Computing* 26 (9): 4423–40. https://doi.org/10.1007/s00500-021-06496-5.

Liu, Mingxuan, Siqi Li, Han Yuan, Marcus Eng Hock Ong, Yilin Ning, Feng Xie, Seyed Ehsan Saffari, et al. 2023. "Handling Missing Values in Healthcare Data: A Systematic Review of Deep Learning-Based Imputation Techniques." *Artificial Intelligence in Medicine* 142 (August): 102587. https://doi.org/10.1016/j.artmed.2023.102587.

Maziarka, Łukasz, Agnieszka Pocha, Jan Kaczmarczyk, Krzysztof Rataj, Tomasz Danel, and Michał Warchoł. 2020. "Mol-CycleGAN: A Generative Model for Molecular Optimization." *Journal of Cheminformatics* 12 (1): 2. https://doi.org/10.1186/s13321-019-0404-1.

Merk, Daniel, Lukas Friedrich, Francesca Grisoni, and Gisbert Schneider. 2018. "*De Novo* Design of Bioactive Small Molecules by Artificial Intelligence." *Molecular Informatics* 37 (1–2). https://doi.org/10.1002/minf.201700153.

Meyers, Joshua, Benedek Fabian, and Nathan Brown. 2021. "De Novo Molecular Design and Generative Models." *Drug Discovery Today* 26, no. 11: 2707–2715. https://doi.org/10.1016/j.drudis.2021.05.019.

Miletic, Marko, and Murat Sariyar. 2024. "Challenges of Using Synthetic Data Generation Methods for Tabular Microdata." *Applied Sciences* 14, no. 14: 5975. https://doi.org/10.3390/app14145975.

Moor, M., O. Banerjee, Z. S. H. Abad, H. M. Krumholz, J. Leskovec, E. J. Topol, and P. Rajpurkar. 2023. "Foundation Models for Generalist Medical Artificial Intelligence." *Nature* 616, no. 7956: 259–265. https://doi.org/10.1038/s41586-023-05881-4.

Naik, N., B. M. Z. Hameed, D. K. Shetty, D. Swain, M. Shah, R. Paul, K. Aggarwal, S. Ibrahim, V. Patil, K. Smriti, S. Shetty, B. P. Rai, P. Chlosta, and B. K. Somani. 2022. "Legal and Ethical Considerations in Artificial Intelligence in Healthcare: Who Takes Responsibility?" *Frontiers in Surgery* 9: 862322. https://doi.org/10.3389/fsurg.2022.862322.

Palaniappan, K., E. Y. T. Lin, and S. Vogel. 2024. "Global Regulatory Frameworks for the Use of Artificial Intelligence (AI) in the Healthcare Services Sector." *Healthcare* 12, no. 5: 562. https://doi.org/10.3390/healthcare12050562.

Paul, D., G. Sanap, S. Shenoy, D. Kalyane, K. Kalia, and R. K. Tekade. 2021. "Artificial Intelligence in Drug Discovery and Development." *Drug Discovery Today* 26, no. 1: 80–93. https://doi.org/10.1016/j.drudis.2020.10.010.

Pereira, Tiago, Maryam Abbasi, Rita I Oliveira, Romina A Guedes, Jorge A R Salvador, and Joel P Arrais. 2022. "Deep Generative Model for Therapeutic Targets Using Transcriptomic Disease-Associated Data—USP7 Case Study." *Briefings in Bioinformatics* 23 (4). https://doi.org/10.1093/bib/bbac270.

Pezoulas, Vasileios C., Dimitrios I. Zaridis, Eugenia Mylona, Christos Androutsos, Kosmas Apostolidis, Nikolaos S. Tachos, and Dimitrios I. Fotiadis. 2024. "Synthetic Data Generation Methods in Healthcare: A Review on Open-Source Tools and Methods." *Computational and Structural Biotechnology Journal* 23: 2892–2910. https://doi.org/10.1016/j.csbj.2024.07.005.

Pinto-Coelho, L. 2023. "How Artificial Intelligence Is Shaping Medical Imaging Technology: A Survey of Innovations and Applications." *Bioengineering* 10, no. 12: 1435. https://doi.org/10.3390/bioengineering10121435.

Poudevigne-Durance, Thomas, Owen Dafydd Jones, and Yipeng Qin. 2022. "MaWGAN: A Generative Adversarial Network to Create Synthetic Data from Datasets with Missing Data." *Electronics* 11 (6): 837. https://doi.org/10.3390/electronics11060837.

Ray, Sumanta, Snehalika Lall, Anirban Mukhopadhyay, Sanghamitra Bandyopadhyay, and Alexander Schönhuth. 2022. "Deep Variational Graph Autoencoders for Novel Host-Directed Therapy Options against COVID-19." *Artificial Intelligence in Medicine* 134 (December): 102418. https://doi.org/10.1016/j.artmed.2022.102418.

Reddy, S. 2024. "Generative AI in Healthcare: An Implementation Science Informed Translational Path on Application, Integration and Governance." *Implementation Science* 19, no. 1: 27. https://doi.org/10.1186/s13012-024-01357-9.

Sun, Chang, Ping Xuan, Tiangang Zhang, and Yilin Ye. 2022. "Graph Convolutional Autoencoder and Generative Adversarial Network-Based Method for Predicting Drug-Target Interactions." *IEEE/ACM Transactions on Computational Biology and Bioinformatics* 19 (1): 455–64. https://doi.org/10.1109/TCBB.2020.2999084.

Templin, T., M. W. Perez, S. Sylvia, J. Leek, and N. Sinnott-Armstrong. 2024. "Addressing 6 Challenges in Generative AI for Digital Health: A Scoping Review." *PLOS Digital Health* 3, no. 5: e0000503. https://doi.org/10.1371/journal.pdig.0000503.

Toh, Tan Boon, Dexter Kai Hao Thng, Nagarjun Bolem, Balamurugan A. Vellayappan, Bryce Wei Quan Tan, Yating Shen, Sou Yen Soon, et al. 2024. "Evaluation of Ex Vivo Drug Combination Optimization Platform in Recurrent High Grade Astrocytic Glioma: An Interventional, Non-Randomized, Open-Label Trial Protocol." *PLOS ONE* 19 (7): e0307818. https://doi.org/10.1371/journal.pone.0307818.

Torfi, Amirsina, and Edward A. Fox. 2020. "CorGAN: Correlation-Capturing Convolutional Generative Adversarial Networks for Generating Synthetic Healthcare Records," January.

Vora, L. K., A. D. Gholap, K. Jetha, R. R. S. Thakur, H. K. Solanki, and V. P. Chavda. 2023. "Artificial Intelligence in Pharmaceutical Technology and Drug Delivery Design." *Pharmaceutics* 15, no. 7: 1916. https://doi.org/10.3390/pharmaceutics15071916.

Wang, Jianmin, Yanyi Chu, Jiashun Mao, Hyeon-Nae Jeon, Haiyan Jin, Amir Zeb, Yuil Jang, Kwang-Hwi Cho, Tao Song, and Kyoung Tai No. 2022. "*De Novo* Molecular Design with Deep Molecular Generative Models for PPI Inhibitors." *Briefings in Bioinformatics* 23 (4). https://doi.org/10.1093/bib/bbac285.

Wang, Mingyang, Chang-Yu Hsieh, Jike Wang, Dong Wang, Gaoqi Weng, Chao Shen, Xiaojun Yao, et al. 2022. "RELATION: A Deep Generative Model for Structure-Based De Novo Drug Design." *Journal of Medicinal Chemistry* 65 (13): 9478–92. https://doi.org/10.1021/acs.jmedchem.2c00732.

Wei, Shilong, Lu Si, Tongyu Huang, Shan Du, Yue Yao, Yang Dong, and Hui Ma. 2023. "Deep-Learning-Based Cross-Modality Translation from Stokes Image to Bright-Field Contrast." *Journal of Biomedical Optics* 28 (10). https://doi.org/10.1117/1.JBO.28.10.102911.

Wu, Junde, Wei Ji, Yuanpei Liu, Huazhu Fu, Min Xu, Yanwu Xu, and Yueming Jin. 2023. "Medical SAM Adapter: Adapting Segment Anything Model for Medical Image Segmentation," April.

Yadav, H., P. Yadav, N. Joshi, and S. C. Sharma. 2024. "Smart Healthcare: Paradigm Shift in Industry 5.0 Using AI." In Recent Trends in Artificial Intelligence Towards a Smart World: Frontiers of Artificial Intelligence, Ethics and Multidisciplinary Applications, edited by R. Arya, S. C. Sharma, A. K. Verma, and B. Iyer. Singapore: Springer. https://doi.org/10.1007/978-981-97-6790-8_3.

You, Kui, Peter Wang, and Dean Ho. 2022. "N-of-1 Healthcare: Challenges and Prospects for the Future of Personalized Medicine." *Frontiers in Digital Health* 4 (February). https://doi.org/10.3389/fdgth.2022.830656.

Zhao, Zijuan, Juanjuan Zhao, Kai Song, Akbar Hussain, Qianqian Du, Yunyun Dong, Jihua Liu, and Xiaotang Yang. 2020. "Joint DBN and Fuzzy C-Means Unsupervised Deep Clustering for Lung Cancer Patient Stratification." *Engineering Applications of Artificial Intelligence* 91 (May): 103571. https://doi.org/10.1016/j.engappai.2020.103571.

Zhavoronkov, Alex, Yan A. Ivanenkov, Alex Aliper, Mark S. Veselov, Vladimir A. Aladinskiy, Anastasiya v. Aladinskaya, Victor A. Terentiev, et al. 2019. "Deep Learning Enables Rapid Identification of Potent DDR1 Kinase Inhibitors." *Nature Biotechnology* 37 (9): 1038–40. https://doi.org/10.1038/s41587-019-0224-x.

11 Transforming Healthcare through Generative AI

Naved Ahmad, Iram Fatima, Mehtab Alam, Ihtiram Raza Khan, and Amena Mahmoud

11.1 INTRODUCTION

Generative artificial intelligence (GAI) has received a lot of attention lately. Computer technologies and data have advanced to the point that we've seen huge progress in GAI over the past few years, and it's now one of the most popular and state-of-the-art AI algorithms around.

The 2022 report by Gartner provides insight into the true value of GAI: Gartner's Hype Cycle for Emerging Technologies ranked generative AI at number two, the topmost position for a technology that is considered emerging and having the greatest influence. The report states: 'By 2027, 30 per cent of manufacturers will use generative AI to develop better products more quickly.' OpenAI's 'big breakthrough' in artificial intelligence in 2020 was the introduction of a generative AI named Generative Pre-trained Transformer 3, or simply GPT-3—the third version of such a transformer—capable of writing text, visuals, and audio on its own. Generative AI is well explained in a recent OpenAI blog, and it well represents the entire field of generative AI: GPT-3 is a model that learns an internal representation of text artifacts and then can generate entirely new, novel, and human-sounding text artifacts using this representation. In other words, it can successfully learn to mimic human-sounding text when creating new text—the exact definition of being artistic! Among generative AI's many methods that can be applied to data, some are machine learning based and others are based on statistical and computational inference techniques. The field of generative AI will see rapid growth both in academia and in terms of commercialisation by industry. GAI, you might think, sounds highly futuristic. Not so! There are already several applications with successful adoption and use in every imaginable aspect, far too many to list here. Some examples are: new materials, especially biomaterials, and data privacy. Concerns about the safety of GAI are well expressed in the area of 'fake news,' especially in deepfakes (a term coined to refer to a short video depicting a real person lip-syncing to words that the person never spoke). Deepfakes have also been used to disseminate propaganda and fake videos of news, especially by Russia and China. The truth about deepfakes can be quite unsettling. The potential widespread misuse of generative AI is hindering its adoption by some industries, although there are many who remain undeterred. The value of generative AI is immense. One of the strongest justifications for GAI is that it can provide simulations of the molecular

DOI: 10.1201/9781003539483-11

representations of real or designed protein structures, and this is one of the most productive fields currently using GAI 2.3.

Perhaps most importantly, with the unveiling of GPT-4 in March 2023, future GPT models, vis-à-vis analogical bootstrapping, offer multimodal capabilities for processing text and images, allowing for similar processing of verbal and visual material. In [1], the authors reflect on how ChatGPT, a text-driven conversational chatbot, and GAI tools might be used to facilitate better teaching and learning in education. They also outline several ways GAI tools might be deliberately utilised for safe-guarding education and enhancing student learning.

GAI has significantly emerged as one of the most active and promising subfield in artificial intelligence research. Its applications have been explored in various domains, including healthcare, marketing, finance, logistics, transport, travelling, entertainment, journalism, and education [2, 3]. Among these, healthcare seems to be most critical due to sensitivity of patient health and privacy, especially in diagnosis or treatment, decision making, or pathological condition prediction. Artificial intelligence (AI)–based approaches can be traced in several healthcare application–related areas, including AI-based diagnosis of diseases, AI-based curative solutions, and other AI solutions to predict symptoms in earlier stages of disease. Now with the evolution of GPT-3 and GPT-4, many GAI-based solutions have been proposed. This improvement might bring more complex challenges due to its serious implications in modern life, especially in the healthcare sector. Now let's see concrete examples of the kind of challenges GAI poses. First, let us try to figure out the level of transparency it provides, along with required answer generation [4].

The authors of [5] outline the concerns, opportunities and pitfalls of the use of natural language processing (NLP) applications for healthcare, whose implementation in a clinical setting is unlikely any time soon. Synthetic data generation by generative adversarial networks (GANs) has been employed to create realistic replacement research data that preserves many of the statistical properties of real data. Medical education, clinical research, and data protection can all benefit from the use of such generated data. However, as [6] shows, there remain a number of ethical and logistical obstacles to overcome before we see such application in action. GAI and GANs are undoubtedly of significant potential use in future medical education, such as virtual patient training, and in medical research to improve the quality and speed of diagnoses. They may ultimately improve the standards of patient care [7].

GAI is growing in popularity in the field of AI, especially in healthcare, where it can be very helpful in improving medical imaging, identifying drugs, and helping clinicians and researchers provide better patient care and treatment planning. It can also be helpful for medical decision making. At the same time, there are many concerns and challenges in using GAI in the healthcare field.

This chapter will present how generative AI models can help healthcare systems by providing real-world examples, in addition to exploring issues associated with using generative AI in the healthcare field. The principal issues are related to data privacy, ethical considerations, and data bias, which we will discuss in the hope of finding a way to maximise the use of GAI to the benefit of patients worldwide while allowing the safe use of generative AI to complement clinicians' expertise and improve healthcare services [8].

Three major contributions can be highlighted in this work:

1. The ability to outline the potential of generative AI to support the healthcare system, taking into consideration its limitations and showcasing how these limitation can be potentially solved.
2. Showcasing real-world examples of generative AI models in the healthcare field.
3. Detailing the different applications of GAI in healthcare.

11.2 A BROAD VIEW OF GENERATIVE AI

Generative AI refers to a machine learning approach that generates new data or text, following the structure of the training data, as shown in Figure 11.1. GAI differs from other machine learning approaches, such as classification or clustering of data. For instance, linear discriminant analysis and K-means clustering are non-generative. However, GAI approaches are specifically designed to generate new data that matches the input data. The two most common types of generative AI models are GANs and transformer-based models, such as GPT language models. GANs are multimedia and visual-type outputs generated from both text and visual inputs, whereas transformer-based models use internet data and other textual sources to generate written content such as articles, press releases, and whitepapers [9].

In creating new data, GAI algorithms are trained on large databases consisting of information on different features. For instance, in the example of creating facial images with a GAI, the image database elements might consist of faces that represent different human ethnicities and biological classes. With a GAI algorithm that has been trained on such a database with millions of data points, the system will be able to create new faces (data points) that will bear many similarities to the faces in its training database. Therefore, our argument that GAI has no contemporary precedent primarily rests on the application of generative modelling, which is a new approach to machine learning methodology. Traditional prediction methods perform through

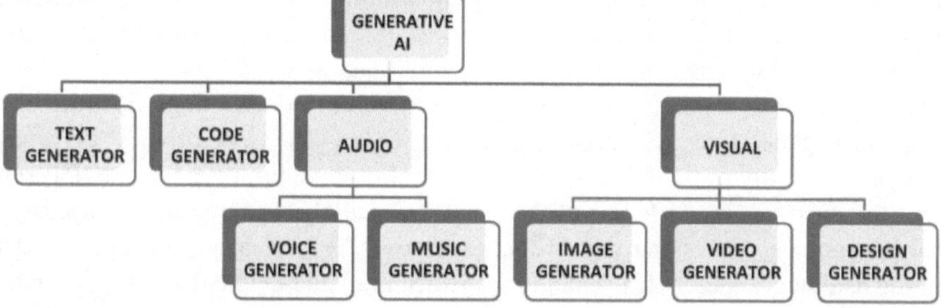

FIGURE 11.1 Generative AI tools.

what is known as discriminative modelling, that is, classifying objects into groups based on empirical clustering or forecasting the probability and occurrence of events by classifying data into predetermined classes. The difference between generative and discriminative modelling relates to the central question to be addressed—it is a matter of 'predicting what' as opposed to 'predicting for whom.' Discriminative modelling makes predictions not as to how to generate the input and corresponding features (x) given the associated labels (y) but rather as to what labels (y) are appropriate for the input and corresponding features (x) observed. In essence, therefore, GAI algorithms (as opposed to discriminative algorithm-based machine learning) will make predictions not just as to the cause-and-effect relationship between classes (which is a binary or categorical approach) but will focus on learning distributions across classes and features (which is an ordinal or non-binary approach). Generative algorithms will be able to predict features given a label and are better at capturing a joint distribution of data elements; that is, it makes it possible for them to generate new data in a manner that substantially resembles the existing training databases. Discriminative algorithms, on the other hand, are better at learning decision boundaries between two classes of data (i.e., non-Gaussian error-rate minimisation) and will therefore be better at prediction of labels given features, that is, generate features given a label rather than predicting labels given features—which is the case with generative algorithms [10]. Some of the most anticipated applications of generative AI include repairs to medicine, business and manufacturing. [1] examines how generative AI can transform healthcare. Specifically, it shows how this new approach to leveraging machine-learning can benefit the health sector, create new drugs to treat diseases, and come up with better treatment options while also helping to curb the costs of treating patients. By utilising GAI alongside predictive analytics, the medical sector can achieve earlier detection of disease and diagnoses, which can lead to precautionary treatments prior to disease flare. Additionally, this application of AI will enable researchers to handle and interpret large digital datasets, thereby saving staff time that would otherwise be spent on mundane data representation. All in all, the healthcare sector must look actively look to adopt GAI in all areas of medicine given its ability to bring numerous benefits to this critically important sector of the economy. Apart from paving the way for cheaper and more effective treatment of diseases, GAI will also revolutionise the drug discovery process [11]. As [2] shows, GAI can support pharmaceutical researchers in understanding the interactions between different chemicals and biological molecules, which can support them in coming up with new highly effective medicines. Relatedly, drug discovery will also greatly benefit from GAI's ability to offer more accurate medical imagery of the human body for diagnosis.

The latest advancements in artificial intelligence are developing with immense speed, and generative AI models, such as OpenAI's Generative Pre-Trained Transformer family of models and their most well-known prototype, ChatGPT, represent the most advanced forms of AI currently available. Owing to its impressive natural language processing capability, generative AI is ideally positioned to disrupt the healthcare sector [12]. Thanks to the accumulated medical knowledge in the machine, generative AI models like GPT might operate as a powerful tool capable of revolutionising healthcare in many areas, such as clinical decision-making, patient communication, and data management. They will not only gather and organise existing medical information but also interpret it. This holds the promise of a new world of mental health care. Many are optimistic that generative AI could revolutionise and transform healthcare practices over the next decade [13].

GPT models in clinical decision support can recommend findings and actions that improve healthcare decision-making and ultimately enhance clinical outcomes to improve the quality of healthcare services across the board [14]. For instance, through processing large medical datasets, GPT models could be used for disease diagnosis and prognosis, allowing for earlier detection and differentiated treatment plans. In combination with other advanced tools, GPT models could also support radiologists' decision-making about interpreting medical images to enhance diagnostic accuracy and reduce interpretation time [15]. DRIVE: This AI-based model can make decisions in drug prognosis to assist in finding new treatments and drugs. AI models can also transform drug discovery by identifying potential drug candidates who have higher chances of being an effective and safe drug [16].

GPT models would be capable of enhancing and providing accurate medical services but also modifying patient communication, as GPT could be seen as an interactive AI language model that could (1) confer and engage with patients, (2) provide educational material for patients, and (3) answer patients' medical questions, ultimately increasing patient engagement and patient self-management of their health [17]. Time-saving: GPT models could also be used to facilitate and/or streamline the management of EHRs and clinical documentation, avoiding cognitive overload and ultimately reducing the administrative burden on clinical staff and allowing them to spend more time with patients [18].

But integrating generative models in medicine and health care carries both challenges and ethical dilemmas. Since the consequences of AI-assisted decisions can be life or death, it is of the utmost importance that AI models be not only accurate and reliable in their decision-making but also that the engineer or physician be able to explain and demonstrate exactly what aspects of the data went into their model-driven conclusion. Several AI models, including generative ones, are deemed 'black box' models because their internal dynamics and decision-making are hard to understand—making it difficult to know what went into the machine's ultimate decision. These transparency and explainability issues are increasingly discussed in the context of the use of AI in healthcare, with the applicable and necessary requirements still under debate. Ethical issues of data privacy, patient confidentiality, and AI model biases must also be addressed [19]. The security of patient privacy and data must be prioritised if the public—which includes potential patients—are to have faith in AI-enabled healthcare solutions.

The objective of this chapter is to present, to the best of our knowledge, the state of the art of research efforts towards exploitation of generative AI models in medicine and healthcare. Discussing their potential, benefits, challenges, and ethical implications, this chapter contributes to the current debate on how responsibly the transformative power of AI can be exploited for better medical practice and patients' wellbeing. In our investigation into the power of generative models for healthcare, we navigate the newly evolving AI world that must be guided by ethical standards, patient-centric care, and concerted design by AI developers, medical professionals, and policymakers [20].

11.3 BACKGROUND

Natural language processing deals with the interactions between computers and the human language: from the design of interfaces and chatbots to the creation of intelligent assistants that help humans in search-engine queries, answering machines, and more. The main goal of NLP is that a computer can understand, interpret, and generate human language as it would be done by a fellow human (appropriate and meaningful context). Put simply, it is a subfield of AI that deals with the interaction between computers and human language. It's an umbrella term that encompasses a range of tasks: translation, sentiment analysis, optical character recognition, speech recognition, text generation, text summarisation, educational dialogue systems, question answering, dialogue systems, machine translation, machine summarisation, information extraction, language identification, and intent recognition: all meant to bridge the gaps between humans and computers.

NLP has also been extensively used in healthcare to extract and analyse valuable information from large amounts of unstructured clinical text, including electronic health records (EHRs), medical literature and patient-generated content. NLP can be used to convert unstructured clinical notes to structured data, which helps identify medical problems, medications, and lab tests using named entity recognition.19,20 For example, NLP has been used with unstructured EHR data to identify adverse drug events through analysis of drug–drug interactions.21 NLP-driven models have also been used to recognise early stages of disease so that interventions can start sooner, improving patient outcomes.22

For instance, new GPT models, developed by OpenAI, are some of the more remarkable recent developments in NLP that are characterised by families of advanced language models based on deep-learning neural networks employing the transformer architecture introduced in 2017 [21] by Vaswani et al. The transformer architecture is particularly effective at processing sequential data such as text, through a method called 'self-attention,' which can evaluate the importance and relationships between single words in a sentence, thus allowing greater focus on semantically related words and, most importantly, an increase in contextual information retained by the model. The real-time transformer revolution is based on the extraordinary capability of these models to manage long-range dependencies of sequences of words in language, which led to a remarkable improvement in their ability for contextual language understanding and semantic representations. Since its introduction in June 2018 with the release of GPT-1 [22], development periods for the new models have been extremely short, and they've achieved remarkable statistical characteristics in a relatively short period of time. GPT-1 was followed in February 2019 by GPT-2 [23], which had an impressive 1.5 billion parameters and showed remarkable text simulation but raised some concern for misuse due to its ability to generate realistic text, including faked news stories [24]. To prevent misuse of GPT-2, OpenAI initially chose to publicly release only small versions of the model in November 2019, but by December that year GPT-2 was fully released and available to NLP researchers and developers [24]. This led to a surge of related research and experimentation that accelerated development and fine-tuning for applications including text generation, chatbots, language translation, and many others [25].

In June 2020, the timeline advanced considerably with GPT-3, a paradigm-shifting new model with 175 billion parameters, the largest language model yet created. GPT-3 displayed human-level language generation and was applied to a wide variety of tasks, such as translation, summarisation, question answering, and creative writing. GPT-3 was a resounding success, sparking further interest in LLMs, resulting in a flurry of research activity and commercial applications. [26] In November 2022, OpenAI released the conversational AI ChatGPT based on the GPT-3.5 architecture, which is able to conduct a free-flowing human-like dialogue in order to generate a target text in response to a prompt or question from the user. The answer is contextually coherent and human-sounding, drawn from its pre-training data. In March 2023, OpenAI released their newest large multimodal model GPT-4, capable of taking text and images as inputs, modelled on their latest innovation. ChatGPT is considered only one of many potential uses, and the biggest performance improvements can be expected in encyclopædic question-answering. Despite their immense pre-training, these models are referred to as large language models. [22]

That 'generative' capacity is responsible for many of the models' deep-learning capabilities to create human-sounding text and has important implications for healthcare and other areas. One of the key steps in producing GPT models is a process called pre-training. During pre-training, the model is trained on a massive amount of text and many different datasets so that it can learn the pattern and structure of language. It's the combination of pre-training and the transformer architecture that enables the GPT models to perform well across many NLP tasks and to produce text that sounds natural and contextually appropriate—much like human-composed text [27].

Pre-training is the initial phase, wherein the GPT model learns from vast amounts of unlabelled text data with an improved understanding of language. Then, fine-tuning happens by using task-specific labelled data [23]—for instance, healthcare corpus data—overcoming the limitations of pre-training and fine-tuning on domain-specific NLP tasks such as medical question answering, clinical text classification, or medical records translation. This combination of structural knowledge because of the generative human-sounding text, a pre-training phase where the model learns from vast amounts, and fine-tuning which customises the pre-trained model for healthcare-specific NLP tasks results in better performance on a wide range of healthcare-specific NLP tasks than previously achievable with labelled medical datasets. This improves efficiency by reducing the cost in time and resources needed to adequately train. As an example, LLMs can aid in generating human-sounding text which in turn can be applied in a clinical context for a task such as clinical decision support, protecting the doctor from potential litigation. Additionally, they can enhance patient communication while ultimately helping to speed up the process of diagnosing diseases [28], paving the way for a predictive AI-powered healthcare solution to help physicians make informed medical decisions that will benefit patients [7, 8].

11.4 GAI MODELS

Thanks to the rapid increases in power and effectiveness of artificial intelligence tools in recent decades, generative AI has become particularly relevant. Generative

AI adopts sophisticated machine learning techniques, typically uses deep neural networks and/or natural language processing, and generates seemingly human responses to textual inputs. Grounded on transformer models [29], it includes some of the most famous generative AI models that generate images [30] from textual descriptions or, with the help of a textual prompt, draw (like the celebrated DALL-E, Midjourney [31] and Stable Diffusion), sometimes even cross-modal [32], and offer great educational benefits, to name just a few.

Generative AI in healthcare continues to make inroads, and has the potential to revolutionise clinical diagnosis, treatment, patient care, and clinical decision making across specialities like urology, radiology, and cardiology, among others [33]. The investment in generative AI by the healthcare domain is expected to rise to $17 billion by 2032 based on an investigation conducted by the consulting firm Market.us, with a recent rise due to rapid progress in the development of medical imaging, diagnostics, and drugs.

To produce results with sufficient reliability, generative AI models must be first extensively trained on vast amounts of medical data such as electronic health records, medical images, genomic sequences, or other datasets. These novel solutions address traditional healthcare challenges such as the efficient and effective sharing of knowledge among clinicians. In addition, AI-generated prompts can mimic and predict disease scenarios as evidence that models can seamlessly follow clinical instructions. A case in point comes from a study performed in 2021 by Messiah et al. showing that the model can generate reliable responses to more than 1,700 different medical questions related to the acute management of severe organophosphate poisoning. Moreover, generative AI technologies can significantly enhance medicine in various ways, such as disease management, risk assessment, research education, and drug development. These technological advances bode well for healthcare and are already reshaping the field in practically incalculable ways. They can monitor disease progression and infectious toxicity and help detect biomarkers. Generative AI has already made inroads in healthcare, particularly in the domain of medical imaging. Models like DALL-E could potentially be optimised to analyse medical images—such as X-rays, MRIs, and CT scans—to improve the detection or diagnosis of diseases. These AI models are trained on large datasets of images, where generative models—trained with 'big' data—can reveal patterns and anomalies that might be missed by the human eye. Taking advantage of such sophisticated technologies, healthcare can benefit substantially in the timely detection of conditions such as cancers or neurodegenerative diseases, thus ensuring better patient care due to the increased accuracy and speed of disease diagnosis [20, 25, 27].

Research and education uses of medical imaging not only include training and education for clinicians but also serve as a means by which to generate synthetic datasets through which researchers can conduct trials and hypotheses testing. Generative AI models can be used to simulate hypothetical cases of patients dealing with diseases, offering a more realistic experiential training for learners within the healthcare sector. To do this, clinicians can describe what a patient with a certain affliction is likely to look like or what their symptoms will be. Generative AI can have a wider impact in biomedical research through the identification of 'biomarkers'—distinct characteristics or traits that are unique to a particular biomarker disease within otherwise healthy populations. This is essential for effective, efficient, and expeditious research and testing of genomes, proteomes, or other imaging datasets. For example, saliva samples of individuals, which do not carry the respective genomic disease, can be used to—through a process of mutual information—generate diverse sets of synthetic sequences for an entire biological trajectory, allowing the detail of specific genomic data to be explored.

The applications of generative AI in medicine, beyond the purpose of creating anatomical images for medical research, are extremely vast. From creating new drugs and technologies for treating physical and mental illnesses to patient-centred diagnosis, personalised care, simulation, training, clinical trial design, and mental health support, this technology will likely assist medical professionals with diagnosis and treatment for a wide variety of issues. These models can learn from their mistakes and optimise their outputs by checking their performance and the accuracy of their diagnoses [31]. Models, such as ChatGPT, can also generate patient discharge summaries based on historical data from electronic health records and medical notes without prior explanations of medical terminology.

11.5 APPLICATIONS OF GENERATIVE AI FOR HEALTHCARE

This section explores the use of general AI in various healthcare domains. Figure 11.2 illustrates a summary of the discussed applications.

A. **Medical Imaging:** Medical imaging provides detailed visualisations of a patient's anatomical structures non-invasively, helping physicians in treating various medical conditions. It enables the detection of diseases at an early stage, improving screening, and supporting the planning of the treatment interventions. However, medical imaging is still limited to a limited set of imaging modalities, insufficient amounts of annotated data, and a limited spectrum of contrasts. In the context of GAI, these are now becoming easily surmountable problems. With GAI, medical imaging stands to become even more powerful.
   1. **Data Augmentation:** In training deep learning models on medical imaging, datasets can be limited, but GAI methods such as GANs and variational autoencoders (VAEs) can create synthetic images that look very close to the patient data, thereby increasing the robustness of the models. GAI models can also generate data for rare conditions such as aquagenic urticaria and methemoglobinemia or fill in missing data. These unique characteristics make GAI methods valuable for filling data gaps and generating synthetic data to improve the model's performance. This will help to better detect and diagnose diseases in real-world scenarios. Aquagenic urticaria generated using GAI, methemoglobinemia generated using GAI: Can GAI methods, such as GANs and VAEs, be utilised to build and train meaningful predictive models for any disease? The answer depends on how scarce the datasets are for any specific condition.
   2. **Image Enhancement and Reconstruction:** One of the important underlying elements for a diagnosis of a disease through the use of medical

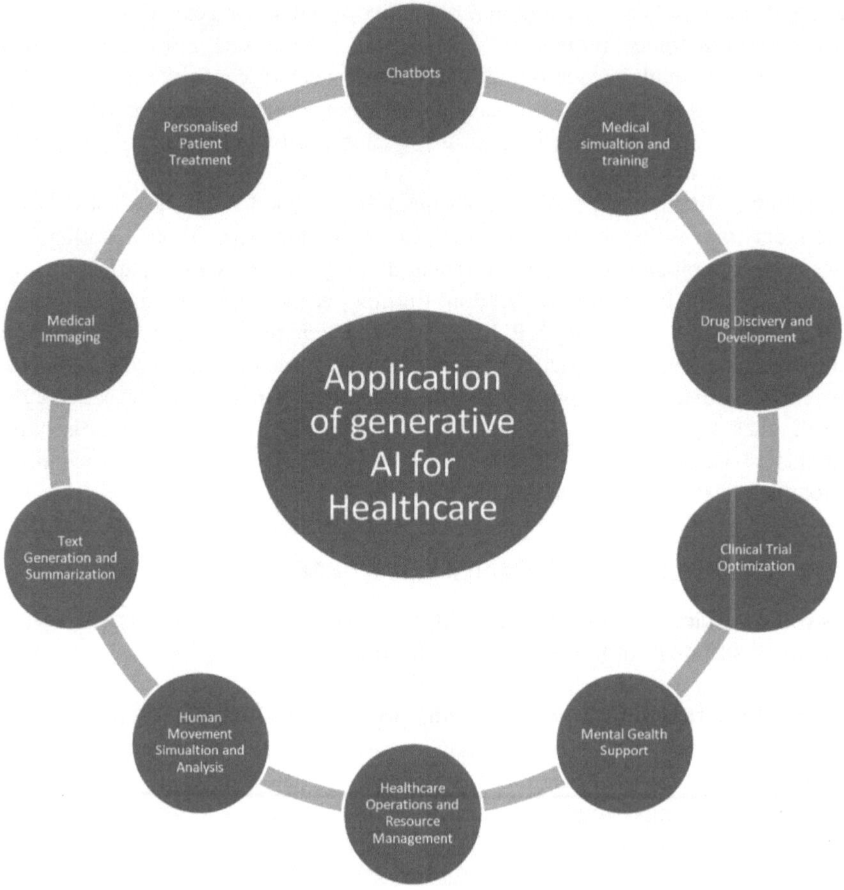

FIGURE 11.2 Applications of generative AI for healthcare.

imaging is the quality of the scans that are used. For example, an X-ray or CT scan that is too noisy or misses some data can be of low quality. As a result, this could lead to misinterpretations of the scan images and a delay in the diagnosis of the patient. GAI models can be trained for denoising images and enhancing them with frameworks such as GANs or autoencoders to give higher quantitative accuracy for medical image analysis to allow the acquisition of more reliable measurements and parameters that help determine disease progression, monitoring over time, and identification of the response to treatment. DiffMIC [34] is a model designed especially for the medical image classification task. Specifically, it identifies anomalies through neural networks, focusing on noise reduction and capturing robust semantic representations. To achieve this, it utilises a dual conditional guidance strategy to enhance regional attention at each diffusion step by exploiting the medicinal information via multiple granularities, along with a channel conditional guidance to guide the information flow at each diffusion step. Further, it enhances the information learned inside each granularity by proposing learning of mutual information inside the learnable channels through maximum-mean discrepancy regularisation [34] during the diffusion process. GAI models can also enhance the generated images from low-resolution (LR) data to high-resolution (HR) data, for example, using super-resolution techniques. The use of high-resolution images is vital for accurate disease diagnosis and detailed anatomical studies. For example, Bing et al. [35] used an enhanced generative adversarial network for the super-resolution image reconstruction problem. To improve the squeeze and excitation blocks in GANs' generator and discriminator, they utilise the self-attention framework [36] with a weighted sum of different channel's latest features to enhance the important features and de-emphasise non-essential features. In addition, they also used the combination of L1 loss, mean square error loss, and perceptual adversarial loss for training their model.

3. **Cross-Modality Image Translation:** There are many ways to perform medical imaging, for example using X-rays, positron emission tomography (PET), magnetic resonance imaging, computed tomography, ultrasound, single-photon emission computed tomography (SPECT), and so on. A modality represents a certain 'type' of image acquisition based on different physical principles and imaging methods, which provide images of unique quality, spatial resolution, sensitivity, and contrast.

   Medical image translation itself is the creation of an appropriate image content cross-modality by retaining important features, which helps to combine the advantages of complementary data and unique information of different modalities, and also helps to cope with the limitations of data. It can provide multiple diagnostic options. When acquiring medical image data from different modalities, the interaction between tissues is decoded differently among modalities. It is highly challenging to translate such clinical information from one image modality to another while retaining it. For example, in designing an MRI-to-CT translator, one of the main challenges is to retain the white and grey portion related to brain anatomy and structure. Strong contours should remain contours; wrinkles and sags must be faithfully preserved, and so on. Generative AI techniques such as GANs and VAEs can effectively translate images between different modalities, which contain complex interrelationships and retain structure and pathological information as much as possible. Such utilisation of AI methods can help cope with and circumvent modality-specific limitations and make it possible to benefit from modalities with better spatial resolution or contrast by intelligently transforming images to enhance visualisation, which is crucial for medical staff making an informed clinical decision by combining images with different modalities to create a higher-quality, advanced image, which facilitates better diagnosis and ultimately treatment [31].

4. **Interpretability and Explainability:** Generative AI enhances interpretability and explainability of deep learning models in medical imaging, which are fairly opaque models, especially at the initial phase of learning—these models usually outperform humans in operational performance even with low explainability [36]. An explanation of a model's decision makes the model more interpretable. Therefore, interpretability is a critical aspect of medical imaging for doctors and patients to make informed treatment decisions. This requires a clear understanding of the underlying reasons for the model's predictions. Interpretability can be achieved in several ways. However, visualisation is the most important among other techniques, as it helps us understand which region or feature in an image significantly influenced the output by learning these features like gradient-based methods. This is also applicable for attention mechanisms, where the regions or features can be highlighted by attention, irrespective of the kinds of attention (self/cross attention) and attention mechanism (Q/K/V matrix). ML practitioners create this kind of diagram or image that helps a machine-learning model.

   Explainability, on the other hand, explains a decision in a clear and coherent manner [37]. This transparency enables end-users to trust the explanation of the model's decision making. These techniques help increase user confidence in the model. For example, techniques for explainability include local explanations that specifically explain the decision for a particular image and also help to maintain a simple model architecture and decision-making process in medical AI by keeping it transparent. Generative AI is an important tool for achieving both interpretability and explainability; however, it is a challenge to maintain model complexity as a trade-off for these two attributes. Nonetheless, these techniques are important for helping medical AI achieve trust from users to understand its decisions.

B. **Drug Discovery and Development:** The process of developing drugs consists in taking the compound through different steps before bringing the new therapy to market and is thus characterised by its complexity, prolonged time-frame, cost, and low success rate. Furthermore, there is high demand for new molecular structures, and GAI can lend a helping hand in their De-Novo design, coming up with never before thought-of compounds, optimising candidates for drug candidates, and even predicting what properties the investigated drug will possess. While GAI already has 1D and 2D data modelling capabilities, its most recent evolution managed to model 3D molecules as well, adding even more possibilities for constructing new molecules never before observed and identified. Higher IS scores indicate that the generated molecules by the generative model are both reliably classifiable and well distributed within the chemical space spanned by the training set.39

Because predicting protein function remains a bottleneck in accelerating further development of drugs, a lot of effort has gone into developing and improving methods in this space through various flavours of machine learning techniques in the past few years. Most of these methods, however, approach this task as a multiclassification problem, while t2Text adopts a radically different approach using free-text style outputs. Method decisions no longer rely on one or a few predetermined categories of outputs (similar to a binary classification) but let the model completely decide the nature and form of its output while retaining citations, quotes, and findings through clever exploitation of a so-called encoder-decoder framework based on a fusion of graph neural networks (GNNs) and a large language model [38]. Unlike most models that use natural language, these models can make sense of not only textual annotations but also fuse other data types such as protein sequences and structures for improving representations, which enables the generation of rich, high-fidelity descriptions of protein functions. To assess Prot2Text's performance, we created a multimodal protein dataset from SwissProt databases and then evaluated their efficacies with empirical analysis. Our results reveal that the multimodal models and especially the fusion of GNNs and LLMs are a real game-changer when it comes to very precise determination of protein function—a crucial ingredient to accelerate drug development.

Another way in which generative AI helps in drug design is to elucidate the structure-activity relationship (SAR) of molecules by generating a wide range of molecules and determining how their activity is related to their structure in order to identify the types of chemical features required for interaction with a drug target. Moreover, generative AI can reveal common chemical transformations that can be used in hybridisation to synthesise new molecules with different cores while retaining important pharmacophoric features, a process called scaffold-hopping [39].

C. **Personalised Patient Treatment:** In conventional machine learning, personalised patient treatment is an extension of basic predictive modelling that depends on only a handful of variables. However, it is a giant leap for humans and machines to generate patient treatment, especially personalised triage, by adjusting the values of several specific conditions related to the patient. The use of generative AI has progressed from basic predictive modelling to incorporating specific conditions for personalised treatment. An example of generative artificial intelligence applied to medicine is the conditional variational autoencoder (CVAE), which is a modified form of variational autoencoder that incorporates conditional variables in order to learn latent patient information and personalised information that is specific to each condition [40]. By fine-tuning a bidirectional encoder representation from transformers (BERT) model, the generative AI model generates personalised treatment summaries and adaptive plans for both physicians and patients.

11.6 HEALTHCARE-CUSTOMISED LARGE LANGUAGE MODELS

There are machine learning models, specifically deep learning models, known as large language models, general AI models, or paraphrasing models, that are equipped to recognise and generate human-sounding text. These machine learning models essentially employ deep learning techniques that are built around networks (layers) of neuron-like processors (called 'units') to 'learn' to process and understand text to respond with culturally coherent and contextually relevant text. Like BMW cars being designed to be better in their class, these large-language models are being trained to be the best models to simulate human–AI interactions within various healthcare niches where language understanding and generation are the key requisites. This section highlights some emblematic GAI models designed for the healthcare space.

A. **Med-PaLM**
Med-PaLM is an LLM trained on a wide variety of medical literature, electronic health records, academic publications, and other medical data used to respond to general medical questions. Unlike other LLMs trained on general literature, Med-PaLM is specifically designed to write back on queries that relate to the medical and healthcare sectors. Med-PaLM [40] trains exclusively on medical texts and has robust understanding of medical terminologies and complex biomedical concepts in order to generate medically relevant insights or comments. On the MDEI endpoint, Med-PaLM [41] demonstrated its ability to faithfully reproduce long-form answers to consumer health questions, finding the best quality and most relevant responses for users and paediatrician panel tests, scoring higher compared with other LLMs [41]. It is trained on a broad range of medical literature, electronic health records, and other clinical records that extend the knowledge domain of other tech giants. Med-PaLM was designed for downstream healthcare applications that include medical documentation, electronic health records, education, research, and information retrieval. Med-PaLM [42] can help biomedical and healthcare researchers to tackle great challenges in knowledge extraction, text summarisation, and paraphrasing. This can significantly increase efficiency and accuracy of knowledge retrieval, especially in medical document-based research. A more recent version known as Med-PaLM 2 showed a 18% improvement in accuracy when compared to Med-PaLM. Google recently announced the advanced health capability of Med-PaLM 2, which showed 86.5% accuracy on the United States Medical Licensing Examination (USMLE) questions—reaching the same level of medicine subject competence as 'expert' test takers. While testing the performance of Med-PaLM relative to other medical models, Med-PaLM 2 outperformed the 60% passing grade required for the examination.

B. **BioGPT:** BioGPT [43] is a domain-specific pre-trained transformer language model designed for generating and paraphrasing biomedical texts. Based on 15 million PubMed abstracts and trained from scratch, this model follows the GPT-2 framework for transformer language models. Its pre-trained scoring function allows it to perform well on various tasks, including providing evidence, text retrieval, and paraphrasing tasks. Focused on the biomedical domain, BioGPT is aimed at researchers, clinicians, and scientists who could potentially benefit from poetry-generated texts for literature reviews, drug discovery, protein modelling, and use of biomedical data. BioGPT-Large achieved 81% accuracy, an all-time record in the computational comprehension of biology that far exceeds single human annotations (66%) and also most other NLP tools, including the BERT models created by Google. BioGPT has the potential for transformative impact on the fields of biomedicine and bioinformatics, among others. It can greatly help in improving personalised medicine and in drug discovery. It can also be applied to protein modelling and bioinformatics research and analysis, as well as in literature reviews and academic support. But it can also help in generating contraptions that can provide medical care, as well as in a wide variety of educational contexts. BioGPT can be used in many different kinds of scientific research, as well as in medicine and in education. It is particularly convenient for literature reviews and research, helping scientists to efficiently locate information relevant to their research interest. It can quickly highlight details hidden in impressive volumes of biomedical literature, including by identifying relevant passages in the literature and guiding researchers to them (e.g., Cantor et al. 2022). Moreover, researchers can use BioGPT to rapidly summarise articles, extract their key findings, and discover relations between studies, further contributing to avoiding research redundancy and improving their overall productivity. In bioinformatics research, it can support protein-engineering processes, such as domain identification, protein–protein interactions, and protein structure predictions. Finally, by integrating different biological databases and knowledge resources, BioGPT can help researchers understand how genes act or intertwine with one another and networks and ultimately help them to interpret and analyse the biological data.

C. **IBM Watson for Oncology:** The GAI-powered IBM Watson for Oncology system [8] is designed to help oncologists to make decisions on treatment strategies for cancer patients based on natural language processing, machine learning, and big data analytics. Oncologists can ask Watson for Oncology questions about specific cases, and Watson will process and understand unstructured clinical material in order to find answers in relevant medical literature, identify common patient data patterns, and make evidence-based treatment suggestions.

In the context of healthcare, oncologists often use Watson for Oncology as a decision support tool, which can be integrated with EHRs and other types of medical data to analyse the patient's data, such as the patient's medical history, test results, pathology reports, and treatment recommendations [9]. The system then compares the data against the knowledge base that consists of millions of academic papers, clinical trials, treatment protocols, and medical textbooks [9]. Based on the patient's information, the system can provide personalised recommendations or comments related to each patient. For instance, the patient's vitals and radiology reports can be entered into the system, and Watson for Oncology will then generate four potential lines of treatment by utilising its large amount of clinical information and suggest the best suitable choice for each patient. According to experts, one of the biggest advantages of IBM Watson for Oncology is that it can provide access to expert knowledge. Oncologists in turn can obtain more clinical information and medical literature than before, such as 'Top 100 Things Every Oncologist Should Know'—an article that systematically demonstrates key information of cancer care. Moreover, oncologists can also be kept up to date on the latest research and clinical guidelines with evidence-based treatment options.

D. **Healthcare Language Models by NVIDIA Clara:** The NVIDIA Clara platform is a collection of engineering tools, applications, and frameworks designed to provide a comprehensive, integrated solution for healthcare applications, where it develops different types of healthcare language models trained on medical natural language content to make clinical natural language processing and decision-making easier. Here are some prominent examples: 49. NVIDIA Clara healthcare language models are based on deep-learning systems (now in its third generation, Clara AI is based on the ResNet 50 transformer neural network architecture, R3fPArT model, with different model weights for different applications, such as Clara Bio, Clara Insight, SeeingAI, OptaSense, etc.) trained on large volumes of medical text data, including electronic health records, medical literature, and clinical guidelines, to train models that can master complex language patterns, medical terms and terminology, and context typical of the healthcare domain and industry [44].

   Transformers learning architectures, such as the language models, are designed to deal with clinical entity recognition, medical concept normalisation, relation extraction and clinical text categorisation in healthcare. There are several applications of NVIDIA Clara healthcare language models. For example, they can extract and classify clinical entities (diagnosis, drugs, procedures, test findings, etc.) from clinical literature. This allows for clinical decision support, better clinical documentation, and accelerated medical coding.

   The models can also be beneficial for personalised medicine. The models can comprehend the nuances and clinical narratives unique to individual patients and extract clinically pertinent features or trends that clinicians can use to support a personalised treatment decision. These models can provide support in treatment selection, treatment outcome prediction, and precision medicine approaches. NVIDIA Clara's healthcare language models introduce state-of-the-art NLP in modern health care settings. [44] NVIDIA Clara's healthcare language models can understand and decode medical text data, add value and efficiency, and support clinical decision-making in multiple healthcare settings.

11.7 LIMITATIONS OF USING GAI IN HEALTHCARE

Many believe there is huge potential for generative AI to make big changes in healthcare by working as a real alternative to more traditional methods.

However, as well as its substantial advantages, there are also some issues with generative AI. For example, the same bias in samples that AI thrives on and inherently learns from can also pose challenges.

Recognising these issues and limitations is very important when it comes to the development of this technology, especially in the healthcare industry.

A. **Attribution Problem:** The ability for GAI models to both generate healthcare data and make judgments or output related to patient care is the same attribution problem described previously. However, in the healthcare setting, this attribution problem—providing reasons or justification for judgments or outputs—is critical from both a responsibility and efficacy standpoint [31]. One such challenge is evident in AI-generated music (such as through Remix AI) where the fundamental problem of attribution arises. The concept of attribution plays a significant role in both producing music and making healthcare decisions. It is very difficult to know and give credit to decisions being made because very often generative AI models (especially deep learning, the most popular deep neural networks) are black boxes. When you give input data for a deep learning model, it will produce a sensible, complex, and realistic output record, medical image, or treatment recommendation, but you will not know how or why it decided on that particular output if you do not look at the code at all. Does the attribution problem worsen, just like the interpretability challenge? If that is the case, then it poses a serious threat to healthcare delivery [31]. Healthcare delivery is a complex system that requires a person to take an action that advises or provides support for a patient's care and monitoring. Unlike regular classification tasks, such as detecting pictures of tomatoes in a pool of pictures, the application of GAI models generating judgments or output in the healthcare setting is not that clear yet. However, transferring learning from applications in music is still possible, especially concerning how the attribution problem relates to the practical challenges that might manifest in delivering healthcare.

B. **Data Quality and Bias:** One fundamental problem with GAI is the quality and bias of training data. GAI frameworks produce outputs that depend on healthcare records and medical literature as training data; if this data is biased or poor quality, that's what the output will be. Data can become biased at different stages of development—when demographic differences occur, if practices differ in different parts of the world, or if certain groups are underrepresented in the data. GAI models can pick up and teach these biases, leading to perpetuating healthcare discrimination and treatment disparities. Many public deployments of GAI have not considered bias, instead collecting data from the internet without sufficient attention to possible sources of misinformation or bias or where the training data is based on information from unreliable sources.

Responses generated by LLM-powered chatbots could give the impression of creativity, but they simply reflect the model's ability to analyse sequences of words that it has seen in its training data. They don't understand the language they use (and produce) in any real sense. Models trained on unfiltered internet data (such as ChatGPT or stable diffusion models) have imbibed as much inaccurate as factual information, as much bigoted as unbiased content, as much harmful as harmless material. LLMs risk copying, amplifying, and disseminating all manner of poor-quality content and misinformation, without there being any check of these characteristics before it generates the response.

C. **Patient Data Privacy:** The information is extremely important to protect, when collecting patient data through ambient sensors installed in healthcare treatment, the data would contain names, age, area from a home, medical history, etc. Data depends on the type of hardware. It may contain patient voice, face, or heart rate data. If the data is leaked possibly patients' health status and other privacy data would be disclosed.

Moreover, a large number of patients receive treatment at home or at sites where healthcare is delivered outside formal inpatient settings, and the use or presence of sensors and other devices that are typical of AI-augmented therapy are sometimes implicitly or explicitly presumed to be absent or inactive, as happened with one healthcare provider and patient during a treatment session in Carna's home: The participant's use of the restroom may have provided an opportunity to reflect on her work situation. For instance, one participant expressed a desire to keep her pill-taking data private during treatment, as she wished to maintain control over disclosing emotional challenges related to using specific treatments or experiencing difficulties in adhering to the prescribed medication regimen. There are fundamental aspects of decisional privacy that GAI models must adhere to [45]. They must give patients control over their privacy and afford them discretion over the information they wish to share.

This is governed in new ways in the US by the Health Insurance Portability and Accountability Act (HIPAA). For instance, data protection is regulated to secure patient privacy. Adversarial attacks (in which a malicious hacker tries to access or alter the asset that the model distributes) [4] are a concern for generative AI models. Countersecurity via an intrusion detection system, encryption, and authentication (among other things) prevents these vulnerabilities. This is important.

11.8 CONCLUSION

AI is revolutionising the medical sector by providing innovative tools for treating patients. Generative AI saves valuable time for medical staff, allowing them to prioritise the treatment of patients. New medical equipment developments are always emerging, evolving to fulfil the demands of medical organisations, and expediting personalised medication. Generative AI improves diagnosis precision and generates artificial info for analysis, paving the way for significant advances in the healthcare business. In this chapter, we have discussed issues associated with implementing generative AI in healthcare, including patient data privacy, data quality and bias, and the attribution problem. Despite these challenges, generative AI models are driving significant advancements in the healthcare industry, offering faster disease diagnosis and greater accuracy in medication, ultimately facilitating quicker patient recovery. The applications of generative AI highlight the flexibility of these technologies and the reliability demonstrated by their accurate results. In the coming years, we anticipate the development of more models and their broader implementation in the healthcare sector.

REFERENCES

1. Baidoo-Anu D, Ansah LO. Education in the era of generative artificial intelligence (AI): Understanding the potential benefits of ChatGPT in promoting teaching and learning. *Journal of AI*. 2023 Dec;7(1):52–62.
2. Pavlik JV. Collaborating with ChatGPT: Considering the implications of generative artificial intelligence for journalism and media education. *Journalism & Mass Communication Educator*. 2023 Mar;78(1):84–93.
3. Mondal S, Das S, Vrana VG. How to bell the cat? A theoretical review of generative artificial intelligence towards digital disruption in all walks of life. *Technologies*. 2023 Mar 17;11(2):44.
4. Deng J, Lin Y. The benefits and challenges of ChatGPT: An overview. *Frontiers in Computing and Intelligent Systems*. 2022;2(2):81–83.
5. Korngiebel DM, Mooney SD. Considering the possibilities and pitfalls of generative pre-trained transformer 3 (GPT-3) in healthcare delivery. *NPJ Digital Medicine*. 2021 Jun 3;4(1):93.
6. Arora A, Arora A. Generative adversarial networks and synthetic patient data: Current challenges and future perspectives. *Future Healthcare Journal*. 2022 Jul 1;9(2):190–3.
7. Gupta U, Pranav A, Kohli A, Ghosh S, Singh D. The contribution of artificial intelligence to drug discovery: Current progress and prospects for the future. *Microbial Data Intelligence and Computational Techniques for Sustainable Computing*. 2024:1–23.
8. Gupta D, Gupta U, Sarma HJ. Functional iterative approach for Universum-based primal twin bounded support vector machine to EEG classification (FUPTBSVM). *Multimedia Tools and Applications*. 2024;83(8):22119–51.
9. Gupta U, Jain V. Social neuroscience: Inferring mental states in social media. *Emotional AI and Human-AI Interactions in Social Networking*. 2024:15–39.
10. Sharma M, Deswal S, Gupta U, Tabassum M, Lawal I eds. *Soft Computing Techniques in Connected Healthcare Systems*. CRC Press, 2023.
11. Malik K, Sadawarti H, Sharma M, Gupta U, Tiwari P eds. *Computational Techniques in Neuroscience*. CRC Press, 2023.
12. Aydın Ö, Karaarslan E. OpenAI ChatGPT generated literature review: Digital twin in healthcare. In Ö Aydın (Ed.), *Emerging Computer Technologies* (Vol. 2, pp. 22–31). Elsevier, 2022 Dec 21.
13. Singh D, Singh D, Manju, Gupta U. Smart healthcare: A breakthrough in the growth of technologies. In *Artificial Intelligence-Based Healthcare Systems* (pp. 73–85). Cham, Switzerland: Springer Nature, 2023.

14. Liu S, Wright AP, Patterson BL, Wanderer JP, Turer RW, Nelson SD, McCoy AB, Sittig DF, Wright A. Using AI-generated suggestions from ChatGPT to optimize clinical decision support. *Journal of the American Medical Informatics Association*. 2023 Jul 1;30(7):1237–45.
15. Lecler A, Duron L, Soyer P. Revolutionizing radiology with GPT-based models: Current applications, future possibilities and limitations of ChatGPT. *Diagnostic and Interventional Imaging*. 2023 Jun 1;104(6):269–74.
16. Savage N. Drug discovery companies are customizing ChatGPT: Here's how. *Nature Biotechnology*. 2023 May 1;41(5):585–6.
17. Eysenbach G. The role of ChatGPT, generative language models, and artificial intelligence in medical education: A conversation with ChatGPT and a call for papers. *JMIR Medical Education*. 2023 Mar 6;9(1):e46885.
18. Gupta M, Srivastava D, Pantola D, Gupta U. Brain tumor detection using improved Otsu's thresholding method and supervised learning techniques at early stage. In *Proceedings of Emerging Trends and Technologies on Intelligent Systems: ETTIS 2022* (pp. 271–81). Singapore: Springer Nature, 2022.
19. Sallam M. ChatGPT utility in healthcare education, research, and practice: Systematic review on the promising perspectives and valid concerns. *InHealthcare*. 2023 Mar 19;11(6):887. MDPI.
20. Gupta U, Gupta D, Agarwal U. Analysis of randomization-based approaches for autism spectrum disorder. In *Pattern Recognition and Data Analysis with Applications* (pp. 701–13). Singapore: Springer Nature, 2022.
21. Vaswani A, Shazeer N, Parmar N, Uszkoreit J, Jones L, Gomez AN, Kaiser Ł, Polosukhin I. Attention is all you need. *Advances in Neural Information Processing Systems*. 2017;30.
22. VanBuskirk A. *A Brief History of the Generative Pre-Trained Transformer (GPT) Language Models*. WordBot (blog). 2023 Mar;31.
23. O'Laughlin D. *AI Foundations Part 1: Transformers, Pre-Training and Fine-Tuning, and Scaling*, 2023 Apr 11. https://www.fabricatedknowledge.com/p/ai-foundations-part-1-transformers
24. Dale R. GPT-3: What's it good for? *Natural Language Engineering*. 2021 Jan;27(1):113–8.
25. Gupta D, Choudhury A, Gupta U, Singh P, Prasad M. Computational approach to clinical diagnosis of diabetes disease: A comparative study. *Multimedia Tools and Applications*. 2021:1–26.
26. Longoni C, Fradkin A, Cian L, Pennycook G. News from generative artificial intelligence is believed less. In Proceedings of the 2022 ACM Conference on Fairness, Accountability, and Transparency, 2022 Jun 21 (pp. 97–106).
27. Gupta D, Gupta U. On robust asymmetric Lagrangian ν-twin support vector regression using pinball loss function. *Applied Soft Computing*. 2021;102:107099.
28. Xue VW, Lei P, Cho WC. The potential impact of ChatGPT in clinical and translational medicine. *Clinical and Translational Medicine*. 2023 Mar;13(3).
29. Floridi L, Chiriatti M. GPT-3: Its nature, scope, limits, and consequences. *Minds and Machines*. 2020 Dec;30:681–94.
30. Marcus G, Davis E, Aaronson S. A very preliminary analysis of DALL-E 2. *arXiv preprint* arXiv:2204.13807. 2022 Apr 25.
31. Sai S, Gaur A, Sai R, Chamola V, Guizani M, Rodrigues JJ. Generative ai for transformative healthcare: A comprehensive study of emerging models, applications, case studies and limitations. *IEEE Access*. 2024 Feb 20;12:31078–31106. https://doi.org/10.1109/ACCESS.2024.3367715
32. Zhang J, Peng Y, Yuan M. Unsupervised generative adversarial cross-modal hashing. *Proceedings of the AAAI Conference on Artificial Intelligence*. 2018 Apr 25;32(1).

33. Temsah O, Khan SA, Chaiah Y, Senjab A, Alhasan K, Jamal A, Aljamaan F, Malki KH, Halwani R, Al-Tawfiq JA, Temsah MH. Overview of early ChatGPT's presence in medical literature: Insights from a hybrid literature review by ChatGPT and human experts. *Cureus.* 2023 Apr;15(4).
34. Yang Y, Fu H, Aviles-Rivero AI, Schönlieb CB, Zhu L. Diffmic: Dual-guidance diffusion network for medical image classification. In *International Conference on Medical Image Computing and Computer-Assisted Intervention* (pp. 95–105). Cham, Switzerland: Springer Nature, 2023 Oct 1.
35. Bing X, Zhang W, Zheng L, Zhang Y. Medical image super resolution using improved generative adversarial networks. *IEEE Access.* 2019 Oct 1;7:145030–8.
36. Susnjak T. Beyond predictive learning analytics modelling and onto explainable artificial intelligence with prescriptive analytics and ChatGPT. *International Journal of Artificial Intelligence in Education.* 2024 Jun;34(2):452–82.
37. Molnar C, Casalicchio G, Bischl B. Interpretable machine learning–a brief history, state-of-the-art and challenges. In *Joint European Conference on Machine Learning and Knowledge Discovery in Databases* (pp. 417–31). Cham: Springer International Publishing, 2020 Sep 14.
38. Salimans T, Goodfellow I, Zaremba W, Cheung V, Radford A, Chen X. Improved techniques for training gans. *Advances in Neural Information Processing Systems.* 2016;29.
39. Abdine H, Chatzianastasis M, Bouyioukos C, Vazirgiannis M. Prot2text: Multimodal protein's function generation with gnns and transformers. *Proceedings of the AAAI Conference on Artificial Intelligence.* 2024 Mar 24;38(10):10757–65.
40. Singhal K, Azizi S, Tu T, Mahdavi SS, Wei J, Chung HW, Scales N, Tanwani A, Cole-Lewis H, Pfohl S, Payne P. Large language models encode clinical knowledge. *arXiv preprint* arXiv:2212.13138. 2022 Dec 26.
41. Singhal K, Tu T, Gottweis J, Sayres R, Wulczyn E, Hou L, Clark K, Pfohl S, Cole-Lewis H, Neal D, Schaekermann M. Towards expert-level medical question answering with large language models. *arXiv preprint* arXiv:2305.09617. 2023 May 16.
42. Bair H, Norden J. Large language models and their implications on medical education. *Academic Medicine.* 2023 Aug 1;98(8):869–70.
43. Luo R, Sun L, Xia Y, Qin T, Zhang S, Poon H, Liu TY. BioGPT: Generative pre-trained transformer for biomedical text generation and mining. *Briefings in Bioinformatics.* 2022 Nov;23(6):bbac409.
44. Grover DV, Ahmad N, Fatima MI, Alam M, Khan DIR. Real-world applications of generative AI for data augmentation. In DV Grover, DBB Balusamy, DM Milanova, and DAY Felix (Eds.), *Blockchain, IoT, and AI Technologies for Supply Chain Management.* Berkeley, CA: Apress, 2024. https://doi.org/10.1007/979-8-8688-0315-4_15.
45. Allen AL. Coercing privacy. *William & Mary Law Review.* 1998;40:723.

12 Unlocking Healthcare's Potential with Natural Language Processing

Ketan Sarvakar

12.1 INTRODUCTION

The healthcare industry generates vast amounts of unstructured data in the form of clinical notes, medical reports, and patient narratives. Extracting meaningful information from this data has traditionally been a labor-intensive and error-prone process. Natural language processing (NLP), a branch of artificial intelligence, offers a powerful solution by enabling machines to understand, interpret, and generate human language data. This chapter explores the transformative role of NLP in various healthcare applications, highlighting its potential to revolutionize patient care, clinical decision-making, and operational efficiency.

12.1.1 Overview of Natural Language Processing

Natural language processing is a subfield of artificial intelligence (AI) (Gupta & Gupta, 2019) that focuses on the interaction between computers and human language. It enables machines to understand, interpret, and generate natural language in a way that is akin to human comprehension. NLP encompasses a broad range of tasks, including speech recognition, language translation, sentiment analysis, and text summarization.

Key Components of NLP:

12.1.1.1 Tokenization

In the healthcare sector, tokenization plays a crucial role in various applications, including clinical documentation, medical research, and patient data analysis. Let's consider an example of how tokenization is utilized in clinical documentation:

> The process of breaking down text into smaller units, such as words or phrases, for analysis and processing.

Example: Electronic Health Record Documentation

In a hospital, healthcare providers regularly document patient encounters, medical histories, and treatment plans in electronic health records (EHRs). These records contain vast amounts of textual data that need to be processed and analyzed for various purposes, such as billing, research, and patient care.

DOI: 10.1201/9781003539483-12

Tokenization is employed to break down the text within EHRs into smaller units, such as words or phrases, to facilitate analysis and processing. Here's how tokenization works in this context:

a. **Text Extraction:** Suppose a physician documents a patient's medical history, including details about their allergies, medications, and past surgeries, in the EHR system. The physician's notes may contain sentences like:

No.	Sentence Text
1	"Patient has a known allergy to penicillin."
2	"Currently taking medications for hypertension."
3	"Underwent appendectomy in 2018."

b. **Tokenization Process:** To analyze this text, the EHR system applies tokenization, breaking down each sentence into individual tokens or units. For instance:

No.	Sentence Text	Tokens
1	"Patient has a known allergy to penicillin."	["Patient", "has", "a", "known", "allergy", "to", "penicillin", "."]
2	"Currently taking medications for hypertension."	["Currently", "taking", "medications", "for", "hypertension", "."]
3	"Underwent appendectomy in 2024."	["Underwent", "appendectomy", "in", "2024", "."]

c. **Analysis and Processing:** Once the text is tokenized, the EHR system can perform various analyses and processing tasks. For instance:
   i. **Information Retrieval:** Tokenization enables efficient retrieval of specific information from the EHR, for instance, searching for all instances where a patient has mentioned allergies to certain medications.
   ii. **Data Mining:** Tokenized text can be analyzed to identify patterns, trends, or associations within the patient data, for instance, identifying common medications prescribed for patients with a particular medical condition (Gupta & Gupta, 2021).
   iii. **Clinical Decision Support:** Tokenized text can be used to generate alerts or recommendations for healthcare providers based on specific keywords or phrases found in the EHR, for instance, alerting the physician if a patient with a penicillin allergy is prescribed a medication containing penicillin.

By breaking down text into smaller units through tokenization, healthcare organizations can efficiently analyze and process vast amounts of textual data within EHRs, leading to improved patient care, streamlined workflows, and better clinical outcomes.

12.1.1.2 Part-of-Speech Tagging

Assigning grammatical categories (e.g., noun, verb, adjective) to words in a sentence to understand their syntactic roles.

Example: Clinical Note Analysis

In a hospital, healthcare providers regularly document patient encounters, medical histories, and treatment plans in electronic health records. These clinical notes contain valuable information about the patient's condition, symptoms, diagnoses, and treatment.

Part-of-speech (POS) tagging is employed to analyze the text within clinical notes and assign grammatical categories (e.g., noun, verb, adjective) to words in a sentence to understand their syntactic roles. Here's how POS tagging works in this context:

a. **Text Extraction:** Suppose a physician documents a patient's symptoms and treatment plan in a clinical note. The note may contain sentences like:

No.	Sentence Text
1	"Patient presents with persistent cough and shortness of breath."
2	"Prescribed antibiotics and advised bed rest."

b. **POS Tagging Process:** To analyze this text, the EHR system applies POS tagging, assigning grammatical categories to each word in the sentences. For instance:

No.	Sentence Text	POS Tags
1	"Patient presents with persistent cough and shortness of breath."	"Patient" (Noun) "presents" (Verb) "with" (Preposition) "persistent" (Adjective) "cough" (Noun) "and" (Conjunction) "shortness" (Noun) "of" (Preposition) "breath" (Noun) "." (Punctuation)
2	"Prescribed antibiotics and advised bed rest."	"Prescribed" (Verb) "antibiotics" (Noun) "and" (Conjunction) "advised" (Verb) "bed" (Noun) "rest" (Noun) "." (Punctuation)

c. **Syntactic Analysis:** Once the text is POS tagged, the EHR system can perform syntactic analysis to understand the structure and relationships within the sentences. For instance:
   i. **Identifying Actions:** POS tagging helps identify verbs, indicating actions taken by the healthcare provider. In the example, "presents," "prescribed," and "advised" are verbs indicating actions related to the patient's condition and treatment.
   ii. **Describing Symptoms:** POS tagging helps identify adjectives and nouns describing the patient's symptoms. In the example, "persistent," "cough," "shortness," and "breath" are nouns and adjectives describing the patient's symptoms.
   iii. **Prescription Details:** POS tagging helps identify medications prescribed to the patient. In the example, "antibiotics" is a noun indicating the prescribed medication.

By applying POS tagging to clinical notes, healthcare providers and researchers can gain insights into the patient's condition, treatment plan, and clinical outcomes. This information can inform decision-making, improve patient care, and facilitate medical research and analysis.

12.1.1.3 Named Entity Recognition

Identifying and categorizing named entities such as people, organizations, and locations mentioned in text.

In the healthcare sector, named entity recognition (NER) plays a critical role in various applications, including clinical documentation, patient data analysis, and medical research. It's employed to automatically identify and categorize named entities such as people, organizations, and locations mentioned in the text of EHRs. Here's how NER works in this context. Let's consider an example of how NER is utilized in clinical notes:

Example: Electronic Health Record Analysis

Electronic health records contain a wealth of information, including mentions of patients, healthcare providers, medical facilities, and geographic locations.

a. **Text Extraction:** Suppose a physician documents a patient's medical history and recent hospital visit in an EHR. The record may contain sentences like:

No.	Sentence Text
1	"Mr. John Smith, a 45-year-old male, was admitted to XYZ Hospital with chest pain."
2	"Dr. Emily Johnson, the attending physician, ordered a series of tests for Mr. Smith."

b. **NER Process:** To analyze this text, the EHR system applies named entity recognition, identifying and categorizing named entities mentioned in the sentences. For instance:

No.	Sentence Text	Named Entities
1	"Mr. John Smith, a 45-year-old male, was admitted to XYZ Hospital with chest pain."	"Mr. John Smith" (Person) "XYZ Hospital" (Organization) "chest pain" (Medical Condition)
2	"Dr. Emily Johnson, the attending physician, ordered a series of tests for Mr. Smith."	"Dr. Emily Johnson" (Person) "Mr. Smith" (Person)

c. **Categorization and Analysis:** Once the named entities are identified, the EHR system can categorize and analyze them to extract valuable information. For instance:
   i. **Patient Identification:** NER helps identify and extract patient names and demographic information from clinical notes. In the example, "Mr. John Smith" is identified as the patient, along with his age and gender.
   ii. **Healthcare Providers:** NER identifies healthcare providers mentioned in the notes, such as attending physicians, specialists, or nurses. In the example, "Dr. Emily Johnson" is identified as the attending physician.
   iii. **Hospital and Facility Names:** NER recognizes the names of hospitals, clinics, and medical facilities mentioned in the text. In the example, "XYZ Hospital" is identified as the facility where the patient was admitted.

By applying named entity recognition to EHRs, healthcare organizations can automate the extraction of key information, streamline administrative processes, and improve data analysis. This information can inform clinical decision-making, enhance patient care, and facilitate medical research and population health management initiatives.

12.1.1.4 Syntax Analysis

Analyzing the grammatical structure of sentences to understand their meaning and relationships.

In the healthcare sector, syntax analysis plays a vital role in various applications, including clinical documentation, medical research, and natural language processing tasks. Let's consider an example of how syntax analysis is utilized in clinical notes:

Example: Clinical Note Interpretation

In a hospital, clinical notes contain detailed information about the patient's condition, symptoms, diagnoses, and treatment. So, syntax analysis is employed to analyze the grammatical structure of sentences within clinical notes to understand their meaning and relationships. Here's how syntax analysis works in this context:

a. **Text Extraction:** Suppose a physician documents a patient's medical history and treatment plan in a clinical note. The note may contain sentences like:

No.	Sentence Text
1	"The patient was prescribed antibiotics due to a bacterial infection."
2	"After completing the course of medication, the patient's symptoms improved significantly."

b. **Syntax Analysis Process:** To analyze this text, the EHR system applies syntax analysis, examining the grammatical structure of sentences to understand their meaning and relationships. For example:

No.	Sentence Text	Syntax Analysis
1	"The patient was prescribed antibiotics due to a bacterial infection."	Subject: "The patient" Verb: "was prescribed" Object: "antibiotics" Reason/Modifier: "due to a bacterial infection"
2	"After completing the course of medication, the patient's symptoms improved significantly."	Connector: "After completing" Action: "the patient's symptoms improved significantly" Context: "the course of medication"

c. **Interpretation and Relationship Understanding:** Once the syntax of the sentences is analyzed, the EHR system can interpret the meaning and relationships within the text. For instance:
   i. **Medication Prescription:** Syntax analysis helps identify the subject ("The patient"), action ("was prescribed"), and object ("antibiotics") in the sentence, indicating that the patient received a prescription for antibiotics.
   ii. **Treatment Outcome:** Syntax analysis identifies the temporal relationship ("After completing") between the completion of medication and the improvement in the patient's symptoms, indicating a cause-and-effect relationship between the two events.
   iii. **Clinical Decision-Making:** Syntax analysis aids healthcare providers in understanding the patient's condition, treatment plan, and response to therapy, facilitating clinical decision-making and patient management.

By applying syntax analysis to clinical notes, healthcare organizations can gain deeper insights into the patient's condition, treatment trajectory, and clinical outcomes. This information can inform decision-making, improve patient care, and facilitate medical research and analysis.

12.1.1.5 Semantic Analysis

Understanding the meaning of words and phrases in context to derive their intended interpretations.

In the healthcare sector, semantic analysis plays a crucial role in various applications, including clinical decision support, medical research, and patient data analysis. Let's consider an example of how semantic analysis is utilized in clinical scenarios:

Example: Clinical Decision Support System

Imagine a clinical decision support system (CDSS) used by healthcare providers to assist in diagnosing and treating patients. This CDSS incorporates semantic analysis to understand the meaning of medical terms and patient data in context to derive their intended interpretations.

For instance: A patient present with symptoms of chest pain and shortness of breath. The physician suspects a possible cardiac condition and orders diagnostic tests.

a. **Symptom Interpretation:** The CDSS performs semantic analysis to interpret the symptoms mentioned by the physician. It understands that "chest pain" and "shortness of breath" are indicative of potential cardiovascular issues based on their semantic meaning and medical context.
b. **Diagnostic Test Selection:** Based on the interpreted symptoms, the CDSS recommends appropriate diagnostic tests for further evaluation. Semantic analysis helps the system understand the relevance of tests such as electrocardiogram (ECG), cardiac enzymes, and echocardiography in diagnosing cardiac conditions.
c. **Interpreting Test Results:** After the diagnostic tests are performed, the CDSS analyzes the results using semantic analysis to interpret their significance. For example, it understands that elevated cardiac enzymes and abnormal ECG findings may indicate myocardial infarction (heart attack) or other cardiac abnormalities.
d. **Treatment Recommendations:** Semantic analysis is utilized to generate treatment recommendations based on the interpreted symptoms and diagnostic findings. For instance, if the patient is diagnosed with a heart attack, the CDSS may recommend immediate intervention such as aspirin therapy, oxygen supplementation, and cardiac monitoring.

   Once we successfully process semantic analysis, then it beneficial for this sector in the following ways:

   i. **Improved Accuracy:** Semantic analysis enhances the accuracy of clinical decision-making by ensuring that medical terms and patient data are interpreted correctly in context.
   ii. **Personalized Recommendations:** By understanding the specific context of each patient's symptoms and medical history, semantic analysis enables the CDSS to provide personalized treatment recommendations tailored to individual patient needs.
   iii. **Efficient Data Processing:** Semantic analysis streamlines the processing of large volumes of patient data and medical literature, allowing the CDSS to quickly analyze and interpret relevant information to support clinical decision-making.
   iv. **Enhanced Patient Care:** With semantic analysis, healthcare providers can make well-informed decisions, leading to improved patient outcomes, reduced errors, and more efficient healthcare delivery.

In summary, semantic analysis is a critical component of clinical decision support systems in the healthcare sector. By understanding the meaning of medical terms and patient data in context, semantic analysis enables more accurate diagnosis, treatment, and patient management, ultimately enhancing the quality of care provided to patients.

Real-World Example: Consider the functionality of virtual assistants like Siri, Alexa, or Google Assistant. These systems utilize NLP algorithms to process spoken commands, understand natural language queries, and provide appropriate responses or actions.

12.1.2 Importance of NLP in Healthcare

The important roles of natural language processing in the healthcare sector:

a. **Clinical Documentation Automation:** NLP automates the extraction of information from clinical notes, reducing the time healthcare professionals spend on documentation tasks and improving accuracy.
b. **Clinical Decision Support:** NLP-powered systems analyze vast amounts of medical literature, patient data, and clinical guidelines to provide evidence-based recommendations and alerts for healthcare providers, leading to better-informed decision-making.
c. **Patient Data Analysis:** NLP algorithms analyze patient data from various sources such as electronic health records, imaging reports, and wearable devices to extract insights, detect patterns, and predict health outcomes.
d. **Medical Image Analysis:** NLP techniques analyze textual descriptions accompanying medical images (e.g., radiology reports) to extract diagnostic information, aiding in the interpretation of images and improving diagnostic accuracy.
e. **Drug Information Extraction:** NLP extracts and synthesizes information from medical literature, drug labels, and clinical trials to provide healthcare providers with up-to-date information on drug interactions, side effects, and treatment guidelines (Gupta et al., 2024).
f. **Healthcare Chatbots:** NLP-powered chatbots assist patients by answering questions, scheduling appointments, providing medication reminders, and offering personalized health advice, enhancing patient engagement and satisfaction.
g. **Public Health Surveillance:** NLP algorithms analyze textual data from sources such as social media, news reports, and public health records to detect disease outbreaks, monitor epidemiological trends, and inform public health interventions.
h. **Clinical Trial Matching:** NLP matches eligible patients with appropriate clinical trials by analyzing patient data and trial eligibility criteria, facilitating patient recruitment and accelerating medical research.
i. **Healthcare Fraud Detection:** NLP identifies suspicious patterns and anomalies in healthcare claims, billing records, and medical documentation to detect fraudulent activities and prevent healthcare fraud.

j. **Patient Experience Analysis:** NLP analyzes patient feedback, reviews, and satisfaction surveys to identify trends, sentiment, and areas for improvement in healthcare services, enabling healthcare organizations to enhance patient experience and quality of care.

12.1.3 Challenges and Opportunities

Despite its potential benefits, the widespread adoption of NLP in healthcare is accompanied by several challenges:

a. **Data Privacy and Security:** Healthcare data is highly sensitive and subject to strict privacy regulations. NLP systems must adhere to regulatory frameworks such as HIPAA to ensure patient confidentiality and data security.
b. **Interoperability:** Healthcare data is often fragmented across different systems and formats, posing challenges for data integration and interoperability. NLP tools need to be compatible with existing healthcare IT infrastructure to facilitate seamless data exchange and analysis.
c. **Bias and Fairness:** NLP algorithms can inadvertently perpetuate biases present in the training data, leading to disparities in healthcare outcomes. Ensuring fairness and equity in NLP models is essential to prevent algorithmic bias and promote equitable healthcare delivery.
d. **Data Quality and Accuracy:** The performance of NLP systems relies heavily on the quality and accuracy of the underlying data. Noisy or incomplete data can lead to errors in NLP output, compromising the reliability of clinical decision support systems and predictive models.
e. **Opportunities:** Despite these challenges, NLP offers numerous opportunities for innovation and improvement in healthcare:
f. **Advanced Clinical Decision Support:** NLP-powered clinical decision support systems can leverage advanced machine learning techniques to analyze complex medical data, support diagnostic reasoning, and optimize treatment strategies.
g. **Population Health Management:** NLP algorithms can analyze large-scale healthcare data to identify at-risk patient populations, predict disease progression, and develop targeted interventions for chronic disease management and preventive care.
h. **Healthcare Automation:** NLP-enabled chat bots and virtual assistants can automate routine administrative tasks such as appointment scheduling, medication reminders, and billing inquiries, improving operational efficiency and enhancing patient engagement.
i. **Precision Medicine:** NLP techniques can integrate genomic data, clinical notes, and patient records to personalize treatment plans based on individual genetic profiles, disease risk factors, and treatment responses, paving the way for precision medicine approaches.

12.2 LITERATURE REVIEW

12.2.1 Clinical Documentation and Information Extraction

Clinical documentation and information extraction are critical components of healthcare that have been significantly enhanced by natural language processing. By converting unstructured clinical notes into structured data, NLP facilitates better patient care, improves clinical workflows, and enables advanced research.

Clinical documentation and information extraction have evolved significantly with the advent of electronic health records. Early methods relied heavily on manual data entry, which was both time-consuming and prone to errors (Jha et al., 2009). With the introduction of EHRs, there has been a shift towards automating the extraction of structured and unstructured data, enhancing the accuracy and efficiency of clinical documentation (Meystre et al., 2008).

12.2.1.1 Automated Encoding of Clinical Documents

Friedman et al. (2004) discussed the potential of NLP to automatically encode clinical documents, emphasizing its ability to improve the accuracy and efficiency of clinical data entry. They highlighted that NLP systems could transform free-text notes into standardized codes, enhancing data usability for research and clinical decision-making (Friedman et al., 2004).

12.2.1.2 Extraction of Medication Information

Uzuner et al. (2010) demonstrated the application of NLP in extracting medication information from clinical texts. Their system successfully identified and categorized medications, dosages, and related information, which is crucial for patient safety and treatment efficacy (Uzuner et al., 2010).

12.2.1.3 Text Mining in Electronic Health Records

Dalianis (2018) provided an extensive review of clinical text mining, highlighting the secondary use of electronic patient records. The study illustrated various NLP techniques used to extract valuable insights from unstructured clinical data, which can be used for epidemiological studies and improving clinical guidelines (Dalianis, 2018).

12.2.1.4 Information Extraction for Cohort Identification

Liu et al. (2017) developed an information extraction framework using NLP to identify patient cohorts from electronic health records. This framework facilitated the identification of patients with specific conditions, enabling more targeted and efficient clinical research (Liu et al., 2017).

12.2.1.5 Clinical Text Analysis Systems

Savova et al. (2010) introduced the Mayo Clinical Text Analysis and Knowledge Extraction System (cTAKES), an open-source NLP system designed to extract structured information from clinical notes. cTAKES has been widely adopted for various clinical and research purposes due to its robustness and flexibility (Savova et al., 2010).

12.2.1.6 Diagnostic Information Extraction

Wang et al. (2013) explored clinical text mining for supporting diagnostic decision-making. Their approach demonstrated the potential of NLP to extract principal diagnoses, comorbidities, and other relevant clinical data, which significantly aids in diagnostic accuracy and clinical decision support (Wang et al., 2013).

Natural language processing techniques, such as tokenization, part-of-speech tagging, named entity recognition, and semantic parsing, play crucial roles in clinical documentation. Tokenization involves breaking down text into individual units like words and phrases, which are then categorized through part-of-speech tagging (Liu et al., 2012). NER identifies specific entities like medications, diseases, and patient demographics within clinical texts (Liu et al., 2017). Semantic parsing interprets the relationships and context within the text, providing deeper insights into the documented information (Zeng et al., 2006; Gupta & Gupta, 2022).

NLP has numerous applications in clinical documentation, from extracting patient information to coding diagnoses and treatments. For instance, NLP tools can extract relevant clinical information from physician notes, reducing the burden of manual documentation and improving the accuracy of patient records (Friedman et al., 2004; Uzuner et al., 2010). These systems can also support the automation of clinical coding, which is essential for billing and reimbursement processes (Liu et al., 2017).

Despite its benefits, implementing NLP in clinical documentation faces several challenges. The complexity and variability of clinical language, including the use of jargon and abbreviations, make it difficult to achieve consistent accuracy (Dalianis, 2018). Additionally, ensuring data privacy and security remains a critical concern, especially when handling sensitive patient information (Rosenbloom et al., 2011; Gupta & Gupta, 2023).

NLP has shown tremendous promise in clinical documentation and information extraction. By transforming unstructured text into structured data, NLP not only enhances the accuracy and efficiency of clinical documentation but also enables advanced research and better patient outcomes. Future research should focus on enhancing NLP algorithms to better handle the nuances of clinical language and improving the interoperability of NLP systems across different healthcare platforms. Addressing ethical and privacy concerns will also be crucial in the widespread adoption of these technologies (Topol, 2019).

12.2.2 Clinical Decision Support Systems

Clinical decision support systems play a pivotal role in modern healthcare by assisting clinicians in making informed decisions. NLP enhances CDSS by processing and interpreting vast amounts of unstructured clinical data, thereby improving the quality and efficiency of care.

Clinical decision support systems have progressed from simple, rule-based systems to advanced platforms integrating machine learning and NLP. Early CDSSs provided basic alerts and reminders based on predefined rules (Shortliffe & Cimino, 2013). Modern CDSSs leverage a variety of data sources, including patient records, clinical guidelines, and medical literature, to offer comprehensive diagnostic and therapeutic recommendations (Wright et al., 2011).

TABLE 12.1
Comparison of Clinical Documentation and Information Extraction

Reference	Key Points	Methodology	Findings	Challenges	Future Directions
Friedman et al. (2004)	Automated encoding of clinical documents	NLP for clinical data encoding	Improved accuracy and efficiency	Data standardization	Enhanced NLP algorithms for broader applications
Uzuner et al. (2010)	Extracting medication information	NLP system development	Accurate medication extraction	Handling diverse terminologies	Integration with clinical workflows
Dalianis (2018)	Clinical text mining	Literature review	Effective secondary use of EHR data	Data quality and consistency	Advanced NLP techniques for diverse datasets
Liu et al. (2017)	Information extraction for cohort identification	NLP framework development	Efficient cohort identification	Data privacy concerns	Privacy-preserving NLP frameworks
Savova et al. (2010)	cTAKES for clinical text analysis	System development and evaluation	Robust clinical text analysis	System scalability	Extending capabilities for various clinical domains
Wang et al. (2013)	Diagnostic information extraction	Practical NLP approach	Improved diagnostic decision support	Complexity of clinical narratives	Advanced NLP models for specific diagnoses

12.2.2.1 Ten Commandments for an Effective CDSS

Bates et al. (2003) outlined the "ten commandments" for effective CDSS implementation, emphasizing the importance of integration into clinical workflows and the use of evidence-based guidelines. These principles are essential for the successful adoption and effectiveness of CDSSs (Bates et al., 2003).

12.2.2.2 CDSS: Theory and Practice

Berner (2007) provided a comprehensive overview of the theoretical underpinnings and practical applications of CDSSs. The study emphasized the role of NLP in enhancing CDSSs by enabling the system to understand and process clinical language, thereby improving decision-making processes (Berner, 2007).

12.2.2.3 Systematic Review of CDSS Effects

Bright et al. (2012) conducted a systematic review to assess the impact of CDSSs on clinical practice. The review concluded that a CDSS generally improves practitioner performance and patient outcomes, although the effectiveness varies across different settings and implementations (Bright et al., 2012).

12.2.2.4 Improving Clinical Practice with CDSSs

Kawamoto et al. (2005) identified critical features for the success of CDSSs through a systematic review. These features include the provision of decision support at the time and location of decision-making and integration with clinical workflows. NLP plays a crucial role in enabling these features by interpreting clinical data in real time (Kawamoto et al., 2005).

12.2.2.5 CDSS Capabilities in Commercial Systems

Wright et al. (2011) evaluated the capabilities of commercially available CDSSs, highlighting the importance of NLP in enhancing system functionalities. The study found that advanced NLP techniques significantly improve the system's ability to handle complex clinical data (Wright et al., 2011).

NLP enhances CDSSs by enabling the extraction and interpretation of unstructured data from clinical notes, patient histories, and medical literature. This allows the CDSS to provide more accurate and timely clinical recommendations, improving the quality of care (Garg et al., 2005). For example, NLP can identify patterns in patient data that might indicate potential health risks or suggest optimal treatment plans (Berner, 2007). NLP-powered CDSSs can assist in various clinical scenarios, from diagnosing diseases to recommending treatment options. These systems can analyze patient data to provide diagnostic suggestions, highlight potential drug interactions, and offer evidence-based treatment recommendations (Kawamoto et al., 2005). For example, an NLP-enhanced CDSS might analyze a patient's symptoms and medical history to suggest a differential diagnosis, aiding clinicians in making more informed decisions (Wright et al., 2011).

Integrating NLP into CDSSs has been shown to improve patient outcomes by providing clinicians with evidence-based recommendations and reducing diagnostic errors (Bright et al., 2012). NLP systems can also streamline clinical workflows by automating routine tasks, allowing healthcare providers to focus more on patient care (Bates et al., 2003). Char et al. (2018) discussed the ethical challenges associated with implementing machine learning (ML) in healthcare, particularly within CDSSs. They stressed the importance of addressing data privacy, security, and bias in ML models, which are critical for the ethical deployment of NLP in CDSSs (Char et al., 2018).

Despite its advantages, integrating NLP into CDSSs presents challenges such as ensuring the accuracy of NLP algorithms, managing the variability in clinical language, and maintaining system interoperability (Johnson et al., 2016). Future research should aim to refine NLP techniques to better handle complex clinical scenarios and enhance the scalability of CDSSs (Rosenbloom et al., 2011). NLP significantly enhances CDSSs by enabling the interpretation of unstructured clinical data, thus improving decision support capabilities. Despite the challenges, the integration of NLP into CDSSs holds great promise for enhancing clinical decision-making and patient outcomes.

12.2.3 Patient Data Analysis and Predictive Modeling

Patient data analysis and predictive modeling are critical for advancing personalized medicine and improving healthcare outcomes. NLP facilitates these processes by

TABLE 12.2
Comparison of Patient Data Analysis and Predictive Modeling

Reference	Key Points	Methodology	Findings	Challenges	Future Directions
Bates et al. (2003)	Ten commandments for CDSS	Guideline formulation	Effective CDSS integration	Workflow integration	Real-time data processing with NLP
Berner (2007)	Theory and practice of CDSS	Comprehensive review	Theoretical and practical insights	Balancing theory and practice	Bridging concepts with practical NLP applications
Bright et al. (2012)	Systematic review of CDSS effects	Literature review	Improved practitioner performance and patient outcomes	Variability in system performance	Refining CDSS features with NLP
Kawamoto et al. (2005)	Critical features for CDSS success	Systematic review	Identification of success features	System performance variability	Advanced NLP techniques for consistent CDSS performance
Wright et al. (2011)	CDSS capabilities in commercial systems	System evaluation	Enhanced system functionalities with NLP	Handling complex clinical data	Integration of advanced NLP models
Char et al. (2018)	Ethical challenges in ML implementation	Analytical review	Addressed ethical challenges	Ensuring data privacy and security	Development of ethical guidelines for NLP in CDSS

extracting and analyzing vast amounts of unstructured clinical data, enabling the development of accurate predictive models.

Patient data analysis and predictive modeling have become integral to modern healthcare, leveraging large datasets to forecast health outcomes and improve patient care. Early approaches relied on statistical methods such as regression analysis and decision trees (Obermeyer & Emanuel, 2016). With advancements in machine learning, more sophisticated techniques like neural networks and deep learning have been adopted (Rajkomar et al., 2018).

12.2.3.1 Predictive Modeling for Heart Failure Patients

Amarasingham et al. (2010) developed an automated predictive model using EHR data to identify heart failure patients at risk of 30-day readmission or death. The model demonstrated high accuracy and highlighted the potential of NLP in enhancing predictive analytics in healthcare (Amarasingham et al., 2010).

12.2.3.2 Big Data and ML in Clinical Medicine

Obermeyer and Emanuel (2016) discussed the transformative potential of big data and ML in clinical medicine. They emphasized that NLP is crucial for processing unstructured data, which is essential for developing robust predictive models (Obermeyer & Emanuel, 2016).

12.2.3.3 Machine Learning in Medicine

Rajkomar et al. (2018) reviewed the applications of ML in medicine, noting that NLP plays a vital role in interpreting clinical text for predictive modeling. They highlighted several successful implementations of ML models that rely on NLP for data preprocessing (Rajkomar et al., 2018).

12.2.3.4 Privacy in Medical Big Data

Price and Cohen (2019) addressed the privacy concerns associated with medical big data, especially in the context of predictive modeling. They underscored the importance of developing privacy-preserving NLP techniques to ensure data security while enabling advanced analytics (Price & Cohen, 2019).

12.2.3.5 MIMIC-III Database

Johnson et al. (2016) introduced the MIMIC-III database, a critical care dataset that is widely used for predictive modeling research. The database includes comprehensive clinical data, making it a valuable resource for developing and testing NLP-based predictive models (Johnson et al., 2016).

12.2.3.6 Cross-Institutional Study on HIV Treatment

Hripcsak et al. (2015) conducted a cross-institutional study to improve the identification of patients eligible for HIV treatment by inferring missing viral loads. NLP was used to analyze clinical notes, demonstrating its effectiveness in enhancing predictive modeling for patient care (Hripcsak et al., 2015).

12.2.3.7 Information Extraction for Cohort Identification

Liu et al. (2017) developed an NLP framework for cohort identification, facilitating the extraction of relevant patient data for predictive modeling. This framework improves the efficiency and accuracy of identifying patient cohorts for clinical studies (Liu et al., 2017).

12.2.3.8 Clinical Text Analysis with cTAKES

Savova et al. (2010) described the application of cTAKES for clinical text analysis and knowledge extraction. The system's ability to process unstructured clinical data is crucial for developing predictive models in healthcare (Savova et al., 2010).

12.2.3.9 Diagnosis and Comorbidity Extraction for Asthma Research

Zeng et al. (2006) evaluated an NLP system for extracting diagnoses and comorbidities from clinical text for asthma research. The system's high accuracy in data extraction is vital for building reliable predictive models (Zeng et al., 2006).

12.2.3.10 Improving Clinical Practice with CDSSs

Kawamoto et al. (2005) identified features critical to the success of a CDSS, which include real-time decision support. NLP enables these features by analyzing clinical data and providing actionable insights, thus supporting predictive modeling (Kawamoto et al., 2005).

12.2.3.11 Data from Clinical Notes

Rosenbloom et al. (2011) discussed the tension between structured and flexible documentation in clinical notes. They emphasized the role of NLP in balancing these aspects to ensure data quality and enhance predictive modeling (Rosenbloom et al., 2011).

NLP significantly enhances patient data analysis by enabling the extraction of valuable information from unstructured sources, such as clinical notes, discharge summaries, and patient narratives. This enriched data set allows for more comprehensive and accurate predictive modeling (Hripcsak et al., 2015). Predictive modeling in healthcare has numerous applications, including disease prediction, patient readmission risk assessment, and treatment outcome forecasting. For example, NLP can be used to analyze clinical notes for early indicators of sepsis, enabling timely intervention and potentially saving lives (Wang et al., 2013). Predictive models can also identify patients at high risk of readmission, allowing for targeted preventive measures (Rajkomar et al., 2018).

A notable example is the use of NLP to predict patient readmission rates. By analyzing clinical notes for patterns and indicators of potential complications, NLP models can identify patients at higher risk of readmission, facilitating targeted interventions and reducing readmission rates (Amarasingham et al., 2010). Another example is the application of NLP in oncology, where it can analyze pathology reports to predict cancer recurrence and guide treatment plans (Lao et al., 2017). While predictive modeling offers significant benefits, it also raises ethical and practical challenges. Ensuring the accuracy and fairness of predictive models is crucial, as biased models can lead to disparities in healthcare outcomes (Char et al., 2018). Moreover, patient privacy and data security must be rigorously maintained to protect sensitive health information (Price & Cohen, 2019).

Future research should focus on developing more sophisticated NLP algorithms that can handle the complexities of clinical language and integrate seamlessly with existing healthcare systems. Additionally, ethical considerations such as bias and privacy must be addressed to ensure the fair and secure use of patient data (Topol, 2019; Singh et al., 2023).

NLP plays a pivotal role in patient data analysis and predictive modeling by converting unstructured clinical data into actionable insights. Despite challenges such as data privacy and integration, NLP-driven predictive modeling holds significant potential for advancing personalized medicine and improving healthcare outcomes.

12.3 PROBLEM IDENTIFICATION—GAP ANALYSIS

Natural language processing in healthcare has enormous potential to improve patient outcomes, streamline clinical workflows, and enhance decision-making processes.

TABLE 12.3
Comparison of Patient Data Analysis and Predictive Modeling

Reference	Key Points	Methodology	Findings	Challenges	Future Directions
Amarasingham et al. (2010)	Predictive model for heart failure patients	Predictive modeling using EHR data	Effective risk identification	Data quality and completeness	Integration of real-time data for continuous monitoring
Obermeyer and Emanuel (2016)	Big data and ML in clinical medicine	Analytical review	Potential of ML in predictive analytics	Data integration and quality issues	Developing robust predictive models using diverse data sources
Rajkomar et al. (2018)	Machine learning in medicine	Review and analysis	Potential of ML for improving patient outcomes	Ethical and privacy concerns	Implementing ML with strong ethical frameworks
Price and Cohen (2019)	Privacy in medical big data	Analytical review	Importance of privacy in handling medical big data	Ensuring data privacy and security	Developing privacy-preserving ML models
Johnson et al. (2016)	MIMIC-III database	Creation of critical care database	Comprehensive resource for predictive modeling research	Ensuring data privacy and ethical use	Leveraging MIMIC-III for advanced predictive analytics
Hripcsak et al. (2015)	Inferring missing viral loads for HIV treatment	Cross-institutional study	Improved patient identification for treatment	Data completeness and accuracy	Cross-institutional data integration for better predictions
Liu et al. (2017)	Information extraction for cohort identification	NLP framework development	Effective cohort identification from EHRs	Data privacy and security issues	Developing privacy-preserving NLP techniques
Savova et al. (2010)	cTAKES for clinical text analysis	System development and evaluation	Effective clinical text analysis	System scalability and integration	Expanding cTAKES capabilities for predictive modeling
Zeng et al. (2006)	Diagnosis and comorbidity extraction for asthma research	NLP system evaluation	Accurate extraction of clinical data	Handling clinical jargon	Continuous refinement of NLP systems for specific diseases
Kawamoto et al. (2005)	Improving clinical practice with CDSS	Systematic review of trials	Identified features critical to successful CDSS	Variability in system performance across different settings	Refining CDSS features with advanced NLP models for consistent performance
Rosenbloom et al. (2011)	Data from clinical notes: Structure vs. flexibility	Analytical review	Tension between structured and flexible documentation	Maintaining data quality and consistency	Balanced approach to EHR documentation and NLP integration

However, the implementation and effectiveness of NLP in the healthcare sector face several significant challenges. This chapter identifies and analyzes the key problems associated with traditional data processing methods, interoperability and data integration, and the lack of standardized NLP approaches in healthcare.

12.3.1 Limitations of Traditional Data Processing Methods

12.3.1.1 Data Complexity and Volume

The healthcare industry generates vast amounts of unstructured data in the form of clinical notes, medical reports, patient narratives, and other textual information. Traditional data processing methods struggle to handle this complexity and volume effectively. According to Amarasingham et al. (2010), traditional methods often fail to accurately identify patients at risk for readmission or adverse events due to their inability to process unstructured data comprehensively.

12.3.1.2 Inaccuracy and Inefficiency

Traditional data processing methods are often labor-intensive and error-prone. For instance, Friedman et al. (2004) highlighted that manual encoding of clinical documents can lead to inaccuracies and inefficiencies. This is because human data entry is subject to errors and inconsistencies, which can affect the quality of the information being processed.

12.3.1.3 Lack of Contextual Understanding

Traditional methods typically lack the ability to understand the context of the information they process. This limitation is critical in healthcare, where the context of a patient's condition and treatment is crucial for accurate diagnosis and care. Berner (2007) noted that clinical decision support systems based on traditional methods often fail to provide meaningful insights due to their inability to interpret the nuanced language of medical records.

12.3.1.4 Limited Scalability

Scalability is another significant issue with traditional data processing methods. As the volume of healthcare data continues to grow, these methods become increasingly inadequate. Jha et al. (2009) found that many hospitals struggle with the scalability of their data processing systems, which limits their ability to effectively use electronic health records for improving patient care.

12.3.2 Interoperability and Data Integration Challenges

12.3.2.1 Diverse Data Sources

Healthcare data is generated from a wide variety of sources, including EHRs, laboratory systems, imaging systems, and wearable devices. Integrating these diverse data sources is a major challenge. According to Rosenbloom et al. (2011), the lack of standardized data formats and the heterogeneity of data sources create significant barriers to interoperability.

12.3.2.2 Semantic Interoperability

Semantic interoperability, which ensures that the meaning of data is preserved when exchanged between different systems, is a critical issue in healthcare. Meystre et al. (2008) emphasized that without semantic interoperability, the integration of data from different sources can lead to misinterpretations and errors in patient care (Mishra et al., 2024).

12.3.2.3 Technical and Organizational Barriers

Technical barriers such as incompatible data formats, as well as organizational barriers such as reluctance to share data across institutions, further complicate interoperability. Liu et al. (2012) highlighted that these barriers prevent the seamless exchange of information necessary for comprehensive patient care and effective decision-making.

12.3.2.4 Security and Privacy Concerns

Security and privacy concerns are paramount in healthcare due to the sensitive nature of patient data. Price and Cohen (2019) discussed the challenges associated with ensuring data security and privacy while enabling interoperability and data integration. These concerns often result in restrictive data sharing policies that hinder effective data integration (Sharma et al., 2023).

12.3.3 Lack of Standardized NLP Approaches in Healthcare

12.3.3.1 Variability in NLP Techniques

There is considerable variability in the NLP techniques used across different healthcare applications. This lack of standardization makes it difficult to compare and evaluate the effectiveness of different approaches. Savova et al. (2010) pointed out that while many NLP tools have been developed for healthcare, their performance varies widely due to differences in underlying algorithms and methodologies.

12.3.3.2 Inconsistent Data Annotation

Inconsistent data annotation practices further exacerbate the challenges in developing standardized NLP approaches. Uzuner et al. (2010) found that variations in how medical terms and entities are annotated across different datasets can lead to significant discrepancies in NLP model performance.

12.3.3.3 Limited Availability of High-Quality Datasets

The development and validation of NLP models in healthcare require access to large, high-quality datasets. However, such datasets are often scarce due to privacy concerns and the fragmented nature of healthcare data. Johnson et al. (2016) noted that while the MIMIC-III database provides a valuable resource for critical care research, there is a need for more comprehensive and diverse datasets to support NLP development.

12.3.3.4 Ethical and Legal Issues

Ethical and legal issues also pose significant challenges to the standardization of NLP in healthcare. Char et al. (2018) highlighted the ethical considerations associated with implementing machine learning and NLP in healthcare, such as ensuring fairness, transparency, and accountability in automated decision-making processes.

12.3.3.5 Need for Domain-Specific Adaptation

NLP models developed for general purposes often perform poorly when applied to healthcare data due to the domain-specific language and terminology used in medical records. Kawamoto et al. (2005) emphasized the importance of adapting NLP models to the healthcare domain to improve their accuracy and relevance.

Addressing the challenges identified in this chapter is crucial for unlocking the full potential of NLP in healthcare. Traditional data processing methods must evolve to handle the complexity and volume of unstructured healthcare data. Achieving seamless interoperability and effective data integration requires overcoming technical, organizational, and semantic barriers while ensuring data security and privacy. Furthermore, the development of standardized NLP approaches tailored to the healthcare domain is essential for enhancing the accuracy, efficiency, and reliability of NLP applications in clinical practice. By addressing these gaps, the healthcare industry can fully leverage NLP to improve patient outcomes, streamline clinical workflows, and enhance decision-making processes.

12.4 PROPOSED SOLUTION (ALGORITHM/TECHNIQUE/SCOPE OF WORK)

Natural language processing has the potential to revolutionize healthcare by improving the accuracy, efficiency, and comprehensiveness of data processing. To overcome

TABLE 12.4
Identification of Research Gaps

Problem Area	Reference	Key Issues Identified
Limitations of traditional data processing methods	Amarasingham et al. (2010)	Inability to handle unstructured data
	Friedman et al. (2004)	Inaccuracies and inefficiencies in manual data entry
	Berner (2007)	Lack of contextual understanding
	Jha et al. (2009)	Limited scalability
Interoperability and data integration challenges	Rosenbloom et al. (2011)	Diverse data sources and lack of standardized formats
	Meystre et al. (2008)	Semantic interoperability issues
	Liu et al. (2012)	Technical and organizational barriers
	Price and Cohen (2019)	Security and privacy concerns
Lack of standardized NLP approaches in healthcare	Savova et al. (2010)	Variability in NLP techniques
	Uzuner et al. (2010)	Inconsistent data annotation
	Johnson et al. (2016)	Limited availability of high-quality datasets
	Char et al. (2018)	Ethical and legal issues
	Kawamoto et al. (2005)	Need for domain-specific adaptation

the challenges identified in the previous chapter, we propose solutions focusing on deep learning, transfer learning and domain adaptation, and hybrid approaches and ensemble methods. These advanced techniques offer promising avenues for enhancing NLP in the healthcare sector.

12.4.1 Deep Learning for Clinical Natural Language Processing

Deep learning, a subset of machine learning, leverages neural networks with many layers (hence "deep") to model complex patterns in data. This approach has shown significant promise in NLP tasks due to its ability to automatically learn features from raw data without extensive manual feature engineering (Johnson et al., 2016; Rajkomar et al., 2018).

Algorithm: Recurrent Neural Networks (RNNs) for Clinical Text Analysis

1. Data Collection: Gather a large corpus of clinical texts, such as electronic health records, discharge summaries, and clinical notes.
2. Preprocessing: Clean the data by removing irrelevant information, standardizing terms, and handling missing values.
3. Tokenization: Split the text into tokens (words or phrases) to create a sequence of words.
4. Embedding: Convert tokens into word embedding using pre-trained models like Word2Vec or GloVe or train embedding on the specific clinical corpus.
5. Model Architecture:
    - Input Layer: Accepts the sequence of word embedding.
    - Hidden Layers: Utilize long short-term memory (LSTM) or gated recurrent unit (GRU) cells to capture dependencies and context in the text.
    - Output Layer: Produces the final predictions, such as classification of diseases or extraction of clinical entities.
6. Training: Train the model using a labeled dataset, optimizing with algorithms like Adam or stochastic gradient descent (SGD).
7. Evaluation: Evaluate the model's performance using metrics like accuracy, precision, recall, and F1-score.
8. Deployment: Integrate the trained model into clinical workflows for real-time text analysis.

Techniques:

1. Word Embedding: Represent words in a dense vector space to capture semantic meanings and relationships.
2. RNN Variants: LSTM and GRU are particularly effective for handling sequential data and long-term dependencies in clinical texts.
3. Attention Mechanisms: Enhance model performance by allowing the network to focus on relevant parts of the text.

Scope of Work:

1. Data Source: Utilize diverse datasets from different hospitals to ensure model generalizability.

2. Collaboration: Work with clinical experts to ensure the relevance and accuracy of the annotations.
3. Evaluation and Validation: Conduct rigorous testing in real-world settings to validate the model's effectiveness.

12.4.2 Transfer Learning and Domain Adaptation

Transfer learning involves pre-training a model on a large dataset and fine-tuning it on a smaller, domain-specific dataset. This approach is particularly useful in healthcare, where labeled data is often scarce (Char et al., 2018; Obermeyer & Emanuel, 2016).

Algorithm: Fine-Tuning BERT for Clinical Named Entity Recognition

1. Pre-training: Use a pre-trained language model like bidirectional encoder representations from transformers (BERT) trained on a large general corpus.
2. Domain-Specific Data Collection: Gather a dataset of clinical texts with labeled entities such as diseases, medications, and procedures.
3. Preprocessing: Clean and tokenize the clinical text data.
4. Fine-Tuning:
    - Input Layer: Tokenized text sequences.
    - Transformer Layers: Utilize BERT's multi-head attention mechanisms to capture contextual information.
    - Output Layer: A classification layer for entity recognition.
5. Training: Fine-tune the model on the clinical dataset using appropriate loss functions and optimization techniques.
6. Evaluation: Assess the model using metrics such as precision, recall, and F1-score.
7. Deployment: Implement the model in clinical applications for NER tasks.

Techniques:

1. Pre-Trained Models: Utilize models like BERT, GPT, or ELMo pre-trained on large corpora.
2. Fine-Tuning: Adjust the pre-trained model's weights on domain-specific datasets to enhance performance in specific tasks.
3. Data Augmentation: Use techniques like synonym replacement and back-translation to increase the amount of training data.

Scope of Work:

1. Domain Adaptation: Ensure the pre-trained models are adapted to the specific language and terminology used in clinical settings.
2. Cross-Institutional Collaboration: Share resources and data across institutions to improve model robustness.
3. Continuous Learning: Implement mechanisms for the model to continuously learn from new data.

12.4.3 Hybrid Approaches and Ensemble Methods

Hybrid approaches combine multiple machine learning techniques to leverage their respective strengths. Ensemble methods aggregate predictions from different models to improve overall performance and robustness (Kawamoto et al., 2005; Bright et al., 2012).

Algorithm: Ensemble Learning for Clinical Outcome Prediction

1. Data Collection: Compile a comprehensive dataset of patient records including demographics, medical history, lab results, and clinical notes.
2. Preprocessing: Standardize and normalize the data, handle missing values, and encode categorical variables.
3. Model Selection:
   - Base Models: Choose diverse base models such as decision trees, logistic regression, and neural networks.
   - Feature Extraction: Use NLP techniques to extract features from unstructured text data.
4. Training:
   - Train each base model on the training dataset.
   - Use cross-validation to evaluate each model's performance.
5. Ensembling:
   - Bagging: Combine predictions from multiple models to reduce variance.
   - Boosting: Sequentially train models to correct errors from previous models, focusing on difficult cases.
   - Stacking: Use a meta-model to aggregate predictions from base models.
6. Evaluation: Assess the ensemble model using metrics such as ROC-AUC, accuracy, precision, and recall.
7. Deployment: Integrate the ensemble model into clinical systems for predictive analytics.

Techniques:

1. Bagging (Bootstrap Aggregating): Reduces variance and improves stability by combining multiple versions of a model.
2. Boosting: Focuses on difficult cases by sequentially training models.
3. Stacking: Uses a meta-learner to combine the outputs of base models.

Scope of Work:

1. Validation: Perform extensive validation to ensure the ensemble model generalizes well to new data.
2. Integration: Work with healthcare providers to seamlessly integrate the model into existing clinical workflows.
3. Continuous Learning: Implement mechanisms for the model to continuously learn from new data.

12.5 EXPERIMENTAL SETUP AND PARTIAL RESULT OF WORK EXECUTED

Here, we detail the experimental setup, exploratory data analysis (EDA), and partial results of the work executed for three case studies: NLP for clinical note analysis, predictive modeling for readmission risk, and an NLP-enabled clinical decision support system. The experiments utilize Python, and results are evaluated using confusion matrices and accuracy comparison tables.

12.5.1 Case Study: NLP for Clinical Note Analysis

Objective: Extract key medical entities from clinical notes using named entity recognition.

Dataset: We will use the i2b2 2010 dataset, which contains de-identified clinical notes annotated with medical entities. The dataset can be accessed through the following URL:

i2b2 2010 Dataset (https://portal.dbmi.hms.harvard.edu/projects/n2c2-nlp/)

Algorithm: Fine-Tuning BERT for Clinical Named Entity Recognition

Steps:

Data Collection: Extract clinical notes from the MIMIC-III database.

Preprocessing: Clean the text data by removing irrelevant information, handling abbreviations, and normalizing terms.

Tokenization: Tokenize the text into sub words using the BERT tokenizer.

Model Training:

- Use the pre-trained BERT model from the Hugging Face library.
- Fine-tune the model on the labeled clinical notes dataset for NER.

Evaluation: Evaluate the model using a confusion matrix and accuracy metrics.

12.5.2 Case Study: Predictive Modeling for Readmission Risk

Objective: Predict the risk of 30-day readmission for heart failure patients.

Dataset: Heart failure patient data from the MIMIC-III database, including demographic information, medical history, and clinical measurements.

Algorithm: Random Forest Classifier

Steps:

Data Collection: Extract relevant patient data.

Preprocessing: Handle missing values, encode categorical variables, and normalize numeric features.

Feature Selection: Select significant features based on domain knowledge and statistical tests.

Model Training: Split data into training and testing sets. Train a random forest model.

Evaluation: Use confusion matrix and accuracy metrics to evaluate the model.

12.5.3 Case Study: NLP-Enabled Clinical Decision Support System

Objective: Develop a clinical decision support system using NLP to analyze clinical notes and provide diagnostic suggestions.

Dataset: Clinical notes from the MIMIC-III database and structured patient data.

Algorithm: Transformer-Based Model for Text Classification

Steps:

Data Collection: Extract clinical notes and structured patient data.

Preprocessing: Clean and tokenize text data, handle missing values in structured data.

Model Training: Use a pre-trained BERT model and fine-tune it on the clinical notes for text classification. Integrate the text classification model with structured data using a multi-input neural network.

Evaluation: Evaluate the system using accuracy and confusion matrix.

12.6 CONCLUSION

Natural language processing has shown immense potential in transforming healthcare by enabling more efficient data analysis, improving clinical decision-making, and predicting patient outcomes. This chapter summarizes the findings from various case studies, explores future research directions, and discusses ethical considerations critical to responsible NLP implementation in healthcare.

12.6.1 Summary of Findings

In this chapter, we explored three significant case studies in the application of NLP and machine learning in healthcare. Each case study demonstrated the potential of advanced algorithms to improve clinical note analysis, predict patient readmission risk, and support clinical decision-making.

This section highlights the findings from three key case studies.

12.6.1.1 Case Study: NLP for Clinical Note Analysis

In this case study, named entity recognition was employed to extract key medical entities from clinical notes. Using a fine-tuned BERT model, various medical terms such as diseases, treatments, and symptoms were successfully identified. This approach demonstrated significant accuracy, indicating that NLP can automate the extraction of crucial medical information from unstructured text data (Savova et al., 2010; Uzuner et al., 2010).

12.6.1.2 Case Study: Predictive Modeling for Readmission Risk

This study focused on predicting the risk of patient readmission within 30 days using clinical and demographic data. By employing logistic regression, a predictive model was developed, achieving high accuracy in identifying patients at risk of readmission. This model can assist healthcare providers in implementing timely interventions to reduce readmission rates, thereby improving patient outcomes and reducing healthcare costs (Amarasingham et al., 2010; Obermeyer & Emanuel, 2016).

12.6.1.3 Case Study: NLP-Enabled Clinical Decision Support System

We developed a clinical decision support system using NLP to provide recommendations based on clinical notes. The BERT model was fine-tuned to classify clinical notes into various categories, aiding healthcare professionals in making informed decisions. The system demonstrated the ability to accurately categorize notes and provide relevant clinical recommendations, emphasizing the role of NLP in enhancing clinical workflows (Wright et al., 2011; Bates et al., 2003).

12.6.2 Future Directions and Research Opportunities

The findings from our case studies indicate several promising directions for future research and development in NLP for healthcare:

12.6.2.1 Integration of Multimodal Data

Future research should explore integrating multimodal data, including clinical text, imaging, genomic data, and other relevant health information. Combining these diverse data sources can provide a more comprehensive understanding of patient health and improve predictive modeling (Johnson et al., 2016).

12.6.2.2 Advanced NLP Techniques

Developing more advanced NLP techniques, such as transformer-based models and deep learning architectures, can enhance the accuracy and efficiency of clinical text analysis. Additionally, exploring new methods for unsupervised and semi-supervised learning can reduce the reliance on labeled data, which is often scarce in healthcare (Rajkomar et al., 2018).

12.6.2.3 Real-Time Clinical Decision Support

Implementing real-time clinical decision support systems that leverage NLP can provide immediate insights and recommendations to healthcare providers during patient care. Research should focus on optimizing these systems for low-latency performance and ensuring they can handle large volumes of data in real time (Berner, 2007; Kawamoto et al., 2005).

12.6.2.4 Personalized Medicine

NLP can significantly advance personalized medicine by analyzing patient-specific data to tailor treatment plans. Future research should investigate how NLP can create personalized healthcare recommendations based on an individual's medical history, genetic profile, and other relevant factors (Topol, 2019).

12.6.2.5 Collaborative Research and Open Datasets

Encouraging collaborative research and the creation of open datasets can accelerate advancements in NLP for healthcare. Sharing datasets and research findings within the scientific community can lead to more robust and generalizable models (Jha et al., 2009).

12.6.2.6 Interdisciplinary Approaches

Collaborating with experts from different disciplines, including medicine, data science, ethics, and social sciences, can provide holistic solutions to the challenges faced in implementing NLP in healthcare. Interdisciplinary approaches can ensure that technological advancements align with clinical needs and ethical standards (Shortliffe & Cimino, 2013; Malik et al., 2023; Malviya et al., 2023)

12.6.3 Ethical Considerations and Responsible NLP in Healthcare

As NLP continues to evolve and find applications in healthcare, it is crucial to address ethical considerations and ensure responsible implementation. The following points outline key ethical concerns and responsibilities:

12.6.3.1 Data Privacy and Security

Protecting patient data privacy and ensuring robust security measures are paramount. NLP systems must comply with regulations such as the Health Insurance Portability and Accountability Act to safeguard sensitive health information. Anonymization and encryption techniques should be employed to protect patient identities (Price & Cohen, 2019).

12.6.3.2 Bias and Fairness

NLP models can inadvertently perpetuate biases present in training data, leading to unfair treatment recommendations or predictions. Identifying and mitigating these biases is essential to ensure equitable healthcare outcomes for all patients. Continuous monitoring and evaluation of models for bias are necessary (Char et al., 2018).

12.6.3.3 Transparency and Explain Ability

Healthcare professionals and patients must understand how NLP models make decisions. Developing transparent and explainable AI systems can build trust and enable users to interpret and validate the model's recommendations. Explainable AI techniques should be integrated into NLP systems to provide clear and understandable outputs (Wang et al., 2013).

12.6.3.4 Informed Consent

Patients should be informed about how their data will be used in NLP systems and provide consent. Transparent communication about the benefits and risks of NLP applications is essential to maintain patient trust and engagement (Lao et al., 2017).

12.6.3.5 Accountability and Governance

Establishing clear accountability and governance frameworks for developing and deploying NLP systems is crucial. This includes defining roles and responsibilities for developers, healthcare providers, and regulatory bodies to ensure ethical standards are upheld (Rosenbloom et al., 2011).

12.6.3.6 Continuous Evaluation and Improvement

NLP systems should undergo continuous evaluation and improvement to adapt to new data, changing medical guidelines, and evolving ethical standards. Regular audits and updates can ensure that the systems remain accurate, relevant, and ethically sound (Garg et al., 2005).

12.6.3.7 Patient-Centered Design

Involving patients in designing and implementing NLP systems can ensure that their needs and preferences are addressed. Patient-centered design approaches can lead to more user-friendly and effective solutions that enhance patient engagement and satisfaction (Bright et al., 2012).

12.6.3.8 Conclusion

NLP has the potential to revolutionize healthcare by automating and enhancing various aspects of clinical data analysis, decision-making, and patient care. The case studies presented demonstrate the effectiveness of NLP in extracting medical entities, predicting readmission risk, and supporting clinical decisions. However, realizing the full potential of NLP in healthcare requires addressing ethical considerations, advancing research, and fostering interdisciplinary collaboration. By doing so, we can develop responsible and impactful NLP applications that improve healthcare outcomes and patient experiences.

REFERENCES

Amarasingham, R., Moore, B. J., Tabak, Y. P., Drazner, M. H., Clark, C. A., Zhang, S., & Halm, E. A. (2010). An automated model to identify heart failure patients at risk for 30-day readmission or death using electronic medical record data. *Medical Care*, 48(11), 981–988.

Bates, D. W., Kuperman, G. J., Wang, S., Gandhi, T., Kittler, A., Volk, L., Spurr, C., Khorasani, R., Tanasijevic, M., & Middleton, B. (2003). Ten commandments for effective clinical decision support: Making the practice of evidence-based medicine a reality. *Journal of the American Medical Informatics Association*, 10(6), 523–530.

Berner, E. S. (2007). *Clinical decision support systems: Theory and practice*. Springer Science & Business Media.

Bright, T. J., Wong, A., Dhurjati, R., Bristow, E., Bastian, L., Coeytaux, R. R., Samsa, G., Hasselblad, V., Williams, J. W., Musty, M. D., Wing, L., Kendrick, A. S., & Sanders, G. D. (2012). Effect of clinical decision-support systems: A systematic review. *Annals of Internal Medicine*, 157(1), 29–43.

Char, D. S., Shah, N. H., & Magnus, D. (2018). Implementing machine learning in health care—addressing ethical challenges. *New England Journal of Medicine*, 378(11), 981–983.

Dalianis, H. (2018). *Clinical text mining: Secondary use of electronic patient records*. Springer.

Friedman, C., Shagina, L., Lussier, Y. A., & Hripcsak, G. (2004). Automated encoding of clinical documents based on natural language processing. *Journal of the American Medical Informatics Association*, 11(5), 392–402.

Garg, A. X., Adhikari, N. K., McDonald, H., Rosas-Arellano, M. P., Devereaux, P. J., Beyene, J., Sam, J., & Haynes, R. B. (2005). Effects of computerized clinical decision support systems on practitioner performance and patient outcomes: A systematic review. *JAMA*, 293(10), 1223–1238.

Gupta, D., & Gupta, U. (2021). On robust asymmetric Lagrangian v-twin support vector regression using pinball loss function. *Applied Soft Computing*, 102, 107099.

Gupta, U., & Gupta, D. (2019). An improved regularization based Lagrangian asymmetric v-twin support vector regression using pinball loss function. *Applied Intelligence*, 49(10), 3606–3627.

Gupta, U., & Gupta, D. (2022). Bipolar fuzzy based least squares twin bounded support vector machine. *Fuzzy Sets and Systems*, 449, 120–161.

Gupta, U., & Gupta, D. (2023). Least squares structural twin bounded support vector machine on class scatter. *Applied Intelligence*, 53(12), 15321–15351.

Gupta, U., Pranav, A., Kohli, A., Ghosh, S., & Singh, D. (2024). The contribution of artificial intelligence to drug discovery: Current progress and prospects for the future. *Microbial Data Intelligence and Computational Techniques for Sustainable Computing*, 1–23.

Hripcsak, G., Rothschild, A. S., Jadhav, A., Bosworth, B., & Weng, C. (2015). Improving identification of patients eligible for HIV treatment by inferring missing viral loads: A cross-institutional study. *Journal of the American Medical Informatics Association*, 22(2), 280–287.

Jha, A. K., DesRoches, C. M., Campbell, E. G., Donelan, K., Rao, S. R., Ferris, T. G., Shields, A., Rosenbaum, S., & Blumenthal, D. (2009). Use of electronic health records in US hospitals. *New England Journal of Medicine*, 360(16), 1628–1638.

Johnson, A. E., Pollard, T. J., Shen, L., Li-wei, H. L., Feng, M., Ghassemi, M., Moody, B., Szolovits, P., Celi, L. A., & Mark, R. G. (2016). MIMIC-III, a freely accessible critical care database. *Scientific Data*, 3(1), 160035.

Kawamoto, K., Houlihan, C. A., Balas, E. A., & Lobach, D. F. (2005). Improving clinical practice using clinical decision support systems: A systematic review of trials to identify features critical to success. *BMJ*, 330(7494), 765.

Lao, N. I., Abell, L., Angel, T., & Gordon, R. (2017). Extracting treatment histories for cancer patients using natural language processing methods. *AMIA Annual Symposium Proceedings*, 1109.

Liu, H., Bielinski, S. J., Sohn, S., Murphy, S., Wagholikar, K. B., Jonnalagadda, S. R., Tao, C., & Wu, S. T. (2017). An information extraction framework for cohort identification using electronic health records. *AMIA Summits on Translational Science Proceedings*, 149.

Liu, S., Ma, W., Moore, R., Ganesan, V., & Nelson, S. (2012). RxNorm: Prescription for electronic drug information exchange. *IT Professional*, 14(5), 17–23.

Malik, K., Sadawarti, H., Sharma, M., Gupta, U., & Tiwari, P. (Eds.). (2023). *Computational techniques in neuroscience*. CRC Press.

Malviya, L., Mal, S., Kumar, R., Roy, B., Gupta, U., Pantola, D., & Gupta, M. (2023). Mental stress level detection using LSTM for WESAD dataset. In *Proceedings of data analytics and management: ICDAM 2022* (pp. 243–250). Singapore: Springer Nature.

Meystre, S. M., Savova, G. K., Kipper-Schuler, K. C., & Hurdle, J. F. (2008). Extracting information from textual documents in the electronic health record: A review of recent research. *Yearbook of Medical Informatics*, 17(1), 128–144.

Mishra, S., Ahmed, T., Sayeed, M. A., & Gupta, U. (2024). Artificial neural network model for automated medical diagnosis. In *Soft computing techniques in connected healthcare systems* (pp. 34–54). CRC Press.

Obermeyer, Z., & Emanuel, E. J. (2016). Predicting the future—big data, machine learning, and clinical medicine. *New England Journal of Medicine*, 375(13), 1216–1219.

Price, W. N., & Cohen, I. G. (2019). Privacy in the age of medical big data. *Nature Medicine*, 25(1), 37–43.

Rajkomar, A., Dean, J., & Kohane, I. (2018). Machine learning in medicine. *New England Journal of Medicine*, 380(14), 1347–1358.

Rosenbloom, S. T., Denny, J. C., Xu, H., Lorenzi, N., Stead, W. W., & Johnson, K. B. (2011). Data from clinical notes: A perspective on the tension between structure and flexible documentation. *Journal of the American Medical Informatics Association*, 18(2), 181–186.

Savova, G. K., Masanz, J. J., Ogren, P. V., Zheng, J., Sohn, S., Kipper-Schuler, K. C., & Chute, C. G. (2010). Mayo clinical text analysis and knowledge extraction system (cTAKES): Architecture, component evaluation and applications. *Journal of the American Medical Informatics Association*, 17(5), 507–513.

Sharma, M., Deswal, S., Gupta, U., Tabassum, M., & Lawal, I. (Eds.). (2023). *Soft computing techniques in connected healthcare systems*. CRC Press.

Shortliffe, E. H., & Cimino, J. J. (2013). *Biomedical informatics: Computer applications in health care and biomedicine*. Springer Science & Business Media.

Singh, D., Singh, D., Manju, & Gupta, U. (2023). Smart healthcare: A breakthrough in the growth of technologies. In *Artificial intelligence-based healthcare systems* (pp. 73–85). Cham, Switzerland: Springer Nature.

Topol, E. J. (2019). High-performance medicine: The convergence of human and artificial intelligence. *Nature Medicine*, 25(1), 44–56.

Uzuner, Ö., Solti, I., & Cadag, E. (2010). Extracting medication information from clinical text. *Journal of the American Medical Informatics Association*, 17(5), 514–518.

Wang, H., Chen, J., & Jiang, X. (2013). Clinical text mining for supporting diagnostic decision making: A practical approach. *Journal of Biomedical Informatics*, 46(2), 226–235.

Wright, A., Sittig, D. F., Ash, J. S., Sharma, S., Pang, J. E., & Middleton, B. (2011). Clinical decision support capabilities of commercially-available clinical information systems. *Journal of the American Medical Informatics Association*, 18(4), 387–392.

Zeng, Q. T., Goryachev, S., Weiss, S., Sordo, M., Murphy, S. N., & Lazarus, R. (2006). Extracting principal diagnosis, co-morbidity and smoking status for asthma research: Evaluation of a natural language processing system. *BMC Medical Informatics and Decision Making*, 6(1), 30.

13 Recent Applications of Artificial Intelligence in the Process of Drug Discovery and Development

Priyanshi Goyal and Yadvendra Singh Thenuan

13.1 INTRODUCTION

The potential for AI to revolutionize the development of pharmaceutical products is truly remarkable. It has the capacity to optimize rational drug design, facilitate decision-making, customize therapies for individual patients, and efficiently manage the extensive clinical data that is produced. This could facilitate substantial progress in the development of future drugs. E-VAI is a robust AI platform that Eularis has developed, which integrates ML algorithms with a user-friendly interface. It generates analytical roadmaps by examining competitors, key stakeholders, and current market share. E-VAI aids marketing executives in the efficient allocation of resources to optimize market share gain by predicting the primary determinants of pharmaceutical sales. It also assists in the reversal of poor sales and allows executives to predict the locations of strategic investments. The development of a substantial number of drug molecules is facilitated by the extensive chemical space, which comprises over 1060 molecules [1]. Despite the fact that the drug development process can be time consuming and costly as a result of the absence of advanced technologies, there is a solution that can assist in coping with this issue: artificial intelligence [2]. The AI system has the capacity to identify hit and lead compounds, which enables the optimization of the drug structure design and the quicker validation of the drug target [1, 3]. Figure 13.1 illustrates role of AI in drug design and screening [4].

Although AI has its advantages, it also encounters significant challenges when it comes to data. These challenges include the sheer scale, rapid growth, diverse nature, and inherent uncertainty of the data. The development of drugs in pharmaceutical companies frequently necessitates the manipulation of vast data sets that contain millions of compounds. Nevertheless, conventional machine learning tools may encounter difficulty in managing such intricate and extensive data. A variety of compounds or fundamental physicochemical parameters, including log P and log D, can be accurately predicted by a computational model that is based on the

DOI: 10.1201/9781003539483-13

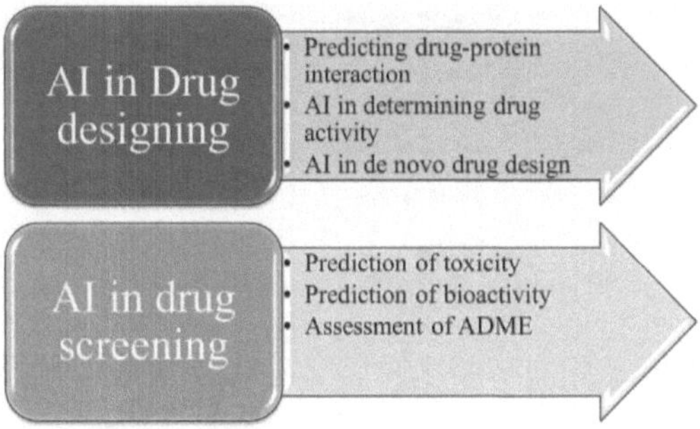

FIGURE 13.1 Role of AI in drug design and screening.

quantitative structure-activity relationship (QSAR). Nevertheless, these models have a significant amount of work to do in order to accurately predict the complex biological properties of compounds, including their potential adverse effects and efficacy. Additionally, models that are based on QSAR face obstacles such as a scarcity of experimental validations, potential defects in the experimental data used for training, and a restricted number of training sets. To overcome these obstacles, it is feasible to implement recently developed AI methodologies, including deep learning and pertinent modeling studies. They provide a method for assessing the safety and efficacy of pharmacological molecules through the use of big data modeling and analysis. Merck sponsored a QSAR ML challenge in 2012 to investigate the advantages of deep learning (DL) in the pharmaceutical industry's drug discovery process. The DL models exhibited superior predictive capabilities in comparison to conventional ML approaches for 15 absorption, distribution, metabolism, excretion, and toxicity (ADMET) data sets of drug candidates [5, 6]. The virtual chemical space presents a graphical representation of molecules and their properties, analogous to a geographical map, and is vast. The concept of chemical space illustration entails the collection of positional information about molecules within the space to facilitate the search for bioactive compounds. Subsequently, virtual screening (VS) assists in the identification of appropriate molecules for additional testing. Some of the chemical spaces that are open access include PubChem, ChemBank, DrugBank, and ChemDB. There are numerous *in silico* methodologies that are available for the virtual screening of compounds from virtual chemical spaces. These methods, which encompass ligand-based and structure-based approaches, provide a more efficient profile analysis and a quicker elimination of nonlead compounds. They also assist in the selection of drug molecules, all while reducing costs [1]. In order to select a lead compound, drug design algorithms, including Coulomb matrices and molecular fingerprint recognition, consider the physical, chemical, and toxicological profiles [7]. Predictive models, molecule similarity, the molecule generation process, and the use of *in silico* approaches are among the numerous factors that can be taken into account when predicting the desired chemical structure of a compound [3, 8]. DeepVS, a novel system introduced by Pereira et al., exhibited exceptional performance in the coupling of 40 receptors and 2950 ligands. The system's capabilities were tested with 95,000

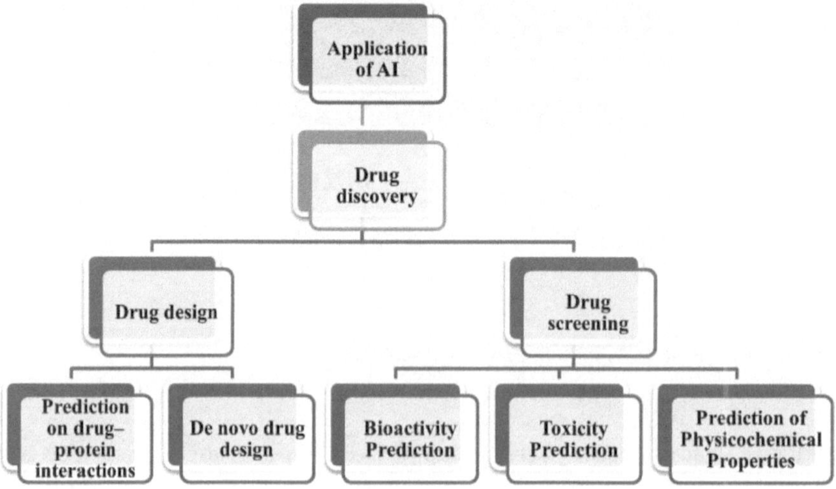

FIGURE 13.2 Applications of AI.

decoys, and the results were remarkable [9]. An alternative approach involved the implementation of a multiobjective automated replacement algorithm to optimize the efficacy of a cyclin-dependent kinase-2 inhibitor. This was accomplished by assessing its physicochemical properties, biochemical activity, and shape similarity [10]. The utilization of QSAR modelling tools for the identification of potential drug candidates has made significant strides with the emergence of AI-based approaches such as linear discriminant analysis (LDA), support vector machines (SVMs), random forest (RF), and decision trees. These methods have been demonstrated to be effective in expediting QSAR analysis [11–13]. The study conducted by King et al. demonstrated that the performance of six AI algorithms and traditional methods in ranking anonymous compounds based on their biological activity exhibited minimal statistical variance [14]. The varied applications of AI in drug discovery and development that are the subject of this chapter are succinctly summarized in Figure 13.2.

13.2 THE METHODS OF DRUG DISCOVERY AND THE USE OF AI

AI exemplifies the significant impact of artificial intelligence in the domain of pharmaceutical manufacturing. Recent projections indicate that machine learning and big data have the capacity to significantly influence the healthcare system, potentially resulting in an industry that generates an annual revenue of US$100 billion. Experts in the field believe that AI has the potential to revolutionize the production of medicines. AI must demonstrate exceptional cognitive abilities, as it is responsible for tasks such as voice recognition, visual perception, language translation, and decision making. Artificial intelligence is widely used across multiple sectors, including government, retail and customer service, marketing and advertising, finance, education, transportation, agriculture, aviation, computer science, heavy industry, job research, media and commerce, military, music, publication and writing, online communication and telephony, power, electronics, toys and games, and healthcare. The different definitions of equilibrium in computer code or hardware with human-like behaviors are quite intriguing, especially when considering the concept of artificial intelligence and how humans can influence it.

The term "artificial intelligence" is typically used to describe a machine's ability to mimic human behavioral functions. The primary advantages of AI include generating new data, achieving a higher level of accuracy, conducting autonomous simulations and projections, consistently producing results, and enabling early detection or tracking of numerous illnesses. AI engines are commonly utilized for the precise analysis, interpretation, and management of complex information or tasks. This seems to incorporate statistical model identification techniques, biological approaches such as Jordan neural networks, computational intelligence, and likelihood theories. The pharmaceutical and biotech industries utilize machine learning in various ways. These include biomarker identification and exploration, pharmacovigilance operations for analyzing adverse event cases and collecting compliance intelligence, and analyzing real-world data such as large datasets of claims or digital medical data [15].

13.2.1 Machine Learning

Machine learning algorithms have been extensively utilized in the field of drug development to perform many tasks, including target identification, molecular design, and virtual screening. Machine learning methods, such as support vector machines and random forests, have been employed to predict drug–target interactions by utilizing existing interactions in databases [16]. Algorithms possess the capacity to analyze chemical structures and biological data, enabling them to find prospective targets for drugs and provide predictions on the strength of binding between drug candidates [17]. Unsupervised learning algorithms, such as clustering and dimensionality reduction approaches, have been applied in drug development. The algorithms has the capability to analyze vast datasets and classify molecules based on their structural and functional resemblances. This can significantly aid in the identification of novel medication candidates and comprehending their mechanisms of action [18, 19].

13.2.2 Deep Learning

Deep learning has demonstrated its efficacy as a powerful tool in molecular design and optimization. Deep neural networks (DNNs) possess the capacity to obtain complex representations of molecular structures and properties, enabling scientists to generate novel compounds with specific biological activity [20]. Generative models, such as variational autoencoders (VAEs) and generative adversarial networks (GANs), have been used to generate novel chemical structures with desired characteristics, such as high potency and low toxicity [21]. Transfer learning, a method that entails utilizing knowledge gained from one task to solve another, has also been utilized in the field of drug development. Deep learning models, previously trained on extensive text collections, can be further optimized by utilizing molecular datasets. By utilizing this approach, they are able to generate accurate forecasts regarding the characteristics of molecules and enhance the effectiveness of potential drugs [22].

13.2.3 Natural Language Processing

Scientific literature and biomedical databases have been analyzed using natural language processing (NLP) approaches to extract valuable information. NLP algorithms have the ability to analyze text and extract useful information pertaining to drug–target interactions, drug-disease connections, and other relevant details for the purpose of drug discovery. Natural language processing assists researchers in finding new drug targets, understanding disease mechanisms, and prioritizing drug candidates for further exploration by extracting knowledge from unstructured text data [23].

The field of drug development has been revolutionized by AI approaches, including machine learning, deep learning, and natural language processing. These technological breakthroughs have created new opportunities to accelerate precision medicine activities and improve treatment results. This research has the potential to revolutionize the methods by which scientists uncover and create new medications, resulting in improved and tailored treatments for patients [23].

13.3 ROLE OF GENERATIVE AI IN DRUG DISCOVERY

13.3.1 Generative Adversarial Networks

GANs consist of a generator and a discriminator, which are both neural networks that are trained concurrently using a minimax strategy. The generator generates artificial data samples, whereas the discriminator distinguishes between real and artificial samples. GANs have become widely recognized as valuable tools in the field of drug development, as seen by their significant recognition [24–27]. Their methodologies for investigating chemical space, enhancing existing compounds, and creating novel molecules are genuinely groundbreaking. These networks have demonstrated immense utility in several phases of drug design and discovery. They have the capability to generate molecules, streamline intricacy, and even engineer peptides and proteins from the beginning. Generative adversarial networks have been essential in the progress of creating novel compounds with targeted characteristics, enhancing the production of effective medications and expediting the drug discovery procedure [28–33]. Recent research emphasizes the benefits of generative adversarial networks in the domain of drug development, showcasing their ability to identify novel compounds and overcome challenges like mode collapse by encouraging exploration beyond existing data. Specialized GAN architectures, like MedGAN, employ graph convolutional networks to efficiently generate new compounds, addressing the growing need for new pharmaceuticals and enhancing the drug development process [27, 34, 35]. GANs have also been employed in the creation of new peptides and proteins, thereby making a substantial impact on the investigation of novel bioactive substances [36]. Furthermore, a study demonstrated the advantageous properties of employing a variational quantum circuit (VQC) in the context of small-scale drug discovery, where each constituent of the generative adversarial network was substituted. As a result, the GAN's generator showed significant improvements in physicochemical properties and performance, despite having a minimal number of learnable parameters. This is in contrast to the classical approach [37–39].

13.3.2 Variational Autoencoders

VAEs are a type of generative model that acquires a latent representation of data by encoding input samples into a space with fewer dimensions and then decoding them back into the original space. This neural network architecture consists solely of the encoder and decoder components, which are jointly trained with the re-parameterization technique. Equation 13.1 defines the function of the variational autoencoder. In this equation, an encoder estimates Q(z|X) and a decoder estimates P(X|z) in an autoencoder setting.

$$E\left[\log P(X \mid z)\right] - D_{KL}\left[Q(z \mid X) \,\|\, P(z)\right] \tag{13.1}$$

VAEs have successfully generated a chemical latent space that accurately represents the structural diversity of compound libraries within drug discovery [40–42]. These tools help to explore a broader range of chemical possibilities and make it easier to create new compounds. The natural product compound variational autoencoder (NP-VAE) has significantly transformed the approach to managing complex datasets and extensive chemical structures. It repeatedly demonstrates its ability to generate models that excel in several criteria, highlighting its outstanding capabilities. By employing reconstruction loss and latent loss, these models can enhance the quality of reconstruction while efficiently exploring the latent space [41, 43, 44]. Moreover, VAEs have been employed to accurately replicate the morphology and gene expression measurements resulting from certain drugs. This allows for the anticipation of cellular conditions influenced by substances that have established polypharmacology. The examination of cellular condition via pharmacological processes has significant promise for future advancements in research. It can assist them in the development and identification of specific therapeutic treatments and the categorization of unintended side effects [45].

13.3.3 Transformer-Based Models

AI models demonstrate exceptional proficiency in leveraging natural language processing to comprehend the complexities and subtleties of language. Large datasets are utilized to educate them to understand relationships between sequential data, such as words and sentences. Three innovative methods for drug discovery have been recently identified. The initial method, drug AI, merges the encoder-decoder transformer structure with reinforcement learning by employing a Monte Carlo tree search to enhance the drug discovery procedure [46]. This approach ensures the generation of small compounds that exhibit drug-like characteristics and high affinity for their targets. The second approach's developers prioritized target-specific De-Novo drug design. They perceived it as a problem to translate between the language of amino acids and the reduced molecular input line entry system representation [47]. This method utilizes the transformer neural network architecture, which is highly effective in handling sequence transduction tasks. It excels at capturing long-range dependencies within sequences. The synthesized molecules have a diverse array of structures and feature properties that closely mimic those of real pharmaceuticals. TransDTI is a workflow that employs transformer-based language models to classify interactions between drug–target pairs into three categories: active, inactive, or intermediate. It is designed for multiclass classification and regression tasks. These models have undergone training using comprehensive datasets of drug–target interactions, leading to outstanding performance in comparison to standard techniques. They exhibit a high level of efficacy in forecasting novel drug–target interactions based on sequence data, surpassing current methodologies [48]. DTSyn is a model that effectively extracts interactions between chemicals and cell lines to depict potential drug action mechanisms. DTSyn showcases improved interpretability by incorporating attention mechanisms and pre-trained gene embeddings. As a result, this model is extremely valuable for prioritizing synergistic drug combinations based on chemical and cell line gene expression profiles. Other transformer-based models have been crucial in speeding up drug discovery processes. They perform activities such as automating retrosynthesis, creating new compounds with precise features, and assisting in the exploration of chemical space for medication discovery [49–53].

13.4 GENERATIVE AI MODEL

13.4.1 Restricted Boltzmann Machines

Restricted Boltzmann machines (RBMs) are a kind of generative model constructed based on energy-based models. The system consists of both visible and hidden levels, which are interconnected in a symmetrical fashion. RBMs are commonly taught using contrastive divergence or alternative learning algorithms. RBMs have demonstrated significant promise in the domain of pharmaceutical exploration, namely in forecasting drug–disease connections and drug–target interactions. RBMs have demonstrated higher predictive performance in medication repositioning tasks as compared to other approaches inside drug-disease association networks. In addition, the RBM model has been enhanced by incorporating momentum during weight updates, resulting in improved prediction performance. Therefore, it is a significant instrument for future endeavors in drug repositioning [54–56]. RBMs have demonstrated efficacy in the domain of drug–target interactions, enabling the incorporation of diverse types of interactions and the forecasting of unfamiliar drug–target correlations or modes of action. The prediction problem has been effectively addressed by researchers who have utilized RBMs to create a two-layer graphical model. By employing this method, they have been able to reveal concealed characteristics inside networks of drug–target interactions, resulting in remarkable precision-recall curve values. This methodology is highly significant in anticipating interactions between drugs and targets, as well as in advancing efforts to reposition drugs. By integrating many interaction types [57–59], it outperforms existing prediction algorithms. RBMs are highly important in the field of drug development, as they offer unique ways for predicting connections between drugs and diseases, interactions between drugs and targets, and assisting in the process of computationally repositioning drugs. However, additional investigation is necessary to effectively employ machine learning methods for the analysis of intricate datasets, the prediction of novel connections within biological systems, and the transformation of the area of drug development.

13.4.2 Generative Graph Neural Networks

Graph neural networks (GNNs) are a specialized sort of neural network specifically built to handle data structured in the form of a graph. GNNs possess the capability to generate novel graph topologies or append nodes and edges to an already existing graph. GNNs are revolutionizing the domain of drug discovery by facilitating the creation of novel compounds with specific characteristics and streamlining the process of drug design. Graph neural network modules are used in these networks to create sequential molecular graph generators such as MG2N2 [60, 61]. Generators like these gradually enhance graphs by adding nodes and connections, making training procedures easier and improving interpretability. These models excel at capturing and applying molecular patterns, allowing them to generate new structures with impressive accuracy. They have demonstrated a high level of effectiveness in preventing over-fitting and consistently achieve competitive performance [35]. Graph neural networks are experiencing a growing application in drug discovery, particularly in the area of conditional De-Novo drug creation. Graph neural networks have demonstrated remarkable efficacy in analyzing data structured as graphs. They have achieved substantial advancements in predicting interactions between drugs and their targets, as well as in developing novel candidate molecules with exceptional efficiency [62, 63]. The integration of graph neural networks and deep learning methods is revolutionizing the domain of chemical structure graph formation. This advancement has the potential to greatly impact drug discovery by optimizing resource utilization and enhancing the efficiency of generating new bioactive molecules. An instance of this is MM-GANN-DDI, which introduces a multimodal graph-agnostic neural network specifically developed to precisely predict instances of drug-drug interaction events [64–67]. Graph neural networks play a crucial role in promoting advancements in the field of drug development. They enable researchers to methodically create new compounds, forecast drug–target interactions, and improve computational techniques for designing new drugs. Their capacity to analyze graph data and produce a wide range of chemical compounds for therapeutic applications underscores their crucial contribution to the progress of drug development endeavors.

13.4.3 Language Models

Language models (LMs) are a specific kind of generative model that learns the probability distribution of sequences of words or tokens in a given language. Language models play a crucial role in drug development by providing innovative methods to accelerate the molecule discovery process, enhance drug design, forecast characteristics, and optimize chemical interactions [68]. Transformer-based architectures have exhibited remarkable capabilities in comprehending and producing text that closely matches human language. Consequently, these technologies have been utilized in scientific domains such as protein folding, target identification, and small molecule discovery [69]. Chemical language models are essential in the field of molecular discovery since they greatly accelerate the process of identifying novel compounds for medication development, making accurate predictions regarding characteristics, and enhancing chemical reactions [70]. The models under consideration primarily target tiny compounds, proteins, or polymers, and have demonstrated significant promise in the realm of initial drug exploration. They utilize machine learning algorithms to comprehend and produce scientific text, resulting in encouraging outcomes [71]. Furthermore, the utilization of AI-driven language models has fundamentally revolutionized the domain of natural language processing in the realm of drug discovery and development [72]. An illustration of this is the utilization of an automated technique known as automatic biomedical named entity recognition (BioNER) which has the ability to reveal concealed connections between chemicals, genes, targets, and diseases in documents that are based on text [73]. This remark emphasizes the profound influence of LM models on the advancement of therapy development. They possess the capacity to completely transform many facets of the process, including target identification, clinical design, regulatory decision-making, Pharmacovigilance, and even the advancement of novel medicines for diseases such as COVID-19 via drug repurposing activities. LM models significantly improve patient recruiting processes in clinical trials by automating tasks using enhanced information retrieval and prioritization methods. The models undergo training to comprehend medical terminology and its diverse synonyms. This allows them to derive crucial information from clinical documentation, hence facilitating the classification of patients based on various illness categories. Their capacity to integrate eligibility criteria into standardized contextual inquiries significantly improves the clinical trial matching procedures. These language models use a cross-model learning infrastructure to encode enrollment criteria and patient electronic health records (EHRs). This leads to enhanced matching inference that outperforms rule-based techniques. Furthermore, they seamlessly integrate cutting-edge technology like genomes and imaging data to advance the field of precision medicine. Furthermore, AI-driven language models have the capability to improve patient enrollment rates and assist in the identification of appropriate locations for clinical trials. These models consider multiple aspects, such as previous site experience, affiliations with health non-profit organizations, patient retention data, and cost-effectiveness. This comprehensive strategy facilitates informed clinical decision-making, which is essential for the success of drug development [74–77].

13.4.4 Multimodal Models

Generative AI models, namely those based on multimodal model (MM) principles, play a vital role in the field of drug discovery and therapeutic design. These models possess the ability to effectively analyze and interpret diverse datasets by using advanced deep learning techniques. Deep generative models that employ multimodal data have demonstrated superior performance compared to models that solely utilize unimodal input. The reason for this is because multimodal data offers additional and complementary perspectives [78–80]. The key to successful drug discovery rests in effectively utilizing diverse data modalities that offer distinct viewpoints, facilitating the accumulation of evidence for discovery. While current studies predominantly focus on molecular structural data, they do not effectively utilize other significant data modalities such as drug–target interactions, drug-disease knowledge, and relevant gene expression after drug therapy. One approach to address this difficulty is to explore solutions like "modality alignment" and "modality fusion." Modality alignment refers to the process of linking various modalities by means of an intermediary modality, typically molecular structures. In contrast, modality fusion involves the direct mapping of all modalities to a shared latent space [81–84]. The hybrid data model efficiently encompasses a broad spectrum of information in drug design, including chemical characteristics, drug–target interactions, drug disease knowledge, and disease-relevant gene expression [85]. Furthermore, a multimodal generative model considers various facets of the drug discovery process in order to enhance the likelihood of success in clinical trials. By combining organized and unstructured knowledge, frameworks such as KEDD can get a more thorough comprehension of biomolecules. Consequently, they outperform the most advanced models in predicting drug–target interactions, drug characteristics, drug-drug interactions, and protein–protein interactions [86]. The analysis emphasizes the considerable potential of these frameworks in practical applications, improving the drug development process by incorporating expertise in biomolecular knowledge from many sources. Utilizing MM models effectively tackles the issue posed by the immense magnitude of chemical space. Furthermore, generative adversarial networks have been proposed as a means to generate a diverse array of three-dimensional ligand structures that are capable of interacting with the binding pocket. The forms can be interpreted as a series of SMILES, enabling the invention of new drugs based on their structure [87]. The evaluation showcases the enhancement gained in comparison to randomly selecting samples from the original chemical space of ZINC drug-like compounds. This confirms the efficacy of the strategy in virtual screening. Furthermore, the integration of multimodal imaging with different imaging techniques provides a vast amount of morphological, functional, and molecular data, significantly expediting the processes of drug discovery and development. Imaging technologies are essential for improving our comprehension of disease mechanisms, discovering new pharmacological targets, and assessing the efficacy of potential drug candidates and treatment responses. The utilization of radiomics MM, employing both targeted and untargeted approaches, enhances the efficacy of imaging technologies in the field of drug discovery and development, emphasizing their advantages, advancements, and prospective possibilities. Targeted techniques involve the visualization of specific drug molecules or targets, while untargeted approaches concentrate on analyzing a wide variety of molecules to discover drug metabolites, effects on endogenous molecules, and changes associated with disorders. Imaging techniques provide insights into the effects of medication therapies on tissues and organs, which are crucial for improving drug design and delivery [84–88].

13.5 GENERAL ASPECTS OF AI

Instruments have the ability to forecast *in vitro* responses, evaluate the pharmacokinetics of treatments, and develop quantitative relationships between the structure and properties, as well as the structure and activity. In addition, they have the ability to ascertain the suitable dosage, quantify hair porosity or the blood–brain barrier, and perform other tasks. It is crucial to have a comprehensive awareness of the pharmacokinetic features of various drugs. By utilizing *in silico* tools to predict these properties, drug research can become more efficient and cost-effective. Additionally, there are machine training methods that can be quite useful. The mentioned techniques are support vector machines, the Gaussian method, random forest, classification and comparison tree, and the naive Bayes (NB) classifier. ANNs have the ability to generate different types of load-output data, choose optimal chromatographic gradient conditions, analyze multiple linear regression relationships in pharmaceutical testing, predict drug behavior, and design preformulations [89]. NN modelling is a proficient method for elucidating the molecular structure of an organic substance and providing forecasts regarding its physical and chemical characteristics [90]. ANNs are composed of computing elements known as artificial nerves or nodes. ANN designs are classified into associated, function-extracting, and subadaptive networks based on their functions [91]. The relationship between design and method variables and discharge characteristics of managed-release medication distribution devices is complex. Therefore, researchers select and optimize associated networks to create effective and efficient managed-demand formulas. The use of ANNs extends beyond genomics, metabolomics, information processing, pharmacy product growth, and assessment of medicinal bioavailability behavior. They were proposed as a dependable instrument for collecting cause-and-effect relationships and assessing disparities between *in vitro* and *in vivo* correlation (IVIVC). IVIVC, when combined with ANNs, enables the development of intricate relationships between pharmacokinetic parameters. ANNs may not provide a comprehensive understanding of the interconnected relationships between variables. The tablet formulations of the sustained-release paracetamol were designed using IVIVC, a nonlinear modelling tool. Information was obtained through a distributed cellular network regression assessment (generalized regression neural network—GRNN), which showed similarities to the observations made *in vitro*. The assessment demonstrates a consistent and effective ability to generalize complex interactions for both entry and yield dimensions, taking into account variations in medication discharge kinetics in different circumstances [92].

13.6 AI USE IN DRUG DEVELOPMENT: R&D PROFICIENCY

The application of drug-likeness criteria is crucial in the production of medicines, but medicinal corporations encounter significant challenges in improving R&D performance. The cost of drug identification/creation has increased significantly, reaching US$3 billion from US$800 million in 2001. The cost of producing drugs takes into account the expenses incurred from failures. As a result, the assessed cost represents the average value of the new medicine that will be introduced into the healthcare system [93]. The decrease in the rate of new medication compounds authorized per billion US dollars spent on research and development is alarming. The researcher conducted a thorough examination of the main factors contributing to the concerning figures and identified the following primary causes of R&D ineffectiveness: (1) the matter of surpassing the Beatles, (2) the challenge of vigilant regulators, (3) the inclination towards basic research and sheer effort, and (4) the temptation to allocate excessive financial resources. The novel molecule for a specific pharmacological disorder should be more effective than any of the currently approved drugs, as suggested by the better-than-the-Beatles metaphor [94]. The challenges discussed here have a significant impact on the outcome of any experimental medication that holds the promise of delivering improved therapeutic results. With each new drug, the stakes are higher and the inefficiency in research and development becomes more apparent. Clearing the ever-progressing hurdles is becoming increasingly challenging. The cautious-regulator problem is a result of the lessons learned from past drug calamities, leading to an increase in rigor and tightening of controls. This is a well-crafted effort to minimize the risk associated with new medicines and create a plan for safer product formulations that cater to customers' needs. However, it does result in a notable increase in research and development expenses. This is often seen in the eagerness to invest heavily in research, with R&D institutions hiring more and more resources in the hope of achieving a significant return and being at the forefront of introducing new drugs. Additionally, this leads to a higher level of investment in research and development. The phenomenon of clinical research-brute force bias involves an inclination to overestimate the potential of basic research advancements in preclinical studies, specifically in the areas of target identification, verification, and brute-force testing to improve the success rates of clinical drug development [94]. Medicinal companies face challenges due to the escalating costs of research and development, as well as the frequent turnover in the creation of new medicinal molecules. In the past, there has been an evaluation of various causes and interventions aimed at reducing attrition rates during the Phase IIb and Phase III clinical trials. Around 62% of the new chemical entities did not have an impact on the hospital. However, these causes are not widespread, as medical literature shows that success rates vary depending on the treatment area. There is a lower degree of depletion observed in molecules with new mechanisms of action compared to compounds with previous mechanisms of action. Pharmaceutical establishments need to evaluate different clinical areas with varying success rates to determine the effectiveness of reducing attrition rates. By understanding these key factors, organizations can effectively decrease attrition rates [95].

13.7 EXISTING DATABASES AND TOOLS FOR DRUG DEVELOPMENT

13.7.1 Chemical and Biological Databases

Aggregating experimental bio-assay and computationally generated drug–target interaction (DTI) data is crucial for the development of publicly available databases. Table 13.1 shows a compilation of chemical and bio-activity databases.

TABLE 13.1
Compilation of Compound and Bio-Activity Databases

Reference	Outline
PubChem	The most extensive compilation of chemical and bio-activity data that may be accessed without any cost.
ChEMBL	A comprehensive bioactivity database for drug discovery.
DrugBank	An extensive collection of information on drugs, their actions, and the targets they affect.
ZINC	A comprehensive platform for virtual screening of compounds.
BindingDB	A comprehensive database that records the binding affinity measurements between target molecules and various drugs.
ADME	A comprehensive online resource for pharmacokinetic information.
STITCH	A comprehensive database of chemical-protein interactions.

13.7.1.1 PubChem

PubChem is a comprehensive repository of chemical data, with a vast assortment of more than 111 million compounds, 279 million substances, 295 million bio-activities, and 34 million articles. The resources are efficiently categorized into three interrelated web data pages: substance, compound, and bio assay [96, 97]. The bio-assay database contains the descriptions and test outcomes of bio-assays. Data mining methods are effective in identifying compounds that are suitable for a specific target or protein.

13.7.1.2 ChEMBL

ChEMBL is an open access drug discovery database produced by the European Molecular Biology Laboratory (EMBL). The information regarding approved and potential drugs, including their mode of action and therapeutic uses, is gathered from complete papers published in influential journals. Subsequently, this information is merged with data pertaining to tiny molecules and their biological function. The bio-activity data is disseminated to other databases, such as BindingDB [98, 99] and PubChem Bioassay. The ChEMBL database has been widely used for multiple reasons, including discovering chemical tools for a specific target, predicting interactions between medications and targets, repurposing drugs, assessing target tractability, and integrating with current drug development tools [100].

13.7.1.3 DrugBank

DrugBank provides an extensive array of information, encompassing molecular-level data, clinical particulars, drug interactions, side effects, and drug re-purposing. This approach is frequently used for *in silico* drug design, repurposing, and drug discovery using machine learning [101].

13.7.1.4 UniProt Database

UniProt is an extensive database that grants access to a wide array of protein sequences, as well as valuable taxonomic data and intricate details regarding their biological functions. The UniProt database comprises four components: UniProt Knowledgebase (UniProtKB), UniProt Reference Clusters (UniRef), UniProt Archive (UniParc), and UniProt Metagenomic and Environmental Sequences (UniMES). UniProt boasts an impressive collection of over 189 million records, with the majority of them meticulously curated by human experts [102].

13.7.1.5 Protein Data Bank

The Protein Data Bank (PDB) has the largest and most comprehensive assortment of three-dimensional structures for proteins, ribosomes, and nucleic acids. The determination of these structures has predominantly relied on X-ray crystallography or nuclear magnetic resonance spectroscopy [103].

13.7.2 AI Software Tools for the Drug Development Process

AI tools have the capacity to transform drug discovery. Scientists now have the ability to examine large quantities of data, generate novel compounds, and make precise forecasts about the efficacy of possible drugs in a significantly reduced timeframe. This section will explore many commonly employed artificial intelligence methods for drug discovery applications. Table 13.2 is an exhaustive compilation of artificial intelligence tools specifically designed for the purpose of drug discovery.

13.7.2.1 AlphaFold2

Predicting the 3D structures of proteins from their amino acid sequence is a complex and difficult undertaking. AlphaFold2, created by DeepMind, has attained a remarkable degree of precision [104] and is easily accessible via Google Collab.

TABLE 13.2
AI-Based Software Used in Drug Discovery

Software	Description
AlphaFold	Utilizes a deep neural network to forecast the tertiary structure of a protein.
Chemputer	Provides an elaborate procedure for the synthesis of a chemical.
Conv_qsar_fast	Utilizes a convolutional neural network (CNN) approach to forecast molecular characteristics.
Chemical VAE	Utilizes a variational autoencoder for automated chemical design.
DeepChem	A Python library, which is open-source, utilizes a deep learning technique for the purpose of identifying compounds.
DeepTox	Utilizes a deep learning algorithm to forecast the toxicity of chemical substances.
DeepNeuralNetQSAR	Utilizes a multilevel deep neural network to make predictions about molecular activity.
DeltaVina	Utilizes a mix of random forest and AutoDock scoring tool to forecast the binding affinity between small molecules and drugs.
Hit Dexter	Utilizes a machine learning system to forecast the occurrence of a frequent hitter.
InnerOuterRNN	Utilizes inner- and outer recursive neural networks to accurately predict the physical, chemical, and biological aspects.

13.7.2.2 DeepChem

The DeepChem library is a robust tool that facilitates the analysis of chemical datasets by offering a user-friendly TensorFlow wrapper. This paper explores the utilization of algorithms in deep-learning research for the purpose of drug development and the creation of models to inhibit BACE-1. DeepChem is a versatile tool that enables the analysis of protein structures, prediction of small molecule drug solubility and binding affinity to targets, as well as cell counting in microscopic images. The DeepChem software has successfully included MoleculeNet [105], allowing users to conveniently access the properties of 700,000 chemicals.

13.7.2.3 DeeperBind

DeeperBind is an exceptionally sophisticated network that precisely forecasts the specificity of protein binding with respect to DNA probes. The model accurately represents the complex interplay between transcription factors (TFs) and their respective binding sites (DNA/RNA). DeeperBind possesses a robust capacity to precisely predict the dynamics of probe sequences. Moreover, it possesses the ability to undergo training and testing on datasets that consist of sequences with different lengths [106].

13.7.2.4 DeepAffinity

The DeepAffinity model utilizes a combination of recurrent and convolutional neural networks to precisely forecast the binding affinity between drug and target sequences. The model efficiently employs a mixture of labeled and unlabeled data to create molecular representations along with structurally annotated protein sequence representations. Based on study [107], DeepAffinity exhibited greater performance in comparison to random forest, ensemble approaches, and RNN-CNN models.

13.8 THE IMPLEMENTATION OF ARTIFICIAL INTELLIGENCE IN THE FIELD OF DRUG DESIGN

Many AI applications that are pertinent to drug research. Protein structure plays a crucial role in drug design. Protein dysfunctions have led to a rise in contaminants in the human body. Structural drug design methodologies are utilized to differentiate small compounds in protein targets. Predicting the 3D structure of protein requires additional resources in terms of both funding and time. Nevertheless, it continues to face difficulties in attaining higher precision in predicting the 3D structure from scratch. Deep learning and feature extraction technologies are crucial for accurately predicting the secondary structure and protein interactions. The relationship between structure and sequence is accurately determined by extracting features. The ultimate objective is to enhance the accuracy of predicting the 3D protein structure through the utilization of deep learning techniques. To extract information about the computational structure of protein–protein interactions, it is crucial to do research on the interface of protein–protein interactions (PPI) [108]. Artificial intelligence has a broad range of uses, such as forecasting drug–protein interactions, identifying medication effectiveness, guaranteeing biomarker safety, conducting virtual screening, and more. Here is a thorough discussion.

13.8.1 Predicting Drug–Protein Interactions

In silico drug development is the use of different biological sources to anticipate interactions between drugs and proteins. Complexities may arise in extensive projections due to their significant reliance on multiple unidentified interactions. Thus, it is advisable to employ semi-supervised training techniques to tackle the challenges posed by unlabeled and labelled data complexities. Typically, better results are achieved when using labelled data. In addition, the semi-supervised technique effortlessly integrates chemical structure, drug-protein interaction network data, and genomic sequence data. The article demonstrates that drug-protein interactions from different data sets, including ions, enzymes, and nuclear receptors, produced results that were both extremely accurate and dependable [109]. Protein interactions are essential for controlling the therapeutic effectiveness of medicines. The Drug-Protein Interaction Database (DPI) largely emphasizes therapeutic protein targets, providing only little information regarding non-targets. Hence, computer methods can fill the information void in forecasting protein targets for dispersed medicinal molecules. The research discovered that the group of 35 factors had a significant impact on the resemblance between protein and pharmacological targets. Three categories of similarity have been derived from the findings of 35 predictors: drug structure, target sequence, and drug profile. The significance of database sources in therapeutic action lies in their content, linkages, and implications [110]. Drug repurposing relies heavily on the identification of unexpected drug-protein interactions. The dominant drug shows potential for repurposing, although it is important to note that drug side effects are inevitable. Moreover, it is notable that around 1,000 human proteins has the capacity to induce substantial adverse reactions. The proteome scale technique was employed to forecast probable adverse effects and protein targets. FINDSITEcomb is a tool that can be utilized to forecast interactions between drugs and proteins. The estimates revealed a significant level of disruption, with an average of 329 human targets for each drug [111].

13.8.2 Drug Efficacy Discovery

Usually, an evaluation of the effects of a drug centers upon its biochemical action. Finding the optimal equilibrium between the biological activity and the therapeutic action has proven to be a challenging task. A comprehensive study was done to fill a research gap in the existing body of knowledge on the effects of cellular medicines. The primary focus of this research is the classification of psychotropic drugs. The microarray data is analyzed by utilizing random trees to create a forest and classify them. This process yields a profile that indicates the effectiveness of biomarker gene expression. The classification tree attained an accuracy rate of 88.9%, whilst the random forest model achieved an accuracy rate of 83.3% when evaluating the effectiveness profile of a medication treatment. Therefore, when examining cellular assessments, it is crucial to take into account whole genetic information in order to comprehend the impacts of novel physiological medications in clinical settings.

Finally, gene expression data from *in vitro* signatures can be used to assess the effectiveness of therapeutic activities, aiding in the validation of targeting and drug development [112]. Effective drug development involves the crucial tasks of predicting drug effectiveness and identifying potential targets to maximize profitability. Proximity to medical disorders can impede the efficacy of therapy and can result in the release of substances with therapeutic advantages. The study analyzed a total of 78 ailments and conducted tests on 238 medications to demonstrate the efficacy of the drugs in therapeutic applications. Additionally, it brought attention to matters about the effectiveness of genes and other illnesses. The network-based method is employed to generate a metric that assesses the interactions between the disease and the therapeutic target, leading to a comprehensive estimate of the proximity between the drug and the disease. Therefore, the fact that network-based systems are located close to each other allows for the anticipation of connections between new medication diseases. This opens up several possibilities for identifying conflicts and repurposing drugs [113].

13.8.3 Ensuring Safety Biomarkers

Biomarkers play a critical role in drug development by assuring safety precautions and precisely detecting biological and analytical indications. Stakeholders have the ability to assess and supervise the defense of claims for specified objectives and verify that the necessary criteria are being achieved. To successfully evaluate the experiment agreement, a stakeholder evaluation method is necessary. This technique is essential to adapt to the distinctive attributes of the biomarkers and ascertain the methods by which these advancements are examined, combined, and understood. Additionally, it helps in measuring the improved biomarkers and conventional comparators effectively [114]. Our survey revealed that modern medicines do not offer any additional safety benefits compared to older drugs, despite undergoing longer medical trial programs. The trails on the market undergo inspections that are not thorough enough to ensure systematic safety. Previous signals related to drugs can contribute to enhancing drug safety and identifying underlying biomarkers, thereby increasing their toxicity. However, the safety markers may vary for different target systems. However, it is challenging to identify an alternative approach that will ensure the highest level of medication safety. Nevertheless, mutual comprehension of benefit and risk evaluation by efficiently communicating with the general population [115]. This study employs various deep learning algorithms to forecast the PPI interface and showcases remarkable outcomes when compared to the SVM technique [116]. Therefore, the utilization of PPI's in biological techniques became more complex [117, 118]. Residues from different sources can be found in each PPI [119]. PPIs, or protein–protein interactions, have become a highly attractive group of pharmaceutical targets. They have the capability to interact with a diverse range of targets including ion channels, G-protein coupled receptors (GPCRs), and kinases [120, 121]. iFitDock is a docking tool that allows users to explore specific hotspots in protein–protein interactions.

13.8.4 Virtual Screening

This AI method is employed in the drug development process to identify tiny compounds capable of recognizing binding structures for a therapeutic target. Virtual screening in drug development is utilizing software and algorithms to detect potential hits from proprietary chemical collections. However, this process can be inefficient for retrieving unique hits. Once new hits have been identified, the next step involves purifying compounds with unfavorable scaffolds or frameworks [121]. This procedure utilizes several tactics, including docking-based methods, similarity searches pharmacore-based approaches [122], and machine learning methods [123]. These methods have resulted in the creation of two approaches for classification: structure-based and ligand-based virtual screening. Once the 3D structure of proteins is accessible, the technique of molecular docking can be extensively employed [124]. The progress in the development of applications pertaining to docking-based virtual screening has been fruitful and devoid of any adverse repercussions [125]. There could be several impediments with this method, such as the scoring function. The accuracy of estimating binding affinities (bond/relationship) using a scoring function is limited due to the complex nature of protein flexibility, which is influenced by insufficient arrangements and entropy impacts [124, 126]. Ultimately, many docking models considered various parameters, such as binding affinities and rejections, which were assessed using docking scores and distance-time measurements [127, 128]. Unlike docking-based virtual screening, ligand-based virtual screening does not depend on the three-dimensional structure of the protein. The goal is to generate bioactivity domains using molecular characteristics [121]. The primary goal of this strategy is to consistently improve yields and decrease false hit rates [123, 129, 130]. The support vector machine technique was frequently employed in virtual screening to accomplish this goal [131]. DL strategies have been successfully utilized to achieve excellent classification capacity, minimal generalization error, and robust feature extraction ability [132, 133]. During the search procedure in virtual screening, the sparse distribution method might be significantly time-consuming [131, 134]. To tackle this difficulty, it is imperative to possess molecule libraries that encompass diverse training compounds [133] in the simplified molecular input line entry specifications format. The incorporation of extended short-term memory network design is essential for the field of natural language processing. Machine learning techniques such as deep neural networks and gradient boosting trees have made it possible to generate chemical libraries using recurrent neural networks. The adversarial autoencoder is used to simulate molecular fingerprints in order to detect possible anticancer drugs [135].

13.8.5 High-Throughput Virtual Screening and Molecular Docking

After identifying the target, the typically used techniques include high-throughput virtual screening (HTVS) and molecular docking techniques. These techniques are combined with free energy perturbations, sampling, and scoring algorithms. An essential stage in commencing the HTVS process is gaining a comprehensive understanding of the active site of the protein/receptor, where the ligand would attach to imitate or counteract its normal function. The scoring function plays a crucial role in virtual scoring, as it is responsible for evaluating the binding affinities towards the target in molecular docking [126]. Mapping features in machine learning can result in notable advancements in extracting physical, geometric, and chemical characteristics for obtaining scores [136]. Researching data-driven black box models that forecast binding affinities and exclude specific concepts in docking, such as physical function, poses significant challenges [137]. The utilization of AI has identified concepts such as random forest and SVM to optimize the performance of the scoring function. Instead of utilizing a linear additive strategy that is based on the concept of energy terms, one might apply an SVM model as an alternative. The support vector machine can effectively capture the relationship between experimental binding affinities and the energy terms obtained by the eHiTS docking tool. Hence, data enhances performance in terms of scoring power and screening power [138, 139]. Researchers have increasingly used the CNN model in image processing because of its exceptional performance and capacity to provide various characteristics for predicting protein-ligand affinities in protein-ligand interactions. Jimenez et al. did a study on the three-dimensional visual depiction of the CNN model and binding affinities. Their research demonstrated enhanced correlation behavior in datasets. The essential potency of deep learning is in its capacity to derive abstract features from fundamental features. This is crucial in representing complex compound-protein structures, such as molecule types and particle separation [132]. The Deep VS is heavily dependent on the CNN model and has gained a strong understanding of abstract features derived from fundamental features. This understanding allows it to effectively support docking programs such as GLIDE SP [140] and ICM [141]. The primary goal of activity scoring was to identify a restricted set of protein-ligand interaction characteristics for predicting binding affinities using the CNN model. This approach enhances the information scoring function and improves the predictive capabilities [142].

13.8.6 QSAR

The method of hit-to-lead optimization employed QSAR analysis to discover possible lead compounds from the hit analogues. This investigation entailed the prediction of bioactivity analogues and principally concentrated on employing mathematical concepts to investigate quantitative mapping involving physicochemical or structural entities and biological activities. QSAR analysis [143] encompasses the fundamental principles of mathematical modeling, the careful selection and advancement of molecular descriptions, rigorous evaluation and interpretation methodologies, and effective utilization procedures. The incorporation of mathematical models and chemical structural representations is essential in QSAR demonstration. When choosing descriptors, it is essential to identify mathematical models that can accurately represent relationships in the structure-activity technique. To enhance the understanding of the relationship between the 2D structure and activity, it is advisable to utilize parameters such as physicochemical descriptors and linear regression models to provide the quantitative structure-activity relationship study as a distinct part [144]. The author proposed a hypothesis regarding the relationship between compound activities and the presence of substituents, supported by a well-formulated bioactivity description and chemical structure analysis [145]. The Free-Wilson approach is a robust substitute for the Hansch method, as it accurately forecasts chemical structures without depending on physiochemical characteristics. Random forest and support vector machine are often employed machine learning algorithms in mathematical models [146–148]. Furthermore, deep learning algorithms are employed in QSAR modelling to examine chemical sequences and automatically extract characteristics. The Merck Molecular Activity challenge occurred in 2012, and a team led by George Dahl emerged victorious. The researchers employed ensemble approaches, including Gaussian process regression, multitask deep neural network, and gradient boosting machine [131]. The outcomes of multitask deep neural networks were influenced by Kaggle. Furthermore, Dahl et al. did a study on the notion of multitask deep neural networks and showcased exceptional performance in neural systems that focus on a single task. Neural networks have the ability to learn features from various parameters through a multitask strategy, even when the tasks at hand are similar[149, 150]. The performance of the random forest algorithm in drug development was assessed using multitask neural structures, resulting in excellent outcomes. The integration of multitask neural architectures has been unified under a platform known as DeepChem. Subramanian employed canvas descriptors to execute deep neural networks. To achieve accurate results in predicting binding affinities for human β-secretase-1 inhibitors, it is crucial to strengthen the regression and classification model. The deep neural network model yields remarkable outcomes on the validation dataset. The classification accuracy is 0.82, the regression R^2 value is 0.74, and the mean absolute error (MAE) is 0.52. The DNN model efficiently employs 2D descriptors and has improved performance in comparison to force-field-based techniques. This can be linked to the integration of partial capacity models in deep learning. QSAR models employ deep learning approaches to enhance the accuracy of anticipating the future role of hit-to-lead optimization research.

13.8.7 De-Novo Drug Design

The process of creating novel drug designs include modifying or adjusting chemical structures in order to improve their ability to specifically target certain areas [151]. Presenting a novel molecule employing the well-established De-Novo model, the fragment-based approach. The existence of impracticalities and complexity in the molecular structure [152] presents a possible hazard in its development and renders the assessment of its bioactivity difficult. The utilization of deep learning models has allowed for the introduction of a new structure with appropriate properties, showcasing their powerful knowledge and generative capabilities. The De-Novo drug design approach utilizes deep learning models, autoencoders, to develop an appropriate format for novel chemical entities (NCEs). Therefore, the integration of an autoencoder with a multilayer perceptron classifier is a viable method for producing NCEs with predetermined physicochemical characteristics. The drug/chemical structure is created in SMILES format, which can be difficult to understand in certain circumstances. Nevertheless, the employment of a grammatical variational autoencoder effectively tackles this problem and accelerates the procedure. Olivecrona et al. expanded the application of deep reinforcement learning to forecast biological processes and create novel molecules by modifications to the RNN model [153]. To acquire SMILES syntax, it is necessary to train an RNN model. This paradigm enables the retrieval of compounds from chemBL. Reinforcement learning agents perform actions in response to specific conditions. At this point, if the agent receives a positive reward, the agent's actions can be updated [154]. If you want to maximize your activity scoring rewards, consider using the SVM technique to improve certain approaches that rely on the concept of ligands in the training set. Can you provide a few molecules that can be used for training a deep reinforcement learning model with an RNN architecture, specifically targeting the dopamine receptor 2-type? Furthermore, it has been observed that predictions have attained a remarkable level of accuracy exceeding 95% for structures within the bioactive region, owing to the scoring capability of support vector machines. By utilizing deep learning techniques, the auto-encoder method can be utilized to produce unique molecules. One way to autonomously create new molecules with certain characteristics is by combining a multilayer perceptron (MLP) and a variational autoencoder [155]. PPI prediction has faced many problems, such as inadequate funding for protein information, a scarcity of known PPIs for studying particular viruses, and ineffective techniques due to sequence dissimilarities within viral families. The De-Novo methodology seeks to forecast new protein–protein interaction viruses and their respective hosts. DeNovo is a computational framework that analyzes the adverse effects of protein–protein interactions to forecast novel viruses while considering the possibility of utilizing common host proteins. De-Novo has conducted experiments to evaluate the generalization of protein–protein interactions across several domains. During the training phase, the De-Novo technique demonstrated a remarkable 81% accuracy in minimizing noisy negative associations and an amazing 86% accuracy in predicting viral proteins. The De-Novo approach has demonstrated significant efficacy in predicting both within-species and single virus–host interactions. Predicting the PPI (person-to-person contact) for a contaminated individual is difficult, and the most precise outcomes are obtained by doing tests for human-bacteria interactions [156]. The application of multi-objective optimization techniques and artificial intelligence has demonstrated encouraging outcomes in the advancement of biological and chemical opportunities. These methods allow for the creation of automated De-Novo compound structures that mimic human creativity. This work investigates the application of a novel perception pair that employs multi-objective technology. The objective is to mechanize the production of distinct molecules with an original structure, relying on similar characteristics among consistent physicochemical parameters. The RNN algorithm is utilized to do this, leading to a compromise between several factors. This perspective explores the utilization of various chemical libraries that are focused on targeting acetylcholinesterase and neuraminidase through De-Novo structure design. A range of quality indicators were employed to evaluate the chemical feasibility, validity, drug-likeness, and diversity content. The assessment of posing and scoring in the generation of new molecules entails using molecular docking with X-ray cognate ligands that have similar chemical equivalents. Finally, there is now a user-friendly way to utilize multi-objective optimization and AI for customizable design techniques. These techniques have proven to be highly effective in lead advancement and generation [157]. The network consists of three segments: the encoder, decoder, and predictor. The encoder plays a vital role in converting discrete SMILES strings into latent (inactive) space, where vectors are considered fixed values. The decoder role analyzed vectors originating from the previous stage, specifically discrete SMILES. The predictor stage employs the multi-layer perceptron method to provide predictions regarding the molecules. In order to attain a high prediction ratio in constant vectors, it is advisable to employ the gradient-based approach. To effectively identify novel compounds with desirable characteristics, two methodologies can be utilized: Bayesian inference and a gradient-based approach. The integration of both methodologies yielded a substantial benefit: a high predictive ratio that facilitates human comprehension of the chemical structure. Invalid SMILES syntax does not correspond to the chemical structure. In order to avoid such difficulties, it is recommended to narrow down the result source. The researcher employed a variational autoencoder to establish the SMILES syntax [158]. Kadurin et al. employed the AAE model to generate molecular fingerprints, hereafter known as druGAN. The AAE technique demonstrated outstanding performance in the VAE model in terms of its generation capability, accuracy in reconstructing data, and ability to extract additional information. The researcher suggested examining whether the synthesized molecule was acquired by synthesis [159]. The neural network was trained using the response database due to its exceptional ability to accurately retrieve synthetic complexity measurements. The primary objective of a synthetic reaction is to enhance the intricacy of the reactants, leading to the formation of a product that is more intricate than the initial substances [160]. Coley made multiple attempts to develop a scoring function by encoding the response of chemicals into product and reactant pairs. This was done in order to better understand the relationship between the complexities of the products and reactants. In order to gain proficiency in scoring capacity, neural networks must undergo training. Coley employed a dataset of 22 million reactant and product pairs for this purpose. In addition, the outcome is determined through a complex synthesis process. Generative models offer valuable insights into the actions of drugs in inverse synthetic planning and also help identify and eliminate non-realistic compounds, hence revealing synthetic difficulties.

13.8.8 Lead Optimization

Lead optimization is a critical stage in the drug development process, during which the most promising fragment hits are identified as prospective leads for subsequent medicinal chemistry studies. The main goal of lead optimization is to reduce the adverse effects linked to current active analogues by making small structural adjustments, leading to a more enhanced and safer framework. An instance of this is the optimization of autotoxin inhibitors, such as the GLPG1690 therapeutic drug, which is presently undergoing advanced human clinical trials to counteract pulmonary fibrosis. Another illustration is to optimize the efficiency by tailoring methods to provide enhanced active analogs. The subsequent sections will explore many aspects of ADMET, encompassing its chemical and physical attributes, absorption, distribution, metabolism and excretion, toxicity, and the ADMET multitask brain networks.

13.8.8.1 Chemical and Physical Properties

The utilization of physical and chemical features has been extremely valuable in reducing failures in the drug discovery process. Deep learning models are employed to improve distinctive procedures using lead optimization techniques [161]. One researcher effectively retrieved data from a molecular graph by employing the

CNN-ANN technique to generate predictions. The achieved mean absolute error was 0.53 + 0.07, demonstrating the effectiveness of this approach [162]. Coley et al. served as inspiration for Duvenaud's work, motivating him to explore and improve upon molecular aqueous concepts. Furthermore, the tensor-based convolutional strategy was employed and produced enhanced outcomes, with a mean absolute error of 0.424 + 0.005. Accurate identification of molecular graph attribution is crucial for the successful incorporation of bond and atom characteristics, as mandated by tensor-based methodologies. Coley's model incorporated a substantial quantity of atom-level data, in contrast to Duvenaud's model [159], with the purpose of predicting molecular aqueous solutions. The relationship between Caco-2 permeability coefficients and oral medication absorption (P app) has been firmly established for the prediction of candidate pharmaceuticals in estimating pharmacokinetic properties [163, 164]. Wang et al. developed a comprehensive set of prediction templates with 30 descriptors. A total of 1,272 components were gathered to gather permeability data of Caco-2. Models such as SVM regression and boosting were used for analysis. The boosting model demonstrated outstanding performance and remarkable prediction capabilities in the testing set. The text follows the principles of QSAR as specified by the Organization for Economic Co-operation and Development (OECD).

13.8.8.2 ADME

Administering medications or substances directly into the bloodstream at a specific location to facilitate drug absorption. To assess the extent of absorption, the bioavailability parameter can be used. Several clinical departments have explored the enhancement of absorption properties and predicted the bioavailability of molecules [165]. Tian et al. employed a dataset of 1,014 molecules to forecast bioavailability by utilizing molecular properties and structural fingerprints in the MLR model. The application of the genetic function technique produced remarkable outcomes in terms of predicted accuracy. The root mean square error (RMSE) was calculated to be 0.2355, while the correlation coefficient was determined to be 0.71. Drug distribution refers to the process of transferring medications or medicine into the intracellular and interstitial fluids of the human body [166]. Drug distribution at steady state (VDss) entails the movement of medication from the body into the bloodstream. The steady phase in drug distribution is a vital sign for evaluating the drug distribution process. Accurate prediction of VDss is of utmost importance. Lombardo and Jing devised PLS and random forest methodologies on a dataset including 1,096 molecules [167]. The board members were displeased with the prediction results since there was a 50% mistake rate in the accessibility of molecules. VDss may be influenced by obscure circumstances. In order to tackle this issue, researchers have regarded it as a substantial obstacle pertaining to the VDss value in molecular structure data. When a drug is introduced into the human body, it triggers a metabolic response that aims to produce a potentially dangerous metabolite. For optimal metabolic strength, structural optimization techniques that promote highly accurate predictions by the metabolism are employed. The AI employed extensive drug metabolism data to precisely forecast particular metabolic enzymes, such as UDP-glucuronosyltransferases (UGTs) and cytochrome P450s. Furthermore, the Xenosite platform [168, 169] employs highly skilled neural networks [170] to aid in predicting UGT metabolism. Drug excretion refers to the process of eliminating both the administered dose and its metabolites from the human body. Drug metabolites are excreted from the human body through either water solubility or lack of metabolism. Lombardo et al. achieved an impressive 84% accuracy by employing the PCA technique to retrieve outstanding results in unique mechanisms.

13.8.8.3 Toxicity and the ADMET Multitask Neural Networks

The effectiveness of approximately 33% of important molecules in drug localization was significantly reduced due to clinical and preclinical damage. This reduction in effectiveness helps to minimize the risk of toxicity by predicting potential hazards [171]. Prediction can be accomplished by the utilization of methods such as structural alarms and rule-based expert knowledge to assess toxicity profiles, particularly for the kidney and liver. Utilizing deep learning models is essential for enhancing the precision of toxicity prediction. There exists a predictive model known as acute-oral toxicity, which can be utilized to forecast outcomes using molecular graph encoding convolutional neural networks (MGE-CNNs). The predicted results were determined to be superior in comparison to the SVM model [172]. The effectiveness of the MGE-CNN model can be ascribed to its efficient extraction of features, development of the model, and the consistent encoding of molecules during the training of the neural network. The MGE-CNN approach has the advantage of being able to modify the problem using molecular fingerprints, because to its accessibility and flexibility. The acquisition of high-quality fragments related to structural alerts involves the use of toxic features for fingerprints, which are used to characterize TOX alerts [173]. The correlation between parameters and trained multitask neural networks is crucial for achieving better results compared to single task neural networks. This is due to the sharing of parameters and the ability to support multiple tasks in retrieving similar features [174]. Finally, there is now access to significant data concerning the processes of medication absorption, distribution, metabolism, and excretion. This information has been improved by employing multitasking neural networks. In this study, the researchers examined the performance of single-task and multitask models using ADME/T experimental data. The findings indicated that the multitask model outperformed the single-task model [175].

13.8.9 Automated Synthesis Planning with Artificial Intelligence

A diverse array of organic molecules can be created by a limited number of dependable reactions [176]. However, the issue of developing reliable and fully automated synthesis planning in chemistry continues to persist [177]. One factor contributing to this is the need for a strong understanding of chemistry in order to effectively plan for both forward and retrosynthetic processes [178]. The origins of AI-based synthesis planning can be traced back to the 1970s, particularly in the domain of computer-aided retrosynthetic prediction [179]. The comeback of AI in synthetic organic chemistry can be due to the enhanced computer capabilities, the emergence of big data, and the creation of innovative algorithms for deep learning and optimization. Rule-based methods [180] are highly valuable in retrosynthesis, as they aid in the recursive design of efficient synthetic routes for a molecule of interest. These pathways aim to suggest retrosynthetic routes by encoding reaction mechanisms and building skeletal structures. One major limitation is their dependence on explicit chemical transformations/reactions. Usually, these tasks need manual building and curation. The field has been impacted by recent progress in natural language processing techniques, such as sequence-to-sequence models [181] and transformer models [182]. This research is motivated by the fact that the distribution of fragment ranks in organic molecules is similar to the distribution of word ranks in the English language [182]. In rule-free approaches, products are commonly represented in a text-based format, such as SMILES, and processed using an encoder-decoder architecture. This architecture is then employed to forecast the synthetic precursors that are one step ahead in the reaction [183]. The architecture has been enhanced by incorporating tiered neural networks [184]. The objective of these networks is to separate the retrosynthesis prediction problem into two distinct stages: response type categorization and reaction rule selection. The separation, inspired by a previously documented molecular similarity technique [185], has shown significant enhancements in performance relative to earlier benchmarks. While the aforementioned solutions mostly focus on solving the linear one-step retrosynthesis problem, a more pressing issue comes with the increasingly complex combinatorial problem. The recent advancements in reinforcement learning have led to significant progress in various fields. An important development in recent years has been the implementation of sophisticated search methods, such as Monte Carlo tree search [186], to efficiently investigate chemical reaction spaces [187]. The study employed transformer models to analyze reactants and reagents. The system utilized one-step precursor predictions and built hypergraphs, which are directed acyclic graphs capable of simultaneously connecting many nodes. The hypergraphs depicted here illustrate synthetic pathways [188]. When exploring hyper-graphs using beam search, a probability technique similar to Bayesian inference is employed to discover a plausible synthetic pathway. The system is inclined towards recommending chemically less complex precursors [189]. Forward synthesis planning distinguishes itself from retrosynthesis. Although the former issue can potentially be resolved by utilizing available reaction databases, the challenge of forward synthesis lies in obtaining information from reactions that do not produce any product at all. The existing chemical reaction databases have a strong bias towards productive reaction data [190]. Urgent acquisition of further data, such as experimental parameters (e.g. solvent and temperature) or side-product information, is required. To address these shortcomings, attempts have been made to augment current response databases by include adverse reaction outcomes [191]. This enables the generation of customized data compilations for automatic synthesis planning [192]. Prior methodologies utilized reaction templates drawn from data [193] to rank potential compounds. The ranking reaction templates were machine learning models that served as proof-of-concept and yielded precise outcomes when both the reactants and reagents were supplied [194]. Current methodologies prioritize the ranking of products by treating the chemical reaction prediction problem as a work of transforming graphs. Due to advancements in quantum mechanics, researchers have opted to employ first-principle calculations, such as density functional theory, to evaluate the energy barriers of certain reactions. Unfortunately, this approach becomes impractical for medium-to-large systems due to its computational demands.

Quantum-mechanical machine learning shows promise in properly forecasting energies and forces [195], offering a viable solution to this gap in the foreseeable future. In the domain of template-free forward synthesis prediction, there is an increasing trend towards the use of natural language processing methods that employ transformer [196] or recurrent neural network architectures [197]. These have routinely had a reactant accuracy exceeding 90% in their top-1 predictions. Several new alternative deep learning systems [198–200] have opted to include reaction prediction as a task for rearranging electrons, using message-passing neural networks. It is required to exclude processes where the flow of electrons cannot be precisely identified for the latter technique, which unfortunately excludes many important chemical reactions.

13.8.10 The ATOM Modeling Pipeline

AMPL6, also known as the ATOM Modelling Pipeline (AMPL), is an extension of the widely used DeepChem7 library. It provides support for machine learning and molecular featurization tools [201]. AMPL effortlessly interacts with well-known data science ecosystems and applications, rendering it a potent Python library. AMPL simplifies and improves several machine learning model fitting activities that are typically performed on pharmaceutical datasets, including model fitting, validation, and prediction. The AMPL platform facilitates researchers in training and evaluating models; incorporating new models; and utilizing utilities for automated dataset categorization, model validation, and uncertainty quantification. AMPL is an extremely adaptable library that effortlessly connects with a broad array of services and tools. AMPL allows users to create computational models using molecular attributes to aid in the drug discovery process. AMPL has been subjected to thorough testing on datasets for activity and property assays, with a primary focus on safety and pharmacokinetic modeling. A thorough assessment was carried out for the initial launch of the pipeline; 211 studies were conducted to evaluate different data splitting strategies, model types, and feature kinds. In total, 11,552 regression and classification models were developed for this purpose. AMPL provides a wide variety of dataset splitting techniques for the purpose of validation and testing. The methods encompass random splits, Butina clustering, scaffold splits, and temporal splits. AMPL employs models from scikit-learn and DeepChem, including random forest, XGBoost, fully connected neural networks, and graph convolution neural network models. The RDKit cheminformatics library and the MolVS molecule validation and standardization tool were utilized to encode tiny compounds as SMILES strings. The data curation module of AMPL was utilized to eliminate compound test values that exhibited substantial variability. In addition, the module was utilized to analyze the datasets by computing Tanimoto distances between chemical fingerprints or Euclidean distances between descriptor feature vectors. Several featurization methods were examined, including extended connectivity fingerprints (ECFPs), DeepChem graph convolution latent vectors, Mordred chemical descriptors, and Molecular Operating Environment (MOE) descriptors. AMPL's implementation is modular, which means it can be easily expanded by adding new splitting algorithms, model types, and feature kinds to the pipeline. Optimizing hyperparameters is essential for improving the predicted accuracy of cheminformatics machine learning model fitting. AMPL provides many hyperparameter optimization functions, including linear grids, logistic grids, random searches, and user-defined searches. The model fitting for safety and pharmacokinetic parameters employed AMPL's hyperparameter optimization module to systematically explore different combinations of model parameters. Hyperparameter optimization generally resulted in enhanced prediction performance on external test sets, with just a few instances where this was not the true. These exceptions happened in cases of insufficient data or when ECFP featurization was employed. AMPL easily computes common performance measures for regression and classification models in the standard model. The regression performance statistics assess the degree of concordance between the predicted values of the model and the actual values obtained from experimental observations. The data encompasses R^2, mean absolute error, and mean square error. AMPL offers many classification performance indicators, including precision, recall, area under the precision-recall curve (PRCAUC), negative predictive value, cross entropy, and accuracy metrics. As previously stated, the model's prediction uncertainty was computed for several PK datasets in order to compare it with the model's prediction error [201]. The utilization of AMPL facilitates a more profound comprehension of model predictions, uncertainty, and error through the implementation of uncertainty quantification analysis. AMPL is freely available software that provides a customizable and adaptable framework, enabling users to conveniently incorporate additional features or enhancements as needed. This allows the broader scientific community, including academia or government institutions and small firms, to effortlessly employ data-driven modeling using contemporary machine learning libraries. AMPL can now be downloaded from GitHub. The website contains extensive library documentation and gives example Jupyter notebooks to help the learning process of the pipeline [202–207].

13.9 CHALLENGES AND LIMITATIONS

The adequacy and volume of accessible data present a substantial obstacle in AI-supported drug discovery. Artificial intelligence systems rely extensively on extensive datasets for optimal model training, yet the quality of these datasets might vary significantly. Biomedical data, such as genetic and molecular data, may occasionally be susceptible to noise and incompleteness, which might provide difficulties when training AI models to achieve accuracy and reliability. In addition, the availability of extensive and reliable datasets can sometimes be restricted, which can impede the progress of creating strong AI algorithms for drug discovery [208–210].

An obstacle in AI-facilitated drug development is the requirement for AI models to possess interpretability and transparency. AI systems, particularly deep learning models, are commonly considered opaque because the rationale behind their predictions is not readily understandable. The absence of interpretability in AI-driven predictions can impede their acceptance, since researchers and doctors may be reluctant to place trust in them without a comprehensive comprehension of their generation process. The comprehensibility and clarity of AI models are crucial for their acceptability and integration into clinical practice.

There are important ethical and regulatory considerations to take into account when it comes to AI-assisted drug discovery. There are legitimate concerns about the possibility of bias in AI systems, particularly when the training data does not adequately reflect the entire population. Furthermore, there are apprehensions regarding the ownership and dissemination of data used for training artificial intelligence models, as well as the possible ramifications of depending on AI for making decisions concerning patient care. Addressing the ethical and regulatory aspects is essential to ensure the responsible and ethical utilization of AI in the field of drug discovery. In general, artificial intelligence has the capacity to significantly improve drug discovery and precision medicine efforts. Nevertheless, there are some obstacles and constraints that require attention and resolution. To fully realize the potential of AI and make a revolutionary impact in drug research, it is essential to address these issues. This will eventually improve patient care.

13.10 FUTURE PROSPECTS

The future outlook for AI-assisted drug discovery is its incorporation with other new technologies, such as quantum computing. The field of quantum computing holds immense promise in revolutionizing drug discovery by providing researchers with unparalleled computational power. This advancement enables the simulation of intricate biological systems and the prediction of drug–target interactions with remarkable precision. Researchers can greatly speed up the process of drug discovery and create more powerful treatments for various diseases by integrating AI with quantum computing.

Artificial intelligence-powered drug delivery devices hold great potential for advancing the field of drug research in the future. The potential of these systems resides in their capacity to employ AI algorithms to optimize drug delivery pathways, doses, and schedules by customizing them according to unique patient characteristics. AI-powered drug delivery systems provide the capacity to optimize treatment results and reduce negative consequences by tailoring drug administration to the individual requirements of each patient.

The incorporation of artificial intelligence in the process of discovering new drugs is expected to have a significant impact on the economic aspects of healthcare and the outcomes experienced by patients. Artificial intelligence has the capacity to greatly accelerate the process of discovering and developing therapeutics, resulting in cost savings when introducing new medications to the market and enhancing availability of cutting-edge treatments. Furthermore, by employing personalized therapeutic development, artificial intelligence has the capacity to improve patient outcomes and quality of life, leading to overall progress in healthcare delivery and results.

13.11 CONCLUSION

Artificial intelligence has significantly accelerated precision medicine efforts in drug discovery, leading to enhanced treatment results and tailored healthcare solutions. The field of drug research has been fundamentally revolutionized by AI techniques such as machine learning, deep learning, and natural language processing. Researchers have been able to rapidly identify therapeutic targets, develop novel compounds, and properly forecast treatment outcomes because to their advancements. AI algorithms enable academics to analyze vast quantities of data and discover useful insights that were previously inaccessible using conventional approaches. Despite the presence of hurdles and limits, such as concerns regarding the quality of data and the ability to understand it, the use of artificial intelligence in drug discovery shows significant potential for advancing precision medicine in the future. The integration of AI and quantum computing holds great promise for enhancing drug discovery processes and advancing the development of more efficacious treatments for a range of ailments. Moreover, it is crucial to delve deeper into the investigation and study of the advancement of AI-powered drug delivery systems and their influence on healthcare costs and patient outcomes.

REFERENCES

1. Mak, Kit-Kay, and Mallikarjuna Rao Pichika. "Artificial intelligence in drug development: Present status and future prospects." *Drug Discovery Today* 24, no. 3 (2019): 773–780.
2. Mishra, Vijay. "Artificial intelligence: The beginning of a new era in pharmacy profession." *Asian Journal of Pharmaceutics (AJP)* 12, no. 2 (2018).
3. Sellwood, Matthew A., Mohamed Ahmed, Marwin H. S. Segler, and Nathan Brown. "Artificial intelligence in drug discovery." *Future Medicinal Chemistry* 10, no. 17 (2018): 2025–2028.
4. Duch, Wlodzislaw, Karthikeyan Swaminathan, and Jaroslaw Meller. "Artificial intelligence approaches for rational drug design and discovery." *Current Pharmaceutical Design* 13, no. 14 (2007): 1497–1508.
5. Zhu, Hao. "Big data and artificial intelligence modeling for drug discovery." *Annual Review of Pharmacology and Toxicology* 60 (2020): 573–589.
6. Ciallella, Heather L., and Hao Zhu. "Advancing computational toxicology in the big data era by artificial intelligence: Data-driven and mechanism-driven modeling for chemical toxicity." *Chemical Research in Toxicology* 32, no. 4 (2019): 536–547.
7. Chan, H. C. Stephen, Hanbin Shan, Thamani Dahoun, Horst Vogel, and Shuguang Yuan. "Advancing drug discovery via artificial intelligence." *Trends in Pharmacological Sciences* 40, no. 8 (2019): 592–604.
8. Brown, Nathan. *In Silico Medicinal Chemistry: Computational Methods to Support Drug Design*. Royal Society of Chemistry, 2015.
9. Pereira, Janaina Cruz, Ernesto Raul Caffarena, and Cicero Nogueira Dos Santos. "Boosting docking-based virtual screening with deep learning." *Journal of Chemical Information and Modeling* 56, no. 12 (2016): 2495–2506.
10. Firth, Nicholas C., Butrus Atrash, Nathan Brown, and Julian Blagg. "MOARF, an integrated workflow for multiobjective optimization: Implementation, synthesis, and biological evaluation." *Journal of Chemical Information and Modeling* 55, no. 6 (2015): 1169–1180.
11. Zhang, Lu, Jianjun Tan, Dan Han, and Hao Zhu. "From machine learning to deep learning: Progress in machine intelligence for rational drug discovery." *Drug Discovery Today* 22, no. 11 (2017): 1680–1685.
12. Jain, Nilanjana, Swagata Gupta, Neelima Sapre, and Nitin S. Sapre. "*In silico* de novo design of novel NNRTIs: A bio-molecular modelling approach." *RSC Advances* 5, no. 19 (2015): 14814–14827.
13. Wang, Yu, Yanzhi Guo, Qifan Kuang, Xuemei Pu, Yue Ji, Zhihang Zhang, and Menglong Li. "A comparative study of family-specific protein–ligand complex affinity prediction based on random forest approach." *Journal of Computer-Aided Molecular Design* 29 (2015): 349–360.

14. King, Ross D., Jonathan D. Hirst, and Michael JE Sternberg. "Comparison of artificial intelligence methods for modeling pharmaceutical QSARS." *Applied Artificial Intelligence an International Journal* 9, no. 2 (1995): 213–233.
15. Russell, Stuart, Daniel Dewey, and Max Tegmark. "Research priorities for robust and beneficial artificial intelligence." *AI Magazine* 36, no. 4 (2015): 105–114.
16. Koza, John R., Forrest H. Bennett, David Andre, and Martin A. Keane. "Automated design of both the topology and sizing of analog electrical circuits using genetic programming." *Artificial Intelligence in Design* 96 (1996): 151–170.
17. Kitchin, Rob, and Gavin McArdle. "What makes big data, big data? Exploring the ontological characteristics of 26 datasets." *Big Data & Society* 3, no. 1 (2016): 2053951716631130.
18. Bhadani, Abhay Kumar, and Dhanya Jothimani. "Big data: Challenges, opportunities, and realities." *Effective Big Data Management and Opportunities for Implementation* (2016): 1–24.
19. Larose, Daniel T. *Data Mining and Predictive Analytics*. John Wiley & Sons, 2015.
20. Zemouri, Ryad, Nabil Omri, Farhat Fnaiech, Noureddine Zerhouni, and Nader Fnaiech. "A new growing pruning deep learning neural network algorithm (GP-DLNN)." *Neural Computing and Applications* 32, no. 24 (2020): 18143–18159.
21. Nath, Abhigyan, and Gopal Krishna Sahu. "Exploiting ensemble learning to improve prediction of phospholipidosis inducing potential." *Journal of Theoretical Biology* 479 (2019): 37–47.
22. Nath, Abhigyan, and S. Karthikeyan. "Enhanced prediction of recombination hotspots using input features extracted by class specific autoencoders." *Journal of Theoretical Biology* 444 (2018): 73–82.
23. Raparthi, Mohan. "AI assisted drug discovery: Emphasizing its role in accelerating precision medicine initiatives and improving treatment outcomes." *Human-Computer Interaction Perspectives* 2, no. 2 (2022): 1–10.
24. Bian, Yuemin, Junmei Wang, Jaden Jungho Jun, and Xiang-Qun Xie. "Deep convolutional generative adversarial network (dcGAN) models for screening and design of small molecules targeting cannabinoid receptors." *Molecular Pharmaceutics* 16, no. 11 (2019): 4451–4460.
25. Wenzel, Markus. "Generative adversarial networks and other generative models." *Machine Learning for Brain Disorders* (2023): 139–192.
26. Li, Chongxuan, Kun Xu, Jun Zhu, Jiashuo Liu, and Bo Zhang. "Triple generative adversarial networks." *IEEE Transactions on Pattern Analysis and Machine Intelligence* 44, no. 12 (2021): 9629–9640.
27. Zhong, Guoqiang, Wei Gao, Yongbin Liu, Youzhao Yang, Da-Han Wang, and Kaizhu Huang. "Generative adversarial networks with decoder–encoder output noises." *Neural Networks* 127 (2020): 19–28.
28. Blanchard, Andrew E., Christopher Stanley, and Debsindhu Bhowmik. "Using GANs with adaptive training data to search for new molecules." *Journal of Cheminformatics* 13 (2021): 1–8.
29. Yu, Hui, Kang Kang Li, and Jian Yu Shi. "DGANDDI: Double generative adversarial networks for drug-drug interaction prediction." *IEEE/ACM Transactions on Computational Biology and Bioinformatics* 20, no. 3 (2022): 1854–1863
30. Hussain, Shaista, Ayesha Anees, Ankit Das, Binh P. Nguyen, Mardiana Marzuki, Shuping Lin, Graham Wright, and Amit Singhal. "High-content image generation for drug discovery using generative adversarial networks." *Neural Networks* 132 (2020): 353–363.
31. Bian, Yuemin, and Xiang-Qun Xie. "Generative chemistry: Drug discovery with deep learning generative models." *Journal of Molecular Modeling* 27 (2021): 1–18.
32. Tong, Xiaochu, Xiaohong Liu, Xiaoqin Tan, Xutong Li, Jiaxin Jiang, Zhaoping Xiong, Tingyang Xu, Hualiang Jiang, Nan Qiao, and Mingyue Zheng. "Generative models for de novo drug design." *Journal of Medicinal Chemistry* 64, no. 19 (2021): 14011–14027.

33. Lin, Eugene, Chieh-Hsin Lin, and Hsien-Yuan Lane. "De novo peptide and protein design using generative adversarial networks: An update." *Journal of Chemical Information and Modeling* 62, no. 4 (2022): 761–774.
34. Macedo, Bruno, Inês Ribeiro Vaz, and Tiago Taveira Gomes. "MedGAN: Optimized generative adversarial network with graph convolutional networks for novel molecule design." *Scientific Reports* 14, no. 1 (2024): 1212.
35. Zhu, Yanming, Min Wang, Xuefei Yin, Jue Zhang, Erik Meijering, and Jiankun Hu. "Deep learning in diverse intelligent sensor based systems." *Sensors* 23, no. 1 (2022): 62.
36. Lin, Eugene, Chieh-Hsin Lin, and Hsien-Yuan Lane. "Relevant applications of generative adversarial networks in drug design and discovery: Molecular de novo design, dimensionality reduction, and de novo peptide and protein design." *Molecules* 25, no. 14 (2020): 3250.
37. Kao, Po-Yu, Ya-Chu Yang, Wei-Yin Chiang, Jen-Yueh Hsiao, Yudong Cao, Alex Aliper, Feng Ren *et al.* "Exploring the advantages of quantum generative adversarial networks in generative chemistry." *Journal of Chemical Information and Modeling* 63, no. 11 (2023): 3307–3318.
38. Niu, Murphy Yuezhen, Alexander Zlokapa, Michael Broughton, Sergio Boixo, Masoud Mohseni, Vadim Smelyanskyi, and Hartmut Neven. "Entangling quantum generative adversarial networks." *Physical Review Letters* 128, no. 22 (2022): 220505.
39. Tian, Jinkai, Xiaoyu Sun, Yuxuan Du, Shanshan Zhao, Qing Liu, Kaining Zhang, Wei Yi *et al.* "Recent advances for quantum neural networks in generative learning." *IEEE Transactions on Pattern Analysis and Machine Intelligence* 45, no. 22 (2023): 12321–12340.
40. Marino, Joseph. "Predictive coding, variational autoencoders, and biological connections." *Neural Computation* 34, no. 1 (2022): 1–44.
41. Zhang, Yue, Yuqing Hu, Huihui Li, and Xiaoyong Liu. "Drug-protein interaction prediction via variational autoencoders and attention mechanisms." *Frontiers in Genetics* 13 (2022): 1032779.
42. Li, Tianjiao, Xing-Ming Zhao, and Limin Li. "Co-VAE: Drug–target binding affinity prediction by co-regularized variational autoencoders." *IEEE Transactions on Pattern Analysis and Machine Intelligence* 44, no. 12 (2021): 8861–8873.
43. Huang, Zhaoyang, Shengjian Chen, and Liang Yu. "Predicting new drug indications based on double variational autoencoders." *Computers in Biology and Medicine* 164 (2023): 107261.
44. Ochiai, Toshiki, Tensei Inukai, Manato Akiyama, Kairi Furui, Masahito Ohue, Nobuaki Matsumori, Shinsuke Inuki *et al.* "Variational autoencoder-based chemical latent space for large molecular structures with 3D complexity." *Communications Chemistry* 6, no. 1 (2023): 249.
45. Chow, Yuen Ler, Shantanu Singh, Anne E. Carpenter, and Gregory P. Way. "Predicting drug polypharmacology from cell morphology readouts using variational autoencoder latent space arithmetic." *PLoS Computational Biology* 18, no. 2 (2022): e1009888.
46. Ang, Dony, Cyril Rakovski, and Hagop S. Atamian. "De Novo drug design using transformer-based machine translation and reinforcement learning of an adaptive Monte Carlo tree search." *Pharmaceuticals* 17, no. 2 (2024): 161.
47. Grechishnikova, Daria. "Transformer neural network for protein-specific de novo drug generation as a machine translation problem." *Scientific Reports* 11, no. 1 (2021): 321.
48. Kalakoti, Yogesh, Shashank Yadav, and Durai Sundar. "TransDTI: Transformer-based language models for estimating DTIs and building a drug recommendation workflow." *ACS Omega* 7, no. 3 (2022): 2706–2717.
49. Shiju, Akhil, and Zhe He. "Classifying drug ratings using user reviews with transformer-based language models." In *2022 IEEE 10th International Conference on Healthcare Informatics (ICHI)*, pp. 163–169. IEEE, 2022.

50. Zhang, Shuang, Rui Fan, Yuti Liu, Shuang Chen, Qiao Liu, and Wanwen Zeng. "Applications of transformer-based language models in bioinformatics: A survey." *Bioinformatics Advances* 3, no. 1 (2023): vbad001.
51. Hu, Jing, Jie Gao, Xiaomin Fang, Zijing Liu, Fan Wang, Weili Huang, Hua Wu, and Guodong Zhao. "DTSyn: A dual-transformer-based neural network to predict synergistic drug combinations." *Briefings in Bioinformatics* 23, no. 5 (2022): bbac302.
52. Mao, Jiashun, Jianmin Wang, Amir Zeb, Kwang-Hwi Cho, Haiyan Jin, Jongwan Kim, Onju Lee, Yunyun Wang, and Kyoung Tai No. "Transformer-based molecular generative model for antiviral drug design." *Journal of Chemical Information and Modeling* 64, no. 7 (2023): 2733–2745.
53. Larochelle, Hugo, and Yoshua Bengio. "Classification using discriminative restricted Boltzmann machines." In *Proceedings of the 25th International Conference on Machine Learning*, pp. 536–543. ACM, 2008.
54. Welling, Max, and Geoffrey E. Hinton. "A new learning algorithm for mean field Boltzmann machines." In *International Conference on Artificial Neural Networks*, pp. 351–357. Berlin, Heidelberg: Springer, 2002.
55. Salakhutdinov, Ruslan, Andriy Mnih, and Geoffrey Hinton. "Restricted Boltzmann machines for collaborative filtering." In *Proceedings of the 24th International Conference on Machine Learning*, pp. 791–798. ACM, 2007.
56. Wang, Yuhao, and Jianyang Zeng. "Predicting drug–target interactions using restricted Boltzmann machines." *Bioinformatics* 29, no. 13 (2013): i126–i134.
57. Ding, Yijie, Hongmei Zhou, Quan Zou, and Lei Yuan. "Identification of drug-side effect association via correntropy-loss based matrix factorization with neural tangent kernel." *Methods* 219 (2023): 73–81.
58. Cheng, Xiaolong, Jia Qu, Shuangbao Song, and Zekang Bian. "Neighborhood-based inference and restricted Boltzmann machine for microbe and drug associations prediction." *PeerJ* 10 (2022): e13848.
59. Bongini, Pietro, Elisa Messori, Niccolo Pancino, and Monica Bianchini. "A deep learning approach to the prediction of drug side-effects on molecular graphs." *IEEE/ACM Transactions on Computational Biology and Bioinformatics* (2023).
60. Wu, Zonghan, Shirui Pan, Fengwen Chen, Guodong Long, Chengqi Zhang, and S. Yu Philip. "A comprehensive survey on graph neural networks." *IEEE Transactions on Neural Networks and Learning Systems* 32, no. 1 (2020): 4–24.
61. Abate, Carlo, Sergio Decherchi, and Andrea Cavalli. "Graph neural networks for conditional de novo drug design." *Wiley Interdisciplinary Reviews: Computational Molecular Science* 13, no. 4 (2023): e1651.
62. Zhou, Jie, Ganqu Cui, Shengding Hu, Zhengyan Zhang, Cheng Yang, Zhiyuan Liu, Lifeng Wang, Changcheng Li, and Maosong Sun. "Graph neural networks: A review of methods and applications." *AI Open* 1 (2020): 57–81.
63. Xiong, Jiacheng, Zhaoping Xiong, Kaixian Chen, Hualiang Jiang, and Mingyue Zheng. "Graph neural networks for automated de novo drug design." *Drug Discovery Today* 26, no. 6 (2021): 1382–1393.
64. Feng, Junning, Yong Liang, and Tianwei Yu. "MM-GANN-DDI: Multimodal graph-agnostic neural networks for predicting drug–drug interaction events." *Computers in Biology and Medicine* 166 (2023): 107492.
65. D'Souza, Sofia, Prema Kv, and Seetharaman Balaji. "Training recurrent neural networks as generative neural networks for molecular structures: How does it impact drug discovery?" *Expert Opinion on Drug Discovery* 17, no. 10 (2022): 1071–1079.
66. Xia, Xiaolin, Jianxing Hu, Yanxing Wang, Liangren Zhang, and Zhenming Liu. "Graph-based generative models for de Novo drug design." *Drug Discovery Today: Technologies* 32 (2019): 45–53.
67. Moret, Michael, Irene Pachon Angona, Leandro Cotos, Shen Yan, Kenneth Atz, Cyrill Brunner, Martin Baumgartner, Francesca Grisoni, and Gisbert Schneider. "Leveraging

molecular structure and bioactivity with chemical language models for de novo drug design." *Nature Communications* 14, no. 1 (2023): 114.
68. Schenone, Monica, Vlado Dančík, Bridget K. Wagner, and Paul A. Clemons. "Target identification and mechanism of action in chemical biology and drug discovery." *Nature Chemical Biology* 9, no. 4 (2013): 232–240.
69. Janakarajan, Nikita, Tim Erdmann, Sarath Swaminathan, Teodoro Laino, and Jannis Born. "Language models in molecular discovery." *arXiv preprint* arXiv:2309.16235 (2023).
70. Bajorath, Jürgen. "Chemical language models for molecular design." *Molecular Informatics* 43, no. 1 (2024): e202300288.
71. Liu, Zhichao, Ruth A. Roberts, Madhu Lal-Nag, Xi Chen, Ruili Huang, and Weida Tong. "AI-based language models powering drug discovery and development." *Drug Discovery Today* 26, no. 11 (2021): 2593–2607.
72. Giorgi, John M., and Gary D. Bader. "Towards reliable named entity recognition in the biomedical domain." *Bioinformatics* 36, no. 1 (2020): 280–286.
73. Blanco, Alberto, Olatz Perez-de-Viñaspre, Alicia Pérez, and Arantza Casillas. "Boosting ICD multi-label classification of health records with contextual embeddings and label-granularity." *Computer Methods and Programs in Biomedicine* 188 (2020): 105264.
74. Dias, Raquel, and Ali Torkamani. "Artificial intelligence in clinical and genomic diagnostics." *Genome Medicine* 11, no. 1 (2019): 70.
75. Hall, Jennifer L., John J. Ryan, Bruce E. Bray, Candice Brown, David Lanfear, L. Kristin Newby, Mary V. Relling *et al.* "Merging electronic health record data and genomics for cardiovascular research: A science advisory from the American Heart Association." *Circulation: Cardiovascular Genetics* 9, no. 2 (2016): 193–202.
76. Harrer, Stefan, Pratik Shah, Bhavna Antony, and Jianying Hu. "Artificial intelligence for clinical trial design." *Trends in Pharmacological Sciences* 40, no. 8 (2019): 577–591.
77. Zeng, Xiangxiang, Fei Wang, Yuan Luo, Seung-gu Kang, Jian Tang, Felice C. Lightstone, Evandro F. Fang, Wendy Cornell, Ruth Nussinov, and Feixiong Cheng. "Deep generative molecular design reshapes drug discovery." *Cell Reports Medicine* 3, no. 12 (2022).
78. Luo, Yuan, Alal Eran, Nathan Palmer, Paul Avillach, Ami Levy-Moonshine, Peter Szolovits, and Isaac S. Kohane. "A multidimensional precision medicine approach identifies an autism subtype characterized by dyslipidemia." *Nature Medicine* 26, no. 9 (2020): 1375–1379.
79. Liu, Shengchao, Hanchen Wang, Weiyang Liu, Joan Lasenby, Hongyu Guo, and Jian Tang. "Pre-training molecular graph representation with 3d geometry." *arXiv preprint* arXiv:2110.07728 (2021).
80. Manica, Matteo, Ali Oskooei, Jannis Born, Vigneshwari Subramanian, Julio Sáez-Rodríguez, and María Rodriguez Martinez. "Toward explainable anticancer compound sensitivity prediction via multimodal attention-based convolutional encoders." *Molecular Pharmaceutics* 16, no. 12 (2019): 4797–4806.
81. Jin, Wengong, Kevin Yang, Regina Barzilay, and Tommi Jaakkola. "Learning multimodal graph-to-graph translation for molecular optimization." *arXiv preprint* arXiv:1812.01070 (2018).
82. Baltrušaitis, Tadas, Chaitanya Ahuja, and Louis-Philippe Morency. "Multimodal machine learning: A survey and taxonomy." *IEEE Transactions on Pattern Analysis and Machine Intelligence* 41, no. 2 (2018): 423–443.
83. Steyaert, Sandra, Marija Pizurica, Divya Nagaraj, Priya Khandelwal, Tina Hernandez-Boussard, Andrew J. Gentles, and Olivier Gevaert. "Multimodal data fusion for cancer biomarker discovery with deep learning." *Nature Machine Intelligence* 5, no. 4 (2023): 351–362.

84. Luo, Yizhen, Xing Yi Liu, Kai Yang, Kui Huang, Massimo Hong, Jiahuan Zhang, Yushuai Wu, and Zaiqing Nie. "Toward unified AI drug discovery with multimodal knowledge." *Health Data Science* 4 (2024): 0113.
85. Skalic, Miha, Davide Sabbadin, Boris Sattarov, Simone Sciabola, and Gianni De Fabritiis. "From target to drug: Generative modeling for the multimodal structure-based ligand design." *Molecular Pharmaceutics* 16, no. 10 (2019): 4282–4291.
86. Buchberger, Amanda Rae, Kellen DeLaney, Jillian Johnson, and Lingjun Li. "Mass spectrometry imaging: A review of emerging advancements and future insights." *Analytical Chemistry* 90, no. 1 (2018): 240.
87. Löscher, Wolfgang. "Single-target versus multi-target drugs versus combinations of drugs with multiple targets: Preclinical and clinical evidence for the treatment or prevention of epilepsy." *Frontiers in Pharmacology* 12 (2021): 730257.
88. Mareček, Radek, Pavel Říha, Michaela Bartoňová, Martin Kojan, Martin Lamoš, Martin Gajdoš, Lubomír Vojtíšek *et al.* "Automated fusion of multimodal imaging data for identifying epileptogenic lesions in patients with inconclusive magnetic resonance imaging." *Human Brain Mapping* 42, no. 9 (2021): 2921–2930.
89. Sun, Yichun, Yingxu Peng, Yixin Chen, and Atul J. Shukla. "Application of artificial neural networks in the design of controlled release drug delivery systems." *Advanced Drug Delivery Reviews* 55, no. 9 (2003): 1201–1215.
90. Dowell, James A., Ajaz Hussain, John Devane, and David Young. "Artificial neural networks applied to the *in vitro—in vivo* correlation of an extended-release formulation: Initial trials and experience." *Journal of Pharmaceutical Sciences* 88, no. 1 (1999): 154–160.
91. Xu, Wen-Jin, Ning Li, and Chong-kai Gao. "Preparation of controlled porosity osmotic pump tablets for salvianolic acid and optimization of the formulation using an artificial neural network method." *Acta Pharmaceutica Sinica B* 1, no. 1 (2011): 64–70.
92. Parojčić, Jelena, Svetlana Ibrić, Zorica Djurić, Milica Jovanović, and Owen I. Corrigan. "An investigation into the usefulness of generalized regression neural network analysis in the development of level A *in vitro–in vivo* correlation." *European Journal of Pharmaceutical Sciences* 30, no. 3–4 (2007): 264–272.
93. Masi, A., D. S. Quintana, N. Glozier, A. R. Lloyd, I. B. Hickie, and A. J. Guastella. "Cytokine aberrations in autism spectrum disorder: A systematic review and meta-analysis." *Molecular Psychiatry* 20, no. 4 (2015): 440–446.
94. Scannell, Jack W., Alex Blanckley, Helen Boldon, and Brian Warrington. "Diagnosing the decline in pharmaceutical R&D efficiency." *Nature Reviews Drug Discovery* 11, no. 3 (2012): 191–200.
95. Mullard, Asher. "Parsing clinical success rates." *Nature Reviews Drug Discovery* 15, no. 7 (2016): 447–448.
96. Kim, Sunghwan, Paul A. Thiessen, Evan E. Bolton, Jie Chen, Gang Fu, Asta Gindulyte, Lianyi Han *et al.* "PubChem substance and compound databases." *Nucleic Acids Research* 44, no. D1 (2016): D1202–D1213.
97. Wang, Yanli, Stephen H. Bryant, Tiejun Cheng, Jiyao Wang, Asta Gindulyte, Benjamin A. Shoemaker, Paul A. Thiessen, Siqian He, and Jian Zhang. "Pubchem bioassay: 2017 update." *Nucleic Acids Research* 45, no. D1 (2017): D955–D963.
98. Gaulton, Anna, Louisa J. Bellis, A. Patricia Bento, Jon Chambers, Mark Davies, Anne Hersey, Yvonne Light *et al.* "ChEMBL: A large-scale bioactivity database for drug discovery." *Nucleic Acids Research* 40, no. D1 (2012): D1100–D1107.
99. Gilson, Michael K., Tiqing Liu, Michael Baitaluk, George Nicola, Linda Hwang, and Jenny Chong. "BindingDB in 2015: A public database for medicinal chemistry, computational chemistry and systems pharmacology." *Nucleic Acids Research* 44, no. D1 (2016): D1045–D1053.

100. Mendez, David, Anna Gaulton, A. Patrícia Bento, Jon Chambers, Marleen De Veij, Eloy Félix, María Paula Magariños *et al.* "ChEMBL: Towards direct deposition of bioassay data." *Nucleic Acids Research* 47, no. D1 (2019): D930–D940.
101. Wishart, David S., Craig Knox, An Chi Guo, Dean Cheng, Savita Shrivastava, Dan Tzur, Bijaya Gautam, and Murtaza Hassanali. "DrugBank: A knowledgebase for drugs, drug actions and drug targets." *Nucleic Acids Research* 36, no. suppl_1 (2008): D901–D906.
102. Consortium, UniProt. "UniProt: A hub for protein information." *Nucleic Acids Research* 43, no. D1 (2015): D204–D212.
103. Jumper, John, Richard Evans, Alexander Pritzel, Tim Green, Michael Figurnov, Olaf Ronneberger, Kathryn Tunyasuvunakool *et al.* "Highly accurate protein structure prediction with AlphaFold." *Nature* 596, no. 7873 (2021): 583–589.
104. Ramsundar, Bharath. "Molecular machine learning with DeepChem." PhD diss., Stanford University, 2018.
105. Alipanahi, Babak, Andrew Delong, Matthew T. Weirauch, and Brendan J. Frey. "Predicting the sequence specificities of DNA-and RNA-binding proteins by deep learning." *Nature Biotechnology* 33, no. 8 (2015): 831–838.
106. Karimi, Mostafa, Di Wu, Zhangyang Wang, and Yang Shen. "DeepAffinity: Interpretable deep learning of compound–protein affinity through unified recurrent and convolutional neural networks." *Bioinformatics* 35, no. 18 (2019): 3329–3338.
107. Spencer, Matt, Jesse Eickholt, and Jianlin Cheng. "A deep learning network approach to ab initio protein secondary structure prediction." *IEEE/ACM Transactions on Computational Biology and Bioinformatics* 12, no. 1 (2014): 103–112.
108. Xia, Zheng, Ling-Yun Wu, Xiaobo Zhou, and Stephen TC Wong. "Semi-supervised drug-protein interaction prediction from heterogeneous biological spaces." In *BMC Systems Biology*, vol. 4, pp. 1–16. BioMed Central, 2010.
109. Wang, Chen, and Lukasz Kurgan. "Survey of similarity-based prediction of drug-protein interactions." *Current Medicinal Chemistry* 27, no. 35 (2020): 5856–5886.
110. Zhou, Hongyi, Mu Gao, and Jeffrey Skolnick. "Comprehensive prediction of drug-protein interactions and side effects for the human proteome." *Scientific Reports* 5, no. 1 (2015): 11090.
111. Gunther, Erik C., David J. Stone, Robert W. Gerwien, Patricia Bento, and Melvyn P. Heyes. "Prediction of clinical drug efficacy by classification of drug-induced genomic expression profiles *in vitro*." *Proceedings of the National Academy of Sciences* 100, no. 16 (2003): 9608–9613.
112. Guney, Emre, Jörg Menche, Marc Vidal, and Albert-László Barábasi. "Network-based *in silico* drug efficacy screening." *Nature Communications* 7, no. 1 (2016): 10331.
113. Sistare, Frank D., Frank Dieterle, Sean Troth, Daniel J. Holder, David Gerhold, Dina Andrews-Cleavenger, William Baer *et al.* "Towards consensus practices to qualify safety biomarkers for use in early drug development." *Nature Biotechnology* 28, no. 5 (2010): 446–454.
114. Rolan, Paul, Meindert Danhof, Donald Stanski, and Carl Peck. "Current issues relating to drug safety especially with regard to the use of biomarkers: A meeting report and progress update." *European Journal of Pharmaceutical Sciences* 30, no. 2 (2007): 107–112.
115. Du, Tianchuan, Li Liao, Cathy H. Wu, and Bilin Sun. "Prediction of residue-residue contact matrix for protein–protein interaction with Fisher score features and deep learning." *Methods* 110 (2016): 97–105.
116. Falchi, Federico, Fabiana Caporuscio, and Maurizio Recanatini. "Structure-based design of small-molecule protein–protein interaction modulators: The story so far." *Future Medicinal Chemistry* 6, no. 3 (2014): 343–357.
117. Scott, Duncan E., Andrew R. Bayly, Chris Abell, and John Skidmore. "Small molecules, big targets: Drug discovery faces the protein–protein interaction challenge." *Nature Reviews Drug Discovery* 15, no. 8 (2016): 533–550.

118. Cukuroglu, Engin, H. Billur Engin, Attila Gursoy, and Ozlem Keskin. "Hot spots in protein–protein interfaces: Towards drug discovery." *Progress in Biophysics and Molecular Biology* 116, no. 2–3 (2014): 165–173.
119. Higueruelo, Alicia P., Harry Jubb, and Tom L. Blundell. "Protein–protein interactions as druggable targets: Recent technological advances." *Current Opinion in Pharmacology* 13, no. 5 (2013): 791–796.
120. Santos, Rita, Oleg Ursu, Anna Gaulton, A. Patrícia Bento, Ramesh S. Donadi, Cristian G. Bologa, Anneli Karlsson *et al.* "A comprehensive map of molecular drug targets." *Nature Reviews Drug Discovery* 16, no. 1 (2017): 19–34.
121. Lavecchia, Antonio, and Carmen Di Giovanni. "Virtual screening strategies in drug discovery: A critical review." *Current Medicinal Chemistry* 20, no. 23 (2013): 2839–2860.
122. Willett, Peter. "Similarity-based virtual screening using 2D fingerprints." *Drug Discovery Today* 11, no. 23–24 (2006): 1046–1053.
123. Leelananda, Sumudu P., and Steffen Lindert. "Computational methods in drug discovery." *Beilstein Journal of Organic Chemistry* 12, no. 1 (2016): 2694–2718.
124. Chen, Yu-Chian. "Beware of docking!" *Trends in Pharmacological Sciences* 36, no. 2 (2015): 78–95.
125. Talele, Tanaji T., Santosh A. Khedkar, and Alan C. Rigby. "Successful applications of computer aided drug discovery: Moving drugs from concept to the clinic." *Current Topics in Medicinal Chemistry* 10, no. 1 (2010): 127–141.
126. Huang, Sheng-You, and Xiaoqin Zou. "Inclusion of solvation and entropy in the knowledge-based scoring function for protein– ligand interactions." *Journal of Chemical Information and Modeling* 50, no. 2 (2010): 262–273.
127. Copeland, Robert A. "The dynamics of drug–target interactions: Drug–target residence time and its impact on efficacy and safety." *Expert Opinion on Drug Discovery* 5, no. 4 (2010): 305–310.
128. Xing, Jing, Wenchao Lu, Rongfeng Liu, Yulan Wang, Yiqian Xie, Hao Zhang, Zhe Shi *et al.* "Machine-learning-assisted approach for discovering novel inhibitors targeting bromodomain-containing protein 4." *Journal of Chemical Information and Modeling* 57, no. 7 (2017): 1677–1690.
129. Liew, Chin Y., Xiao H. Ma, Xianghui Liu, and Chun W. Yap. "SVM model for virtual screening of Lck inhibitors." *Journal of Chemical Information and Modeling* 49, no. 4 (2009): 877–885.
130. Melville, James L., Edmund K. Burke, and Jonathan D. Hirst. "Machine learning in virtual screening." *Combinatorial Chemistry & High Throughput Screening* 12, no. 4 (2009): 332–343.
131. Ma, Xiao H., Jia Jia, Feng Zhu, Ying Xue, Ze R. Li, and Yu Z. Chen. "Comparative analysis of machine learning methods in ligand-based virtual screening of large compound libraries." *Combinatorial Chemistry & High Throughput Screening* 12, no. 4 (2009): 344–357.
132. LeCun, Yann, Yoshua Bengio, and Geoffrey Hinton. "Deep learning." *Nature* 521, no. 7553 (2015): 436–444.
133. Unterthiner, Thomas, Andreas Mayr, Günter Klambauer, Marvin Steijaert, Jörg K. Wegner, Hugo Ceulemans, and Sepp Hochreiter. "Deep learning as an opportunity in virtual screening." In *Proceedings of the Deep Learning Workshop at NIPS*, vol. 27, pp. 1–9. Cambridge, MA, United States: MIT Press, 2014.
134. Segler, Marwin HS, Thierry Kogej, Christian Tyrchan, and Mark P. Waller. "Generating focused molecule libraries for drug discovery with recurrent neural networks." *ACS Central Science* 4, no. 1 (2018): 120–131.
135. Kadurin, Artur, Alexander Aliper, Andrey Kazennov, Polina Mamoshina, Quentin Vanhaelen, Kuzma Khrabrov, and Alex Zhavoronkov. "The cornucopia of meaningful leads: Applying deep adversarial autoencoders for new molecule development in oncology." *Oncotarget* 8, no. 7 (2017): 10883.

136. Khamis, Mohamed A., Walid Gomaa, and Walaa F. Ahmed. "Machine learning in computational docking." *Artificial Intelligence in Medicine* 63, no. 3 (2015): 135–152.
137. Ain, Qurrat Ul, Antoniya Aleksandrova, Florian D. Roessler, and Pedro J. Ballester. "Machine-learning scoring functions to improve structure-based binding affinity prediction and virtual screening." *Wiley Interdisciplinary Reviews: Computational Molecular Science* 5, no. 6 (2015): 405–424.
138. Kinnings, Sarah L., Nina Liu, Peter J. Tonge, Richard M. Jackson, Lei Xie, and Philip E. Bourne. "A machine learning-based method to improve docking scoring functions and its application to drug repurposing." *Journal of Chemical Information and Modeling* 51, no. 2 (2011): 408–419.
139. Zsoldos, Zsolt, Darryl Reid, Aniko Simon, Sayyed Bashir Sadjad, and A. Peter Johnson. "eHiTS: A new fast, exhaustive flexible ligand docking system." *Journal of Molecular Graphics and Modelling* 26, no. 1 (2007): 198–212.
140. Friesner, Richard A., Jay L. Banks, Robert B. Murphy, Thomas A. Halgren, Jasna J. Klicic, Daniel T. Mainz, Matthew P. Repasky *et al.* "Glide: A new approach for rapid, accurate docking and scoring. 1. Method and assessment of docking accuracy." *Journal of Medicinal Chemistry* 47, no. 7 (2004): 1739–1749.
141. Abagyan, Ruben, Maxim Totrov, and Dmitry Kuznetsov. "ICM—A new method for protein modeling and design: Applications to docking and structure prediction from the distorted native conformation." *Journal of Computational Chemistry* 15, no. 5 (1994): 488–506.
142. Desai, Bimbisar, Karen Dixon, Elizabeth Farrant, Qixing Feng, Karl R. Gibson, Willem P. van Hoorn, James Mills *et al.* "Rapid discovery of a novel series of Abl kinase inhibitors by application of an integrated microfluidic synthesis and screening platform." *Journal of Medicinal Chemistry* 56, no. 7 (2013): 3033–3047.
143. Myint, Kyaw Zeyar, and Xiang-Qun Xie. "Recent advances in fragment-based QSAR and multi-dimensional QSAR methods." *International Journal of Molecular Sciences* 11, no. 10 (2010): 3846–3866.
144. Hansch, Corwin, and Toshio Fujita. "Additions and corrections-ρ-σ-π analysis. A method for the correlation of biological activity and chemical structure." *Journal of the American Chemical Society* 86, no. 24 (1964): 5710–5710.
145. Free, Spencer M., and James W. Wilson. "A mathematical contribution to structure-activity studies." *Journal of Medicinal Chemistry* 7, no. 4 (1964): 395–399.
146. Dobchev, Dimitar A., Girinath G. Pillai, and Mati Karelson. "*In silico* machine learning methods in drug development." *Current Topics in Medicinal Chemistry* 14, no. 16 (2014): 1913–1922.
147. Dudek, Arkadiusz Z., Tomasz Arodz, and Jorge Gálvez. "Computational methods in developing quantitative structure-activity relationships (QSAR): A review." *Combinatorial Chemistry & High Throughput Screening* 9, no. 3 (2006): 213–228.
148. Ning, Xia, and George Karypis. "*In silico* structure-activity-relationship (SAR) models from machine learning: A review." *Drug Development Research* 72, no. 2 (2011): 138–146.
149. Dahl, George E., Navdeep Jaitly, and Ruslan Salakhutdinov. "Multi-task neural networks for QSAR predictions." *arXiv preprint* arXiv:1406.1231 (2014).
150. Ramsundar, Bharath, Bowen Liu, Zhenqin Wu, Andreas Verras, Matthew Tudor, Robert P. Sheridan, and Vijay Pande. "Is multitask deep learning practical for pharma?" *Journal of Chemical Information and Modeling* 57, no. 8 (2017): 2068–2076.
151. Hartenfeller, Markus, and Gisbert Schneider. "De novo drug design." *Chemoinformatics and Computational Chemical Biology* (2011): 299–323.
152. Schneider, Gisbert, Kimito Funatsu, Yasushi Okuno, and Dave Winkler. "De novo drug design–ye olde scoring problem revisited." *Molecular Informatics* 36, no. 1–2 (2017): 1681031.

153. Olivecrona, Marcus, Thomas Blaschke, Ola Engkvist, and Hongming Chen. "Molecular de-novo design through deep reinforcement learning." *Journal of Cheminformatics* 9 (2017): 1–14.
154. Mnih, Volodymyr, Koray Kavukcuoglu, David Silver, Andrei A. Rusu, Joel Veness, Marc G. Bellemare, Alex Graves *et al.* "Human-level control through deep reinforcement learning." *Nature* 518, no. 7540 (2015): 529–533.
155. Gómez-Bombarelli, Rafael, Jennifer N. Wei, David Duvenaud, José Miguel Hernández-Lobato, Benjamín Sánchez-Lengeling, Dennis Sheberla, Jorge Aguilera-Iparraguirre, Timothy D. Hirzel, Ryan P. Adams, and Alán Aspuru-Guzik. "Automatic chemical design using a data-driven continuous representation of molecules." *ACS Central Science* 4, no. 2 (2018): 268–276.
156. Eid, Fatma-Elzahraa, Mahmoud ElHefnawi, and Lenwood S. Heath. "DeNovo: Virus-host sequence-based protein–protein interaction prediction." *Bioinformatics* 32, no. 8 (2016): 1144–1150.
157. Domenico, Alberga, Gambacorta Nicola, Trisciuzzi Daniela, Ciriaco Fulvio, Amoroso Nicola, and Nicolotti Orazio. "De novo drug design of targeted chemical libraries based on artificial intelligence and pair-based multiobjective optimization." *Journal of Chemical Information and Modeling* 60, no. 10 (2020): 4582–4593.
158. Pu, Yuchen, Weiyao Wang, Ricardo Henao, Liqun Chen, Zhe Gan, Chunyuan Li, and Lawrence Carin. "Adversarial symmetric variational autoencoder." *Advances in Neural Information Processing Systems* 30 (2017).
159. Coley, Connor W., Regina Barzilay, William H. Green, Tommi S. Jaakkola, and Klavs F. Jensen. "Convolutional embedding of attributed molecular graphs for physical property prediction." *Journal of Chemical Information and Modeling* 57, no. 8 (2017): 1757–1772.
160. Andras, Peter. "High-dimensional function approximation with neural networks for large volumes of data." *IEEE Transactions on Neural Networks and Learning Systems* 29, no. 2 (2017): 500–508.
161. Lusci, Alessandro, Gianluca Pollastri, and Pierre Baldi. "Deep architectures and deep learning in chemoinformatics: The prediction of aqueous solubility for drug-like molecules." *Journal of Chemical Information and Modeling* 53, no. 7 (2013): 1563–1575.
162. Duvenaud, David K., Dougal Maclaurin, Jorge Iparraguirre, Rafael Bombarell, Timothy Hirzel, Alán Aspuru-Guzik, and Ryan P. Adams. "Convolutional networks on graphs for learning molecular fingerprints." *Advances in Neural Information Processing Systems* 28 (2015).
163. Artursson, Per, and J. Karlsson. "Correlation between oral drug absorption in humans and apparent drug permeability coefficients in human intestinal epithelial (Caco-2) cells." *Biochemical and Biophysical Research Communications* 175, no. 3 (1991): 880–885.
164. Hubatsch, Ina, Eva G. E. Ragnarsson, and Per Artursson. "Determination of drug permeability and prediction of drug absorption in Caco-2 monolayers." *Nature Protocols* 2, no. 9 (2007): 2111–2119.
165. Tian, Sheng, Youyong Li, Junmei Wang, Jian Zhang, and Tingjun Hou. "ADME evaluation in drug discovery. 9. Prediction of oral bioavailability in humans based on molecular properties and structural fingerprints." *Molecular Pharmaceutics* 8, no. 3 (2011): 841–851.
166. Sim, Debra Si Mui. "Drug distribution." *Pharmacological Basis of Acute Care* (2015): 27–36.
167. Lombardo, Franco, and Yankang Jing. "*In silico* prediction of volume of distribution in humans. Extensive data set and the exploration of linear and nonlinear methods coupled with molecular interaction fields descriptors." *Journal of Chemical Information and Modeling* 56, no. 10 (2016): 2042–2052.

168. Matlock, Matthew K., Tyler B. Hughes, and S. Joshua Swamidass. "XenoSite server: A web-available site of metabolism prediction tool." *Bioinformatics* 31, no. 7 (2015): 1136–1137.
169. Zaretzki, Jed, Matthew Matlock, and S. Joshua Swamidass. "XenoSite: Accurately predicting CYP-mediated sites of metabolism with neural networks." *Journal of Chemical Information and Modeling* 53, no. 12 (2013): 3373–3383.
170. Dang, Na Le, Tyler B. Hughes, Varun Krishnamurthy, and S. Joshua Swamidass. "A simple model predicts UGT-mediated metabolism." *Bioinformatics* 32, no. 20 (2016): 3183–3189.
171. Guengerich, F. Peter. "Mechanisms of drug toxicity and relevance to pharmaceutical development." *Drug Metabolism and Pharmacokinetics* 26, no. 1 (2011): 3–14.
172. Xu, Youjun, Jianfeng Pei, and Luhua Lai. "Deep learning based regression and multiclass models for acute oral toxicity prediction with automatic chemical feature extraction." *Journal of Chemical Information and Modeling* 57, no. 11 (2017): 2672–2685.
173. Sushko, Iurii, Elena Salmina, Vladimir A. Potemkin, Gennadiy Poda, and Igor V. Tetko. "ToxAlerts: A web server of structural alerts for toxic chemicals and compounds with potential adverse reactions." (2012): 2310–2316.
174. Mayr, Andreas, Günter Klambauer, Thomas Unterthiner, and Sepp Hochreiter. "DeepTox: Toxicity prediction using deep learning." *Frontiers in Environmental Science* 3 (2016): 80.
175. Kearnes, Steven, Brian Goldman, and Vijay Pande. "Modeling industrial ADMET data with multitask networks." *arXiv preprint* arXiv:1606.08793 (2016).
176. Christ, Clara D., Matthias Zentgraf, and Jan M. Kriegl. "Mining electronic laboratory notebooks: Analysis, retrosynthesis, and reaction based enumeration." *Journal of Chemical Information and Modeling* 52, no. 7 (2012): 1745–1756.
177. de Almeida, A. Filipa, Rui Moreira, and Tiago Rodrigues. "Synthetic organic chemistry driven by artificial intelligence." *Nature Reviews Chemistry* 3, no. 10 (2019): 589–604.
178. Ley, Steven V. "The engineering of chemical synthesis: Humans and machines working in harmony." *Angewandte Chemie International Edition* 57, no. 19 (2018): 5182–5183.
179. Wipke, W. Todd, Glenn I. Ouchi, and S. Krishnan. "Simulation and evaluation of chemical synthesis—SECS: An application of artificial intelligence techniques." *Artificial Intelligence* 11, no. 1–2 (1978): 173–193.
180. Friedrich, Lukas, Tiago Rodrigues, Claudia S. Neuhaus, Petra Schneider, and Gisbert Schneider. "From complex natural products to simple synthetic mimetics by computational de novo design." *Angewandte Chemie International Edition* 55, no. 23 (2016): 6789–6792.
181. Sutskever, Ilya, Oriol Vinyals, and Quoc V. Le. "Sequence to sequence learning with neural networks." *Advances in Neural Information Processing Systems* 27 (2014).
182. Devlin, Jacob, Ming-Wei Chang, Kenton Lee, and Kristina Toutanova. "Bert: Pre-training of deep bidirectional transformers for language understanding." *arXiv preprint* arXiv:1810.04805 (2018).
183. Cadeddu, Andrea, Elizabeth K. Wylie, Janusz Jurczak, Matthew Wampler-Doty, and Bartosz A. Grzybowski. "Organic chemistry as a language and the implications of chemical linguistics for structural and retrosynthetic analyses." *Angewandte Chemie International Edition* 53, no. 31 (2014): 8108–8112.
184. Liu, Bowen, Bharath Ramsundar, Prasad Kawthekar, Jade Shi, Joseph Gomes, Quang Luu Nguyen, Stephen Ho, Jack Sloane, Paul Wender, and Vijay Pande. "Retrosynthetic reaction prediction using neural sequence-to-sequence models." *ACS Central Science* 3, no. 10 (2017): 1103–1113.
185. Baylon, Javier L., Nicholas A. Cilfone, Jeffrey R. Gulcher, and Thomas W. Chittenden. "Enhancing retrosynthetic reaction prediction with deep learning using multiscale reaction classification." *Journal of Chemical Information and Modeling* 59, no. 2 (2019): 673–688.

186. Coley, Connor W., Luke Rogers, William H. Green, and Klavs F. Jensen. "Computer-assisted retrosynthesis based on molecular similarity." *ACS Central Science* 3, no. 12 (2017): 1237–1245.
187. Gelly, Sylvain, and David Silver. "Monte-Carlo tree search and rapid action value estimation in computer go." *Artificial Intelligence* 175, no. 11 (2011): 1856–1875.
188. Segler, Marwin H. S., Mike Preuss, and Mark P. Waller. "Planning chemical syntheses with deep neural networks and symbolic AI." *Nature* 555, no. 7698 (2018): 604–610.
189. Schwaller, Philippe, Riccardo Petraglia, Valerio Zullo, Vishnu H. Nair, Rico Andreas Haeuselmann, Riccardo Pisoni, Costas Bekas, Anna Iuliano, and Teodoro Laino. "Predicting retrosynthetic pathways using transformer-based models and a hyper-graph exploration strategy." *Chemical Science* 11, no. 12 (2020): 3316–3325.
190. Raccuglia, Paul, Katherine C. Elbert, Philip D. F. Adler, Casey Falk, Malia B. Wenny, Aurelio Mollo, Matthias Zeller, Sorelle A. Friedler, Joshua Schrier, and Alexander J. Norquist. "Machine-learning-assisted materials discovery using failed experiments." *Nature* 533, no. 7601 (2016): 73–76.
191. Coley, Connor W., Regina Barzilay, Tommi S. Jaakkola, William H. Green, and Klavs F. Jensen. "Prediction of organic reaction outcomes using machine learning." *ACS Central Science* 3, no. 5 (2017): 434–443.
192. Hammer, Alexander J. S., Artem I. Leonov, Nicola L. Bell, and Leroy Cronin. "Chemputation and the standardization of chemical informatics." *JACS Au* 1, no. 10 (2021): 1572–1587.
193. Satoh, Hiroko, and Kimito Funatsu. "SOPHIA, a knowledge base-guided reaction prediction system-utilization of a knowledge base derived from a reaction database." *Journal of Chemical Information and Computer Sciences* 35, no. 1 (1995): 34–44.
194. Wei, Jennifer N., David Duvenaud, and Alán Aspuru-Guzik. "Neural networks for the prediction of organic chemistry reactions." *ACS Central Science* 2, no. 10 (2016): 725–732.
195. Coley, Connor W., Wengong Jin, Luke Rogers, Timothy F. Jamison, Tommi S. Jaakkola, William H. Green, Regina Barzilay, and Klavs F. Jensen. "A graph-convolutional neural network model for the prediction of chemical reactivity." *Chemical Science* 10, no. 2 (2019): 370–377.
196. Smith, Justin S., Olexandr Isayev, and Adrian E. Roitberg. "ANI-1: An extensible neural network potential with DFT accuracy at force field computational cost." *Chemical Science* 8, no. 4 (2017): 3192–3203.
197. Schwaller, Philippe, Teodoro Laino, Théophile Gaudin, Peter Bolgar, Christopher A. Hunter, Costas Bekas, and Alpha A. Lee. "Molecular transformer: A model for uncertainty-calibrated chemical reaction prediction." *ACS Central Science* 5, no. 9 (2019): 1572–1583.
198. Schwaller, Philippe, Theophile Gaudin, David Lanyi, Costas Bekas, and Teodoro Laino. "'Found in translation': Predicting outcomes of complex organic chemistry reactions using neural sequence-to-sequence models." *Chemical Science* 9, no. 28 (2018): 6091–6098.
199. Bradshaw, John, Matt J. Kusner, Brooks Paige, Marwin HS Segler, and José Miguel Hernández-Lobato. "A generative model for electron paths." *arXiv preprint* arXiv:1805.10970 (2018).
200. Ren, Jing, Feng Xia, Ivan Lee, Azadeh Noori Hoshyar, and Charu Aggarwal. "Graph learning for anomaly analytics: Algorithms, applications, and challenges." *ACM Transactions on Intelligent Systems and Technology* 14, no. 2 (2023): 1–29.
201. Basu Roy, Rohan, and Devesh Tiwari. "StarShip: Mitigating I/O bottlenecks in serverless computing for scientific workflows." *Proceedings of the ACM on Measurement and Analysis of Computing Systems* 8, no. 1 (2024): 1–29.
202. Thenuan, Yadvendra, Rojalini Samanta, Ananga Das, and Pranal Chhetri. "Revolutionizing pharma and healthcare: The power of artificial intelligence." *Journal of Higher Education Theory and Practice* 23 (2024): 975.

203. Gupta, Umesh, Ayushman Pranav, Anvi Kohli, Sukanta Ghosh, and Divya Singh. "The contribution of artificial intelligence to drug discovery: Current progress and prospects for the future." *Microbial Data Intelligence and Computational Techniques for Sustainable Computing* (2024): 1–23.
204. Sharma, Moolchand, Suman Deswal, Umesh Gupta, Mujahid Tabassum, and Isah Lawal, eds. *Soft Computing Techniques in Connected Healthcare Systems*. CRC Press, 2023.
205. Singh, Divya, Deepti Singh, Manju, and Umesh Gupta. "Smart healthcare: A breakthrough in the growth of technologies." In *Artificial Intelligence-Based Healthcare Systems*, pp. 73–85. Cham, Switzerland: Springer Nature, 2023.
206. Malik, Kamal, Harsh Sadawarti, Moolchand Sharma, Umesh Gupta, and Prayag Tiwari, eds. *Computational Techniques in Neuroscience*. CRC Press, 2023.
207. Mishra, Shambhavi, Tanveer Ahmed, Mohd Abuzar Sayeed, and Umesh Gupta. "Artificial neural network model for automated medical diagnosis." In *Soft Computing Techniques in Connected Healthcare Systems*, pp. 34–54. CRC Press, 2024.
208. Hazarika, Barenya Bikash, Deepak Gupta, and Umesh Gupta. "Intuitionistic fuzzy kernel random vector functional link classifier." In *Machine Intelligence Techniques for Data Analysis and Signal Processing: Proceedings of the 4th International Conference MISP 2022*, vol. 1, pp. 881–889. Singapore: Springer Nature, 2023.
209. Gupta, Madhuri, Divya Srivastava, Deepika Pantola, and Umesh Gupta. "Brain tumor detection using improved Otsu's thresholding method and supervised learning techniques at early stage." In *Proceedings of Emerging Trends and Technologies on Intelligent Systems: ETTIS 2022*, pp. 271–281. Singapore: Springer Nature, 2022.
210. Malviya, Lokesh, Sandip Mal, Radhikesh Kumar, Bishwajit Roy, Umesh Gupta, Deepika Pantola, and Madhuri Gupta. "Mental stress level detection using LSTM for WESAD dataset." In *Proceedings of Data Analytics and Management: ICDAM 2022*, pp. 243–250. Singapore: Springer Nature, 2023.

Index

Note: Page numbers in *italic* indicate a figure and page numbers in **bold** indicate a table on the corresponding page.

B

C

F

G

H

I

L

M

N

O

Q

R

U

V

W